Therapy for Diabetes Mellitus and Related Disorders

Therapy for Diabetes Mellitus and Related Disorders

Editor   Harold E. Lebovitz, MD

Associate   Ralph A. DeFronzo, MD
Editors   Saul Genuth, MD
                    Robert A. Kreisberg, MD
                    Michael A. Pfeifer, MD
                    William V. Tamborlane, MD

Publisher
Susan Hayes Coughlin

Editorial Director
Peter Banks

Project Manager
Orit Lowy Chicherio

Production Manager
Kim Fawcett

American Diabetes Association, Inc., Alexandria,
Virginia 22314
© 1991 by the American Diabetes Association, Inc.
All rights reserved
First printing June 1991
Printed in the United States of America
ISBN 0-945448-16-3

Table of Contents

Preface

This handbook focuses on the treatment of problems that are of importance in the management of patients with diabetes mellitus. It is part of the continuing effort of the American Diabetes Association (ADA) to assist physicians and other health-care professionals in providing the best care possible for these patients. The book is a companion to the *Physician's Guide to Insulin-Dependent (Type I) Diabetes* and *Physician's Guide to Non-Insulin-Dependent (Type II) Diabetes*.

In contrast to the previously published *Guides*, this manual was not derived by consensus but rather represents the views of the authors. Each expert was asked to focus specifically on the management aspects of his/her subject and to present a concise and practical approach. Each chapter was reviewed by the editorial board and represents currently accepted approaches that are consistent with the guidelines of the American Diabetes Association.

The editors thank the many contributors and ADA staff who have contributed so much of their time to make this manual possible.

Harold E. Lebovitz, MD

Introduction: Goals of Treatment

HAROLD E. LEBOVITZ, MD

Diabetes mellitus is associated with both acute and chronic complications. Acute complications include marked hyperglycemia, ketoacidosis, hyperosmolar nonketotic coma, infections, complications of pregnancy, etc. Chronic complications include microvascular, macrovascular, and neuropathic diseases and become clinically manifest after many years of diabetes (usually >10 yr).

The ideal managment of an individual with diabetes would provide for the following: *1*) no symptoms attributable to diabetes, *2*) prevention of acute complications, *3*) prevention of microvascular and neuropathic disease, and *4*) life expectancy equal to nondiabetic individuals. Ideal management is currently unattainable, but we do strive to achieve management goals that provide for minimal morbidity and mortality for all diabetic patients.

Management goals are defined differently depending on the situation of the patient. For type I (insulin-dependent) diabetic patients, three different levels of treatment have been defined (Table 1). The biochemical indices of metabolic control in type II (non-insulin-dependent) diabetic patients are defined differently (Table 2).

Glycemic control that maintains plasma glucose values at <200 mg/dl (<11.1 mM) will generally eliminate the symptoms of polydipsia, polyuria, polyphagia, weight loss, and increased fatigue. Maintaining plasma glucose levels at 150–165 mg/dl (8–9) mM is usually associated with a sense of well-being and good health. Preventing chronic microvascular and neuropathic complications and eliminating the complication of pregnancy probably require normoglycemic or near-normoglycemic regulation.

Minimizing macrovascular disease requires addressing all of the risk factors, e.g., smoking, hypertension, plasma triglycerides, and

1

Table 1. Levels of Treatment for Type I Diabetic Patients

- Minimal
  - HbA_{1c} 11–13%; glycosylated Hb 13–15%
  - Many self-monitored blood glucose (SMBG) values ≥300 mg/dl (≥16.7 mM)
  - Almost constantly positive urine glucose tests
  - Intermittent spontaneous ketonuria
- Average
  - HbA_{1c} 8–9%; glycosylated Hb 10–11%
  - Premeal SMBG 160–200 mg/dl (8.8–11.1 mM)
  - Intermittent positive urine glucose
  - Rare ketonuria
- Intensive
  - HbA_{1c} 6–7%; glycosylated Hb 10–11%
  - Premeal SMBG 70–120 mg/dl (3.9–6.7 mM); postmeal SMBG <180 mg/dl (<10 mM)
  - Essentially no positive urine glucose or ketones

From *Physician's Guide to Insulin-Dependent (Type I) Diabetes: Diagnosis and Treatment*. Alexandria, VA, Am. Diabetes Assoc., 1988.

serum low-density and high-density lipoprotein cholesterol, as well as blood glucose control.

In defining glycemic treatment goals, alleviation of symptoms and increasing the sense of well-being are realistic goals for all individuals with diabetes. Determining goals to prevent chronic complications requires that *1*) the patient's life expectancy be at least 10–15 yr more, *2*) the patient does not already have significant chronic complications, *3*) the patient does not have an illness that contraindicates intensive treatment, and *4*) the patient is willing and able to follow a regimen for intensive treatment.

Blood-pressure control and regulation of serum lipids in diabetic patients requires somewhat different goals than in the nondiabetic population and are discussed in specific chapters.

Table 2. Biochemical Indices of Metabolic Control in Type II Diabetes

Biochemical Index	Normal	Acceptable	Poor
Fasting plasma glucose (mg/dl)	115 (6.4)	140 (7.8)	>200 (>11.1)
Postprandial (2-h) plasma glucose (mg/dl)	140 (7.8)	200 (11.1)	>235 (>13.1)
HbA_{1c} (%)	6	8	>10
Fasting plasma cholesterol (mg/dl)	200 (5.2)	<240 (<6.2)	>240 (>6.2)
Fasting plasma triglyceride (mg/dl)	150 (1.70)	200 (2.26)	>250 (>2.82)

Values in parentheses are in mM. From *Physician's Guide to Non-Insulin-Dependent (Type II) Diabetes: Diagnosis and Treatment*. 2nd ed. Alexandria, VA, Am. Diabetes Assoc., 1988.

1. Genetic Counseling in Type I Diabetes

FREDDA GINSBERG-FELLNER, MD

To appropriately counsel parents and siblings of individuals with type I (insulin-dependent) diabetes and the patients themselves, a basic understanding of the genetics of this disease is required. In addition to a careful family history, including the age at which insulin was first administered, consider also

1. The putative genes and their penetrance
2. The way in which the disease is inherited, i.e., recessive, dominant, intermediate; single or multiple genes
3. The development of immune-system abnormalities as a prelude to the clinical expression of type I diabetes.
4. The role of pregnancy, both in a mother with and without diabetes, in partially protecting or increasing the risk for diabetes in her offspring
5. Whether the long-term macroangiopathic and microangiopathic complications of diabetes are important, in regard to the decision to have children and whether they too may have genetic components
6. What information is required before counseling and how and where it can be obtained

GENETIC COMPONENT IN TYPE I DIABETES

HLA Linkage

The primary genetic component appears to be linked to the MHC antigens (HLA) located on the short arm of chromosome 6 (Fig.

Dr. Ginsberg-Fellner is Professor of Pediatrics and Director of the Division of Pediatric Endocrinology and Metabolism at the Mount Sinai School of Medicine, New York, NY.

1.1). Close to 90% of all white individuals with type I diabetes have either HLA-DR3 or -DR4. Recent data are consistent with a location close to the DQ locus, perhaps in the direction of DP, with the presence of a non–aspartic acid residue at position 57 of the DQ β-chain and/or an arginine residue at position 52 of the DQ α-chain increasing susceptibility. It remains unclear exactly how these genes function in allowing type I diabetes to develop. In addition, no HLA variants have been found in all individuals with type I diabetes that are also virtually absent in control subjects.

Identical Twins

The concordance rate for diabetes in twin pairs ranges from 20 to 50%, strongly suggesting that genetic factors are required but not sufficient. Studies indicate that

1. If both members will develop diabetes, they usually do so within the first 5 yr after the first twin becomes affected.
2. The concordance rate may be increased in twin pairs with certain HLA antigens, e.g., both HLA-DR3 and -DR4 in whites.
3. The smaller of the twins at birth may be more susceptible.

Because all genes are identical (although immunoglobulin gene rearrangements occur postnatally) in identical twins, the <100% concordance rate for type I diabetes has long been the primary reason for inferring that environmental factors, which are yet to be defined and can affect twins differentially, must play a role.

HLA Relationships and Development of Diabetes

As shown in Table 1.1, siblings who share all HLA antigens (HLA identical for both maternal and paternal haplotypes, where haplotype denotes the entire HLA complex from the A through the D region) with their diabetic sibling have the greatest risk (20–30%),

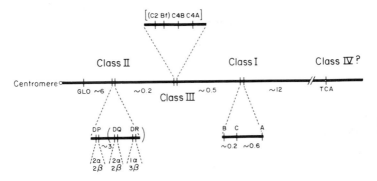

Figure 1.1. Simplification of MHC antigens on short arm of chromosome 6.

Table 1.1. RISK FOR DEVELOPMENT OF TYPE I DIABETES IN SIBLINGS OF PATIENTS WITH DISEASE ACCORDING TO HLA RELATIONSHIP TO PROBAND

HLA Status	Risk (%)
Identical	20–30
Half-identical	5–8
Nonidentical	1–2

whereas those sharing only half the antigens (HLA half-identical or haploidentical) have a much lower risk and, those who share none (HLA nonidentical) have a risk only somewhat greater (1–2%) than that of the general population (0.2–0.3%). Because the assortment of HLA haplotypes in offspring is as expected in a given family, i.e., 25% each HLA identical and nonidentical and 50% half-identical (and there is no deviation from this expected number in families with diabetes), at least 25% of all siblings of patients with type I diabetes can be genetically at risk for the disease. The actual number developing diabetes from the genetically most susceptible group, i.e., HLA identical, is significantly lower, only ~20%.

MODE OF INHERITANCE

Inheritance of type I diabetes seems to be primarily determined by a genetically recessive trait, i.e., one gene must be inherited from each parent. This fact is most important in counseling families because there is often guilt associated with the diagnosis of the disease, particularly when one side of the family already has known clinical diabetes. If the tendency to develop diabetes was inherited as a dominant trait, there would be close to 50% of siblings affected, not the ~8% found. The purported excess of patients with diabetes having both HLA-DR3 and -DR4 and the questionable excess of paternally derived DR4 haplotypes appear to be present in only certain ethnic groups and absent in others. The admixture of type I and type II diabetic patients in the adult-onset group of patients makes genetic analysis even more difficult in families who may have both types of diabetes.

DEVELOPMENT OF IMMUNE SYSTEM ABNORMALITIES

Islet Cell Antibodies

Many tests are available to detect both cytoplasmic (ICA) and surface (ICSA) islet cell antibodies, i.e., antibodies directed against the islets of Langerhans in the pancreas. The antigens responsible for triggering the development of these autoantibodies remain to be thoroughly characterized. Nevertheless, ICA determinations remain an important tool in identifying individuals significantly at risk for the development of type I diabetes, both in families with the disease and in the general population. Note, however, that screening of populations or individuals is discouraged outside the context of defined research studies. Table 1.2 summarizes data on the prevalence of ICA by various techniques.

1. Not all individuals with such antibodies develop diabetes.
2. Individuals with higher titers (i.e., larger amounts) of antibody are probably most at risk.
3. ICA^- individuals, albeit at a lower frequency than ICA^+ ones, can also develop type I diabetes.
4. The time of development of these antibodies is still unclear because, depending on the methodology used, they may be transient.
5. Within 5 yr after the development of diabetes in young individuals (when virtually all the insulin-producing β-cells are dead), <20% of patients will still have these antibodies, and many of these will also have another autoimmune disease.
6. The antibodies may be present for many years (and perhaps even decades) before clinical disease develops.
7. Individuals with other autoimmune diseases, particularly of the thyroid gland, have a higher prevalence of these antibodies.
8. Viral infections may lead to their production (transiently or permanently).
9. Families having more than one member with clinical type I diabetes and those in whom the disease developed before age 21 yr have the most ICA^+ individuals, suggesting that the tendency to develop antibodies could be inherited separately, perhaps even as a dominant trait.

Table 1.2. RISK OVER 5 YR FOR DEVELOPING TYPE I DIABETES ACCORDING TO DETECTION OF ISLET CELL (ICA), ISLET CELL SURFACE (ICSA), AND INSULIN AUTOANTIBODIES

	Risk (%)
High-titer ICA	40–60
Low-titer ICA	5–15
High-titer ICSA	40–70
Low-titer ICSA	3–15
Insulin autoantibodies*	
Age <5 yr	80–90
Age >5 yr	?
No ICA	5–10
No ICSA	2–5

*Most important when combined with insulin responses to intravenous glucose.

Insulin Autoantibodies

Several facts about insulin autoantibodies (IAAs) are clear.

1. The titer is inversely proportional to the age of the subject at the time of diagnosis of type I diabetes, i.e., the younger the individual, the higher the IAA level.
2. In individuals >12 yr old, the antibodies are often undetectable.
3. A combination of testing for ICAs and insulin autoantibodies will probably demonstrate β-cell damage before clinical diabetes develops.

Intravenous Glucose Tolerance Testing as Adjunct to ICA and IAA Determinations

The sum of the 1- and 3-min insulin levels after intravenous glucose challenge may identify individuals most likely to rapidly develop type I diabetes. In fact, nomograms for prediction of the time to decompensation to insulin dependence have been developed. It remains to be determined, however, whether such tests could also identify the subset of non–antibody-positive individuals who will also develop diabetes. In addition, this test is too cumbersome to perform on a populationwide basis, and normal values for children <6 yr of age are still not available.

ROLE OF PREGNANCY IN MOTHER WITH TYPE I DIABETES ON DEVELOPMENT OF DISEASE IN OFFSPRING

Offspring of diabetic mothers have a lower than expected rate of development of type I diabetes (Table 1.3). In contrast, fathers with type I diabetes have about the expected rate of offspring so affected, i.e., similar to the rate for HLA-haploidentical siblings (5–7.5%). The genesis of the maternal protective effect remains unknown.

COMPLICATIONS OF DIABETES AND GENETIC COUNSELING

Although differences exist in the interpretation of the genetic components in long-term complications of diabetes, *1*) familial hyper-

Table 1.3. RISKS FOR DEVELOPMENT OF TYPE I DIABETES IN CHILDREN OF PARENTS WITH DISEASE

	Risk for Offspring (%)
Father	2.5–6.1
Mother	0.5–2.9
Both parents (theoretical)	10–25

Adapted from Warram et al. (5).

Table 1.4. **TESTS AVAILABLE FOR IDENTIFICATION OF INDIVIDUALS AT RISK FOR TYPE I DIABETES**

- Islet cell antibodies
- Insulin autoantibodies
- Rapid intravenous glucose challenge with measurement of serum immunoreactive insulin 1 and 3 min later
- HLA typing to include DQ variants

lipidemia accentuates the risk of cardiovascular complications, and 2) hypertension and kidney disease are more common in individuals with diabetes if there is a family history of high blood pressure.

INFORMATION NECESSARY BEFORE COUNSELING AND WHERE TO OBTAIN IT

Siblings

Risks for siblings of a proband with type I diabetes can be determined with relative ease. Although ICA and insulin-autoantibody determinations plus intravenous glucose tolerance testing are nearly always sufficient, HLA typing can also be done (Table 1.4). HLA typing is expensive, and peripheral blood mononuclear cells must be obtained. Antibody testing is not easy to perform, and thus, serum specimens (2–3 ml is often sufficient) for these autoantibodies and blood samples for HLA tests should be sent to the closest research laboratory. ICA⁺ and/or ICSA⁺ HLA-identical or haploidentical siblings with decreased insulin responses are most at risk. These siblings should be watched carefully, with repeat testing as appropriate.

Children of Parents With Type I Diabetes

Unfortunately, the counseling is much more difficult if a prospective parent alone has type I diabetes. There still is no exact test for the carrier state for the putative genes in the other parent. The absence of HLA-DR3 and/or -DR4 will provide some but not absolute information. Thus, empiric risks can be provided. Nonetheless, note that the protective effect in young diabetic mothers means they have a great chance of having nondiabetic children.

SUGGESTED READING

1. Ginsberg-Fellner F, Witt ME, Franklin BH, Yagihashi S, Toguchi Y, Doberson MJ, Rubinstein P, Notkins AL: Triad of markers for identifying children at risk of developing insulin dependent diabetes mellitus. *JAMA* 254:1469–72, 1985

2. Riley WJ, Maclaren NK, Krischer J, Spillar RP, Silverstein JH, Schatz DA, Schwartz S, Malone J, Shah S, Vadheim C, Rotter JI: A prospective study of the development of diabetes in relatives of patients with insulin dependent diabetes. *N Engl J Med* 323:1167–72, 1990

3. Rubinstein P, Walker M, Mollen N, Carpenter C, Beckerman S, Suciu-Foca N, McEvoy R, Ginsberg-Fellner F: No excess of DR*3/4 in Ashkenazi Jewish or Hispanic IDDM patients. *Diabetes* 39:1138–43, 1990

4. Thomas NM, Ginsberg-Fellner F, McEvoy RC: Strong association between diabetes and displacement of mouse anti-rat insulinoma cell monoclonal antibody by human serum in vitro. *Diabetes* 39:1203–11, 1990

5. Warram JH, Krolewski AS, Gottlieb MS, Kahn CR: Differences in risk of insulin dependent diabetes in offspring of diabetic mothers and diabetic fathers. *N Engl J Med* 311:149–52, 1984

6. Zeigler AG, Herskowitz RD, Jackson RA, Soeldner JS, Eisenbarth GS: Predicting type I diabetes. *Diabetes Care* 13:762–75, 1990

2. Gestational Diabetes Mellitus

DONALD R. COUSTAN, MD

Gestational diabetes is defined as carbohydrate intolerance of variable severity with onset or first recognition during the current pregnancy. Two to 3% of pregnant women are diagnosed with gestational diabetes. The criteria used for diagnosis are specific to pregnancy and differ from those used for the diagnosis of diabetes or impaired glucose tolerance in nonpregnant individuals (Table 2.1).

The American Diabetes Association recommends that all pregnant women undergo screening for gestational diabetes at 24–28 wk gestation via a 50-g 1-h oral glucose challenge, administered without regard to time of day or interval since the last meal. If plasma glucose is ≥140 mg/dl (≥7.8 mM), a 100-g 3-h oral glucose tolerance test (OGTT) should be performed. The OGTT is administered after an overnight fast of 8–14 h and after 3 days of carbohydrate loading. Glucose measurement with test strips and reflectance meters is not recommended for either the 50-g 1-h challenge test or the 100-g 3-h OGTT because of the relatively poor precision of this methodology compared with standard laboratory testing.

PATHOPHYSIOLOGY AND RATIONALE FOR TREATMENT

Objective

Occasionally, a patient will present with diabetic ketoacidosis; these patients probably have previously undiagnosed type I (insulin-dependent) diabetes. Most women with gestational diabetes do not

---

Dr. Coustan is Professor and Chairman of Obstetrics and Gynecology at Brown University Program in Medicine and Gynecologist-in-Chief at Women and Infants Hospital of Rhode Island, Providence, RI.

Table 2.1. CRITERIA FOR DIAGNOSIS OF GESTATIONAL DIABETES

	Time of Testing			
	Fasting	1 h	2 h	3 h
Plasma glucose				
mM	5.8	10.6	9.2	8.1
mg/dl	105	190	165	145

Glucose is measured via glucose oxidase or hexokinase methodology. Gestational diabetes is diagnosed if ≥2 thresholds are met or exceeded.

ordinarily manifest hyperglycemia so severe as to compromise maternal health and well-being. Therefore, the issues of immediate concern center around the health and development of the fetus. Nevertheless, gestational diabetes is a powerful risk factor for the subsequent development of diabetes (Table 2.2).

Fetal Morbidity and Mortality

Recent series of gestational diabetic pregnancies diagnosed and managed in modern perinatal settings report perinatal mortality rates similar to those in the general population. Older studies in which gestational diabetes was not diagnosed and/or treated found significantly increased perinatal death rates. Fetal macrosomia and other morbidities continue to be major problems encountered in these pregnancies.

Pathophysiology

The pathophysiological mechanism underlying the above problems appears to be fetal hyperinsulinemia, or the Pedersen hypothesis, i.e., maternal hyperglycemia → fetal hyperglycemia → fetal hyperinsulinemia → macrosomia/?fetal death/neonatal hypoglycemia. Because glucose readily crosses the placenta by facilitated diffusion,

Table 2.2. LIKELIHOOD OF DEVELOPMENT OF SUBSEQUENT DIABETES 17–23 YR AFTER INDEX PREGNANCY

	Prevalence of Diabetes	
	Previous Gestational Diabetes (%)	Previous Normal Pregnancy (%)
World Health Organization criteria	61	14
National Diabetes Data Group criteria	39	5

Modified from O'Sullivan (2).

even mild degrees of maternal hyperglycemia are transmitted to the fetus. The fetal pancreas can be induced to hypersecrete insulin by hyperglycemia.

THERAPY

Treatment of gestational diabetes is directed toward normalization of maternal glucose levels, detection of maternal hyperglycemia, and assessment of fetal growth and well-being (Fig. 2.1).

Diet

Diet is the cornerstone of therapy for gestational diabetes. The dietary prescription is intended to smooth out the peaks and valleys of circulating glucose levels throughout the day. Specifics are similar to the diet described elsewhere in this book (see chapt. 13) with emphasis on avoidance of refined simple sugars and with an increase in the protein content to reflect the increased protein requirements of pregnancy.

Blood Glucose Monitoring

To ascertain whether the dietary therapy is effective in maintaining euglycemia, circulating blood glucose levels must be monitored regularly. Some health-care providers institute self-monitoring of blood glucose (SMBG) 4–6× daily for women with gestational diabetes, similar to that prescribed for pregnant women with type I or type II (non-insulin-dependent) diabetes. Because the use of daily SMBG by women with gestational diabetes is not necessary to reverse the increased perinatal mortality risk of gestational diabetes, the following approach is generally considered effective:

1. Circulating glucose levels should be measured both fasting and at other times of day throughout the remainder of pregnancy. The frequency and timing of measurements is arbitrary but many measure fasting and 2-h postmeal glucose weekly.
2. Glucose measurements may be performed in any setting (e.g., clinic, hospital laboratory, physician's office, or at home with a reflectance meter). Although not appropriate for diagnostic testing, this technology is acceptable for evaluation of glycemic control in an individual already diagnosed as having gestational diabetes.
3. The goal of the restoration of near euglycemia should be the same as for pregnant women with type I or type II diabetes.
4. Clinical investigations have found that nondiabetic pregnant women maintain circulating plasma glucose levels between 50 and 120–130 mg/dl (2.8 and 6.7–7.3 mM, respectively) throughout the course of the day. Whereas specific goals may vary among centers, insulin is often initiated for fasting plasma glucose >105 mg/dl (>5.8 mM) and/or 2-h postprandial plasma glucose >120 mg/dl (>6.7 mM) on ≥2 occasions within a 2-wk interval.

5. An isolated elevated glucose level can often be attributed to a temporary dietary indiscretion. If the patient is hyperglycemic due to nonadherence to her diet on the day she anticipates glucose measurements, she will probably not display better dietary adherence on other days. A glucose measurement that exceeds the stated goals should prompt either the reassessment of glycemia within the next few days or the institution of insulin therapy.

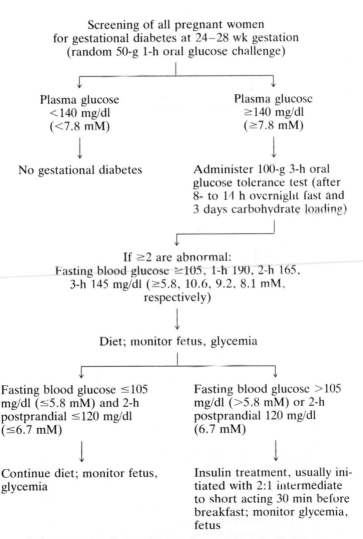

Figure 2.1. Diagnosis and management of gestational diabetes.

Insulin

Different approaches to insulin therapy have been used in gestational diabetes.

1. Patients with fasting hyperglycemia are often initiated on a bedtime dose of intermediate-acting insulin, usually no more than 10 U initially.

2. Patients with postprandial hyperglycemia are often initiated on a mixture of intermediate- and short-acting insulin (2:1), with a common starting dose of 30 U before breakfast. Although hypoglycemia is rare with such doses, all patients should be cautioned about this possibility. Lower starting doses are often administered if the treatment is initiated before the third trimester of pregnancy, i.e., the time of maximal insulin resistance.

Fetal Growth

Because macrosomia is a frequent complication of gestational diabetes, obstetric-care providers often use ultrasound examinations to assess fetal growth. It is important to realize, however, that ultrasound estimates of fetal weight are not perfect. Over- and underestimates of 10–20% are common. Congenital anomalies do not appear to occur more frequently in pregnancies complicated by gestational diabetes.

Assessment of Fetal Well-Being

The obstetric-care provider is generally responsible for determining the mode and frequency of testing of fetal well-being. Several tests exist, and no single approach is superior.

The most widely used approaches are as follows:

- **Fetal activity determinations (kick counts):** The patient notes each perceived fetal movement for a specific time interval each day or notes the amount of time that passes before a predetermined number of movements have occurred each day. A significant decline in the number of movements or an increase in the time it takes to attain the appropriate number of movements prompts the need for one of the tests described below. Fetal activity determinations have a high likelihood of false positives, but the test costs nothing and is convenient for the patient.
- **Contraction stress test:** If at least three uterine contractions occur within 10 min, a fetal monitor can be used to evaluate the fetal response to those contractions. Recurrent late decelerations of the fetal heart rate are evidence of fetal compromise. If contractions are not occurring spontaneously, some specialists may use an oxytocin challenge. This test may become abnormal earlier than many of the other tests and so is considered particularly sensitive.

- **Nonstress test:** The fetal monitor is placed, and the patient notes fetal movements. The presence of accelerations of the fetal heart rate in conjunction with fetal movements denotes fetal well-being.
- **Biophysical profile:** This test combines the nonstress test with ultrasound determination of fetal movement, tone, breathing, and amniotic fluid volume. It is sensitive and specific but requires an ultrasound unit and an experienced operator plus a fetal monitor.

Hypertension in pregnancy is defined as a systolic blood pressure of >140 mmHg, *or* a diastolic blood pressure of >90 mmHg, *or* a 30-mmHg rise in systolic blood pressure, *or* a 15-mmHg rise in diastolic blood pressure on at least two occasions at least 6 h apart. Complications such as hypertension, inadequate diabetes control, or a previous perinatal loss dictate that testing begin sooner and/or be performed more frequently.

Timing and Mode of Delivery

Because gestational diabetes may be associated with delay in fetal pulmonic maturation, amniocentesis is generally performed to assess lung maturity before elective cesarean section or induction of labor. In some centers, this step is omitted if the gestational age is well documented to be 39 or 40 wk, whereas in others, the test is still performed. Gestational diabetes is not an indication for cesarean section.

POSTPREGNANCY TESTING

Because gestational diabetes is a risk factor for the subsequent development of type I or type II diabetes, patients with gestational diabetes should be periodically evaluated for the development of diabetes.

SUGGESTED READING

1. American Diabetes Association: Position statement: gestational diabetes mellitus. *Diabetes Care* 13 (Suppl. 1):5–6, 1990
2. O'Sullivan JB: Subsequent morbidity among gestational diabetic women. In *Carbohydrate Metabolism in Pregnancy and the Newborn*. Sutherland HW, Stowers JM, Eds. New York, Churchill Livingstone, 1984, p. 174–80
3. Pedersen J, Bojsen-Moller B, Poulsen H: Blood sugar in newborn infants of diabetic mothers. *Acta Endocrinol Scand* 15:33–36, 1954
4. Reece EA, Coustan DR (Eds.): *Diabetes Mellitus in Pregnancy: Principles and Practice*. New York, Churchill Livingstone, 1988
5. Second International Workshop-Conference on Gestational Diabetes: Summary and recommendations. *Diabetes* 34 (Suppl. 2):123–26, 1985

3. Management of Pregnant Diabetic Patients

E. ALBERT REECE, MD, and RUBEN QUINTERO, MD

PRECONCEPTIONAL METABOLIC CONTROL AND CONGENITAL MALFORMATIONS

The incidence of congenital anomalies among children of diabetic women (except for women with gestational diabetes) is $4-10\times$ higher than among their nondiabetic counterparts. Glycosylated hemoglobin determinations made early in the second trimester show that the frequency of malformations correlates with the degree of glycemic control rather than with the patient's White's classification.

Evidence suggests that the maternal metabolic milieu has a direct influence on embryogenesis during a critical and vulnerable developmental period. Normalization of blood glucose in the preconceptional period and the maintenance of normal glycemic control throughout this critical phase of organogenesis result in a reduced incidence of anomalies.

Intensive insulin treatment in periconceptional patients improves glycemic control. The goal of preconceptional counseling and control is to achieve glycemic control before becoming pregnant.

MANAGEMENT OF UNCOMPLICATED PREGNANT DIABETIC PATIENTS WITHOUT VASCULOPATHY

Diabetic patients can be classified into two groups, according to the presence or absence of diabetic vasculopathy. The first group in-

Dr. Reece is the Abraham Roth Professor and Chair of Ob/Gyn, Professor of Medicine, and Director of the Division of Maternal-Fetal Medicine, and Dr. Quintero is an Instructor at the Yale University School of Medicine, New Haven, CT.

Table 3.1. CLASSIFICATION OF DIABETES IN PREGNANCY

Class	Criteria
A	Chemical diabetes: abnormal glucose tolerance test
B	Onset after age 20 yr, <10 yr duration
C	Onset between age 10 and 20 yr, duration 10–20 yr
D_1	Onset <10 yr, duration >20 yr
D_2	Duration of diabetes >20 yr
D_3	Calcification of the vessels of the legs
D_4	Benign retinopathy
D_5	Hypertension
F	Nephropathy
R	Proliferative retinopathy
H	Coronary artery disease

Modified from White (12).

cludes White's classes A, A/B, B, C, and D (without hypertension), and the second group consists of classes D (with hypertension), F, FR, and H (Table 3.1). The fundamental differences in the management of the two groups are that patients in group 2 have a more advanced disease, requiring more intense evaluation and surveillance because advanced disease places the pregnancy at a greater risk for complications.

Third-trimester mean maternal blood glucose level correlates linearly with the perinatal mortality rate. Achievement and maintenance of euglycemia requires multiple daily blood glucose determinations, with the frequency of self-monitoring of blood glucose (SMBG) based somewhat on the severity of the disease.

Excellent glucose control in patients with type I (insulin-dependent) diabetes begins to deteriorate when SMBG is less than four determinations a day (10). In patients with gestational diabetes (classes A and A/B), ~20% convert during the course of pregnancy from non–insulin requiring to insulin requiring. Therefore, it is necessary to obtain blood glucose determinations weekly to determine the adequacy of glycemic control.

The recommended management approach for diabetic pregnancy and labor is outlined in Table 3.2.

1. Except for class A patients, glucose should be monitored at least 5×/day (e.g., at fasting, 2 h after lunch, before and after dinner, and at bedtime) throughout the course of pregnancy.
2. An early ultrasound examination should be performed to date the pregnancy and to establish growth parameters against which future examinations can be compared.
3. At 18–20 wk, all type I diabetic patients should receive a fetal echocardiogram to rule out cardiac malformations.
4. Patients should be seen for clinical evaluation every 2 wk until 32 wk, after which they should be seen weekly.

5. Nonstress tests and/or biophysical profiles should be done weekly after the 32nd wk.
6. Fetal lung-maturity studies should be undertaken when elective delivery is planned, because of maternal or fetal indications such as preeclampsia, placenta previa, or poor glycemic control. Otherwise, patients should be allowed to go into labor spontaneously, independent of their White's classification.

Diet

Pregnancy normally demands an additional intake of 300–400 kcal/ day above basal requirements. No additional calories are required for pregnant diabetic patients. The composition of the diet should be ~50% carbohydrate, ~20% protein, and 30% fats (with no more than 10% saturated fat). Sodium restriction is not recommended. Similarly, no weight-loss diets should be prescribed. Three meals a

Table 3.2. MANAGEMENT OF UNCOMPLICATED PREGNANT DIABETIC PATIENTS

Class A and A/B
- Glucose determinations weekly
- Biweekly visits until 34 wk; then weekly
- Ultrasound examinations every 4–6 wk in 3rd trimester
- Nonstress test at 34 wk; then weekly
- HbA_{1c} not necessary
- No 24-h urine, ophthalmologic evaluation, or fetal ECG necessary
- Daily fetal movement counts

Class B and C
- Daily self-monitoring of blood glucose
- Biweekly visits until 34 wk; then weekly
- Ultrasound: level II at ~20 wk, then follow-up every 4–6 wk
- HbA_{1c} monthly
- Nonstress test at 33 wk; then weekly
- Ophthalmologic evaluation, follow-up according to findings
- 24-h urine, initially and in each trimester
- Daily fetal movement counts

Class D–FR
- Above plus ECG initially, uric acid, liver-function test, fibrinogen, fibrin split products: may repeat in each trimester

Delivery time
- Class A and B: ≤42 wk gestation
- Class C–FR: at term or pulmonic maturity

Labor
- Blood glucose to be maintained at ≤100 mg/dl (≤5.5 mM)
- Intravenous D_5W ½ normal saline solution and 10 U short-acting insulin (~1 U insulin/h)
- D_5W ½ normal saline solution piggybacked to the insulin-carrying solution to adjust glycemia
- Hourly fingerstick blood glucose determinations

D_5W, 5% dextrose solution.

day with two or three snacks are usually sufficient for type I diabetic patients. Snacks may be omitted for type II (non-insulin-dependent) diabetic patients, except at bedtime. A weight gain of 22–30 lb is considered acceptable, with 2–4 lb in the first trimester and 0.5–0.1 lb/wk thereafter.

Exercise

The risk/benefit ratio of either occasional or regular exercise in pregnant women with type I, type II, or gestational diabetes is unknown. General guidelines have been recommended by the American College of Obstetricians and Gynecologists (Table 3.3). Exercise should not be prescribed for patients with antecedent hypertension, pregnancy-induced hypertension, macrovascular or microvascular disease, autonomic dysfunction, or lack of counter-regulatory mechanisms. Supervision is necessary with the prescription of exercise to diabetic pregnant women.

Insulin

With multiple daily injections of insulin, two thirds of the total dose for the day is given in the morning, in a 2:1 ratio of intermediate- to short-acting insulin (e.g., NPH:regular). The remaining third is given before dinner in a 1:1 ratio. Alternatively, 3 daily injections may be given: the usual morning dose, a second administration of short-acting insulin at dinner, and a third injection of intermediate-acting insulin at bedtime.

The latter regimen allows for smoother control of fasting blood glucose levels during overnight fasting. Occasionally, patients need to be treated with short-acting insulin before each meal and with intermediate-acting insulin at bedtime.

Insulin can also be administered continuously through the use of battery-operated pumps, which deliver insulin at a defined rate. Although insulin pumps most closely resemble the physiological insulin secretion of the pancreas, clinical studies have failed to show any significant advantages over multiple daily injections in terms of

Table 3.3. EXERCISE IN PREGNANCY

- Maternal heart rate should not exceed 140 beats/min
- Strenuous activities should not exceed 15 min in duration
- No exercise should be performed in the supine position after the 4th mo of gestation
- Exercises with the Valsalva maneuver should be avoided
- Calorie intake should be adequate to meet the extra energy needs of pregnancy and the exercise performed
- Maternal core temperature should not exceed 38°C

From The American College of Obstetricians and Gynecologists: *Exercise During Pregnancy and the Postnatal Period*. Washington, DC, ACOG Home Exercise Programs, © 1985.

fetal outcome, mean blood glucose, glycosylated hemoglobin, or mean amplitude of glycemic excursion.

Adverse effects of insulin therapy include hypoglycemia and ketosis.

Hypoglycemia. Both chemical and clinical hypoglycemic episodes occur during the course of pregnancy and are believed to result, in part, from intensive insulin treatment aimed at achieving good glycemic control. Insulin-clamp studies demonstrate a blunted counterregulatory hormone response in diabetic patients who experience multiple hypoglycemic episodes. Hypoglycemia has been associated with teratogenic effects in rat offspring; however, there are no clinical data to confirm any potential teratogenic effect of hypoglycemia on human fetuses.

Ketosis. The presence of ketone bodies denotes a state of cellular starvation due to hypoglycemia or to a relative lack of insulin with concomitant hyperglycemia. Ketoacidosis has been associated with a 50–90% fetal mortality rate. Therefore, ketosis should be vigorously treated and prevented.

MANAGEMENT OF COMPLICATED PREGNANT DIABETIC PATIENTS WITH VASCULOPATHY

Evidence of vascular complications places pregnant diabetic women in a higher risk category for both maternal and fetal morbidity and mortality. The primary cause of maternal death among pregnant diabetic women is no longer diabetic ketoacidosis but cardiorenal complications. Similarly, fetal mortality is significantly higher in diabetic patients with vasculopathy than in those without vasculopathy. Although many organs can be affected by diabetic vascular complications, the kidneys, eyes, and heart are associated with the most significant clinical consequences.

Diabetic Nephropathy

Diabetic nephropathy (White's class F) is one of the most critical complications affecting the outcome of pregnancy and is the leading cause of death in diabetic patients <40 yr old. It is defined by proteinuria ([+] Albustix, >300 mg/24-h collection), hypertension, reduced glomerular filtration rate (GFR) and end-stage renal disease. Its incidence rises sharply after 10 yr of diabetes. Because of the increase in GFR observed and the decreased tubular reabsorption of protein in pregnancy, the diagnosis of diabetic nephropathy in pregnancy is based on a value of >300–500 mg/day urinary protein during the first half of the pregnancy.

The physician caring for the pregnant woman with diabetic nephropathy should be interested in knowing whether pregnancy will alter the course of the renal damage and how the renal involvement will affect the pregnancy. Normally, the amount of proteinuria increases during pregnancy (due to the combination of factors mentioned above) and subsides after delivery. On the other hand, the expected rise in the creatinine clearance (CrCl) is only observed in 32% of patients. Whether tighter glycemic control allows for the normal expected rise in CrCl is unknown. Overall, the status of diabetic nephropathy will remain stable in most patients, but 20–40% will experience either a permanent or temporary decrease in kidney function. The mean rate of fall of CrCl is 0.81 ml · min^{-1} · mo^{-1}. The presence of hypertension is associated with heavier proteinuria, lower CrCl, and mild azotemia. The perinatal impact of diabetic nephropathy is outlined in Table 3.4.

The risks of preterm labor, stillbirth, neonatal death, and fetal distress are significantly increased among patients with diabetic nephropathy. However, with contemporary means of evaluation and treatment, the perinatal survival in this group can exceed 90% if fetuses are delivered at ≥36 wk.

Management should begin before conception with adequate counseling and glycemic control. Assessment of kidney function, including a 24-h urine collection every trimester to determine CrCl and the rate of protein excretion, is recommended. The treatment of hypertension is indicated; however, experience with antihypertensive drugs in diabetic patients is limited. Angiotensin-converting enzyme inhibitors have been used, but their safety has not been established. β-Blockers may potentially interfere with the vasoactive response to a hypoglycemic episode.

The presence of kidney failure, defined as CrCl <30 ml/min, or creatinine >5 mg/dl (>442 mM), constitutes a particular management problem for patients with diabetic nephropathy. If such patients are seen in a preconception clinic and are seriously contemplating becoming pregnant, they should be advised to consider kidney transplantation or dialysis before pregnancy. On the other hand, if kidney failure develops during pregnancy, peritoneal dialysis or hemodialysis may be used. Patients with uncontrollable hypertension should be advised against conception.

Table 3.4. PERINATAL OUTCOME OF CLASS F DIABETIC PATIENTS COMPARED WITH NONNEPHROPATHIC PREGNANT DIABETIC PATIENTS

- No higher incidence of spontaneous abortions
- No higher incidence of congenital malformations
- Increased incidence of intrauterine growth retardation: 19 vs. 2.2%
- Risk of stillbirth: higher than in diabetic patients without kidney disease
- Risk of neonatal death: double that of diabetic patients without kidney disease
- Preterm labor: 30%
- Fetal distress: 30%
- Superimposed pregnancy-induced hypertension
- Respiratory distress syndrome: 23 vs. 8% of diabetic patients without kidney disease
- Neonatal jaundice: 36 vs. 20%
- 3% of babies have developmental problems in childhood, most do well

Retinopathy

Class R diabetes includes pregnant patients with diabetic retinopathy. There are essentially two types of diabetic retinopathy: background diabetic retinopathy (BDR), which is nonproliferative, and proliferative diabetic retinopathy (PDR). PDR is the most frequent cause of blindness among patients with type I diabetes; whereas macular edema is the primary cause for those with type II diabetes.

Diabetic retinopathy can progress rapidly over short periods. Diabetic patients should have a complete ophthalmologic evaluation at the beginning of pregnancy. Follow-up visits or treatments should be scheduled according to the findings. Although there is no contraindication for laser photocoagulation in pregnancy, not enough data are available regarding the safety of fluorescein use in pregnancy.

Coronary Artery Disease (CAD)

White's class H diabetes is defined as the presence of CAD in pregnant diabetic patients. CAD occurs more commonly at a younger age and with greater severity in diabetic patients than in nondiabetic patients. Patients are defined as class H if they have a history of myocardial infarction (MI) or angina or if they develop these complications during pregnancy. Particular problems in the diagnosis of class H diabetes result from the inability of most pregnant patients to complete a standard stress-tolerance test. Additionally, neither radioisotopes nor angiography may be used safely to confirm the diagnosis. Therefore, clinicians must rely on signs and symptoms of advanced disease such as angina or MI to diagnose CAD in pregnancy. There are few data regarding the outcome of pregnancy in diabetic patients with CAD. Patients with angina seem to have had better prognoses than those whose pregnancies were complicated by either a history of MI or the development of MI during pregnancy.

If CAD is diagnosed before pregnancy, patients should be advised against pregnancy. Patients may elect to undergo bypass surgery to improve their overall medical condition. When CAD is first diagnosed during pregnancy, however, management should depend on whether the patient presents with angina or MI.

Patients with angina can be treated with selective β-blockers (see chapt. 44). In addition, although the use of Ca^{2+}-channel blockers in pregnancy has not been tested, they may be an appropriate therapeutic choice. MI during pregnancy presents a particularly difficult management problem. The coexistence of pregnancy and MI is stressful, whereas patients are at an increased risk of dying if they undergo surgery within 3–6 mo after MI. This 3- to 6-mo period is likely to overlap with the end of the pregnancy. Should the patient require a cesarean section for obstetric indications, the same risk applies. No recommendations can be made as to whether the termination or continuation of pregnancy is preferable.

SUGGESTED READING

1. Coustan DR, Reece EA, Sherwin RS, Rudolph McJ, Bates S, Sockin SM, Holford T, Tamborlane WV: A randomized clinical trial of the insulin pump vs intensive conventional therapy in diabetic pregnancies. *JAMA* 255:631–36, 1986
2. Fuhrmann K. Reiher H, Semmler K, Fischer F, Fischer M, Glockner E: Prevention of congenital malformations in infants of insulin-dependent diabetic mothers. *Diabetes Care* 6:219–23, 1983
3. Goldman JA, Dicker D, Feldberg D: Pregnancy outcome in patients with insulin-dependent diabetes mellitus with preconceptional diabetic control: a comparative study. *Am J Obstet Gynecol* 155:293–97, 1986
4. Kioko EM, Shaw KM, Clarke AD, Warren DJ: Successful pregnancy in a diabetic patient treated with continuous ambulatory peritoneal dialysis. *Diabetes Care* 6:298–300, 1983
5. Kitzmiller JL, Gavin LA, Gin GD, Jovanovic-Peterson L, Main EK, Zigrang WD: Preconception care of diabetes: glycemic control prevents congenital anomalies. *JAMA* 265:731–36, 1991
6. Miller E, Hare JW, Cloherty JP: Elevated maternal hemoglobin A_{1c} in early pregnancy and major congenital anomalies in infants of diabetic mothers. *N Engl J Med* 304:1331–34, 1981
7. Mills JL, Knopp RH, Simpson JL, et al.: Lack of relation of increased malformation rates in infants of diabetic mothers to glycemic control during organogenesis. *N Engl J Med* 318:671–76, 1988
8. Pinter E, Reece EA, Leranth C, Garcia-Segura M, Sanyal MK, Hobbins JC, Mahoney MJ, Naftolin F: Arachidonic acid prevents hyperglycemia-associated yolk sac damage and embryopathy. *Am J Obstet Gynecol* 155:691–702, 1986
9. Reece EA, Hobbins JC: Diabetic embryopathy: pathogenesis, prenatal diagnosis and prevention. *Obstet Gynecol Survey* 41:325–35, 1986
10. Skyler JS: Self-monitoring of blood glucose. *Med Clin North Am* 66:1227–50, 1982
11. Smoak IW, Sadler TW: Embryopathic effects of short-term exposure to hypoglycemia in mouse embryous in vitro. *Am J Obstet Gynecol* 163:619–24, 1990
12. White P: Diabetes mellitus in pregnancy. *Clin Perinatal* 1:331–47, 1974

4. Antepartum and Intrapartum Obstetric Care

GABRIELE ROSSI, MD, and MICHAEL P. DIAMOND, MD

During the last decade, the frequency of perinatal mortality in pregnancies complicated by diabetes mellitus has been dramatically reduced by therapeutic strategies directed toward normalizing maternal circulating glucose levels. However, neonatal morbidity in these pregnancies continues to exceed the levels observed in the nondiabetic population. Intensive antepartum surveillance of diabetic pregnancies is crucial.

PATHOPHYSIOLOGY OF PERINATAL MORBIDITY

The fetal pancreatic response to hyperglycemia induced by elevated maternal glucose levels results in pancreatic islet β-cell hypertrophy and hyperplasia. Support for this hypothesis is provided by observations that macrosomia is related to fetal hyperinsulinemia in the Rhesus monkey and the elevated umbilical cord blood and amniotic fluid insulin levels detected in macrosomic infants of diabetic mothers. Similarly, neonatal hypoglycemia may be explained as a response to high fetal insulin levels. Moreover, experimental data link fetal hyperinsulinemia with chronic hypoxia, resulting in increased fetal erythropoiesis with consequent neonatal polycythemia and hyperbilirubinemia. The precise mechanism whereby fetal insulin and glucose interfere with lung maturation and decrease surfactant production remains unclear.

Dr. Rossi is a Postdoctoral Fellow and Dr. Diamond is an Assistant Professor of Obstetrics and Gynecology at the Yale University School of Medicine, New Haven, CT.

PREPREGNANCY CARE

Organogenetic defects of the infant of the diabetic mother develop at least partly as a consequence of derangements in metabolic control during the period of organogenesis (2–10 wk after conception in the human). Although a direct correlation between the degree of aberration of metabolic regulation and the development of malformations seems to exist, even minor deteriorations in metabolic control may increase the risk of malformation. Additionally, recent animal data have demonstrated the detrimental effect of a poorly controlled metabolic state on oocyte maturation and development of preimplantation embryos. Thus, tight metabolic control before attempts to conceive is important.

At initial visit

- Review menstrual, contraceptive, fertility, social, and reproductive histories.
- Evaluate rubella and thyroid status.
- Do complete blood count.
- Obtain bacterial cultures of urinary and genital tract.
- Advise patient to
  - Institute tight metabolic controls.
  - Use mechanical contraception for 3 mo.
  - Assess ovulatory function by measuring plasma progesterone and basal body temperature.

When pregnancy is suspected

- Measure β-subunit of human chorionic gonadotropin (hCG).
- Follow hCG serially until time for ultrasound.
- Do ultrasound scan to date gestation.

In case of a discrepancy between dates and test results, management of the diabetic pregnancy should be guided by the ultrasound age, supported by ovulatory indices, rather than menstrual age.

STANDARD MANAGEMENT IN PREGNANCY

Table 4.1 summarizes management of the pregnant woman with diabetes. Baseline evaluation can include weight, blood pressure, hematocrit, thyroid function, urinalysis, and urine culture. Urinary cultures may be repeated each trimester and more often if symptoms develop. Urinary tract infections are of concern because of the increased incidence of urinary tract infections in diabetic patients.

Prenatal vitamins are recommended beginning at the initial antepartum visit and should include folic acid. Iron sulfate is recommended, particularly in anemic patients.

Patients should measure fasting, 2-h postprandial, and evening blood glucose levels, with the goal usually of a fasting blood glucose

Table 4.1. **STANDARD MANAGEMENT IN PREGNANCY**

Prenatal visits
- Commence by 8 wk from last menstrual period
- Monthly until 28 wk
- Twice weekly until 36 wk
- Weekly until term

Prenatal vitamins

Metabolic assessment with goal of fasting blood glucose <100 mg/dl (<5.5 mM)

Urinary cultures each trimester to detect urinary tract infection

Creatinine clearance and urinary protein determination to assess preexistent and/or developing kidney damage

Monitor weight gain and blood pressure changes to detect onset of pregnancy-induced hypertension or alteration of cardiovascular or renal status

Maternal serum α-fetoprotein screen to detect neural tube defects

---

of 60–90 mg/dl (3.3–5 mM) and 2-h postprandial levels ≤120 mg/dl (≤6.7 mM). There does not appear to be any difference in metabolic control achievable with continuous subcutaneous pump therapy versus multiple daily injections.

Creatinine clearance and urinary protein from a 24-h collection may be evaluated each trimester of pregnancy (more frequently in hypertensive patients) to assess preexistent and/or developing kidney damage. Weight gain and blood pressure changes should be closely monitored because they may reflect the onset of pregnancy-induced hypertension or alteration of cardiovascular or renal status.

A maternal serum α-fetoprotein (AFP) screen at 16 wk is useful in the pregnancy diabetic woman because the incidence of neural tube defects is increased ~20-fold over nondiabetic pregnancies. Values obtained are then compared to a nomogram, which is based on gestational age. Although it has been suggested that AFP may be 60% lower in the diabetic pregnancy than in the nondiabetic pregnancy at a given gestational age, well-controlled diabetic patients do not need any correction in AFP levels before interpretation. A positive screen requires further evaluation (e.g., a 2nd screen and ultrasound assessment of the fetus) because false-positive values may be related to various factors.

ASSESSMENT OF FETAL WELL-BEING

Whereas assessment of fetal well-being is important in all high-risk pregnancies, it is especially important in diabetic gestations because of the potential for unexplained stillbirths in these pregnancies. Currently, the assessment of fetoplacental function by measurement of placental steroids and proteins (e.g., human placental lactogen) is used rarely if at all for the clinical management of diabetic pregnancy. Biophysical techniques are more useful.

Ultrasound

An ultrasound scan in the first part of a diabetic pregnancy is the most convenient way to concomitantly date the gestation and rule out early growth delay, which is a risk marker associated with poor fetal growth and congenital malformations.

In the middle of the second trimester (18–20 wk), a detailed ultrasonic fetal examination performed by an experienced obstetrician should be performed to identify malformations. Careful fetal echocardiographic assessment is recommended to exclude major structural cardiac abnormalities. Routine ultrasound scans to assess fetal growth can be performed at 20 and 28 wk. When fetal malformation is ruled out, hydramnios is often explained by unsuspected suboptimal maternal metabolic control. Furthermore, fetuses who have an abdominal circumference ≥1 cm above average at wk 28 or 29 have a 77% likelihood of developing macrosomia, whereas fetuses with smaller abdominal circumferences have a 96% likelihood of not becoming macrosomic.

Third-trimester examinations should be directed toward ultrasound parameters that might suggest fetal macrosomia, alerting the physician to the possibility of cephalopelvic disproportion and/or shoulder dystocia. The BPD does not evaluate head-to-body disproportion and subsequent shoulder dystocia; hence, macrosomic indices based on BPD and chest or abdominal diameters have been developed.

Intrauterine growth retardation (IUGR) affects infants born from diabetic mothers with end-organ disease. Symmetrical IUGR may be distinguished from asymmetrical IUGR by head-to-body ratios. However, the lack of precise gestational age creates difficulty in distinguishing fetuses with symmetrical IUGR from fetuses that are appropriately grown but with inaccurate dates. The transverse cerebellar diameter may represent a useful parameter to distinguish these entities because it is not affected by the growth retardation process.

Fetal Heart-Rate Monitoring

After ~30 wk gestation, the fetal heart rate (FHR) can be used to assess fetal well-being. Additionally, more prolonged increases in FHR (called accelerations) are predictive of fetal well-being. The nonstress test (NST), which is based on the presence of FHR accelerations, is a simple and rapid screening procedure that has no contraindications. It should be performed twice weekly beginning no later than 32 wk gestation in diabetic pregnancies. An NST is considered to be reactive (i.e., predictive of fetal well-being) if there are at least two accelerations of the FHR of 15 beats/min for 15 s duration in a 20-min period. If a reactive NST cannot be documented, it can be extended. If the NST is still nonreactive after 40 min of testing, the patient is often given a glucose-containing drink and the test repeated. About 90% of nonreactive NSTs will become reactive after this maneuver. This approach reduces the number of patients requiring more involved evaluation. The latter may be performed by a contraction stress test (CST) or biophysical profile (BPP). A CST is initiated by controlled infusion of a dilute pitocin (oxytocin) solution or by nipple stimulation. A positive (or concerning) CST reveals late decelerations (reduction in FHR after a contraction), indicating placental insufficiency with adequate uterine contraction (3/10 min). A negative CST predicts fetal well-being for 1 wk. An alternative to CST is a BPP, which can include NST, fetal breathing movements, gross body movements, fetal tone, amniotic fluid volume. Some physicians also perform ultrasonographic characterization of the placenta. Each of these parameters is awarded 2 points if normal and 0 points if abnormal. A score of 10 (or 12) indicates fetal well-being, and a repeat test should be done in 3 days. A score of <8 is suspicious; the test should then be repeated earlier. The fetus is considered to be compromised with a score of ≤6, and an accelerated delivery must be seriously considered.

The early surveillance program, starting at 32 wk, may be integrated with maternal evaluation of fetal movements. Pregnant diabetic women should be instructed on fetal movement counts (count to 10 in <2 h twice daily). Although the false-positive rate is considerable and may reach 60%, maternal assessment of fetal activity is a simple and inexpensive screening technique for fetal testing. None of these biophysical techniques is predictive of fetal well-being in the event of abdominal trauma or abruptions.

TIMING OF DELIVERY

The following management scheme may serve as a guide for determination of the time for intervention.

1. Delivery may be mandatory even without documented lung maturity when maternal or fetal compromise is present, which puts the life of either at significant risk (e.g., severe fetal compromise determined by CST, maternal eclampsia, or severe preeclampsia).

2. Delivery is recommended with documented lung maturity in the case of significant maternal or fetal problems that do not pose an immediate risk. Fetal lung maturation must be documented by a mature lecithin-sphingomyelin ratio (L/S) and the presence of phosphatidylglycerol (PG) from an amniotic fluid specimen. Caution should be used in planning the delivery of patients with L/S >2.0 but absent PG. Therefore, in cases of absent PG, a safer L/S of 3.5 should be considered (e.g., poor maternal metabolic control, maternal hypertensive disorder of pregnancy, intrauterine growth retardation, strongly suspected fetal macrosomia, previous classic cesarean section, equivocal antepartum assessment of fetal condition).

3. Elective delivery may be considered at 38 wk in uncomplicated diabetic pregnancy if the cervix is ripe and lung maturity is documented.

Additional considerations:

1. Severe oligohydramnios may be considered in special circumstances to be an indication to proceed with delivery without amniotic fluid studies.
2. Planned repeat cesarean sections can be performed at 38 wk if fetal lung maturity is documented.
3. If the cervix is unfavorable and pregnancy reaches 40 wk, cervical ripening may be attempted as an alternative to primary cesarean section.
4. Under no condition should the diabetic pregnancy be allowed to proceed beyond 42 wk; in fact, rarely will pregnancies progress beyond 40 wk without attempts of delivery.

ROUTE OF DELIVERY

The mode of delivery for diabetic patients remains controversial. In the uncomplicated diabetic pregnancy, vaginal delivery is preferable to cesarean section because diabetes is not an a priori indication for the surgical procedure. Cesarean section is usually indicated before term when fetal distress or maternal compromise are detected.

At term, elective cesarean section should be reserved for cases in which the cervix is not favorable for delivery or when macrosomia is suspected on the basis of clinical signs and ultrasound measurements. An estimated fetal weight >4500 g is an indication for cesarean section; fetuses with estimated weight 4000–4500 g should be delivered based on the evaluation of past maternal history, the maternal pelvis, and progress of labor. A previous history of shoulder dystocia could also be an indication for cesarean section, unless the current fetus has a significantly lower estimated weight.

INTRAPARTUM MANAGEMENT

Spontaneous Labor

The onset of spontaneous labor is most beneficial for the patient because of an increased chance of spontaneous delivery, a shorter labor, and possibly less need for analgesia. To minimize the risk of lower urinary tract infection with catheterization during labor, micturition is encouraged.

Continuous FHR monitoring is performed; after spontaneous rupture of the membranes or amniotomy, a fetal scalp electrode should be attached. If the intensity of contractions is uncertain, an intrauterine pressure catheter should be placed and labor augmented with pitocin as needed.

Despite antepartum attempts to identify patients with fetal macrosomia, cervical dilation and descent of the fetal vertex should be evaluated by an experienced obstetrician, because arrest of dilation or descent should alert the physician to the possibility of cephalopelvic disproportion. A fetus with an ultrasound estimated weight >4000 g should be actively managed with a generous episiotomy in anticipation of possible shoulder dystocia.

The goal of metabolic management during labor is to maintain maternal plasma glucose levels at ~100 mg/dl to minimize the risk of subsequent neonatal hypoglycemia. Maternal glucose levels may be monitored hourly, and an infusion of 100–125 ml/h (of a solution of 10 U of regular insulin added to 1000 ml of 5% dextrose) may be added to maintain good glucose control.

Cesarean Section

- The patient undergoing an elective cesarean section should not eat or drink after midnight.
- Insulin administration should be restricted, often to administration of half the usual regular insulin dose.
- Epidural anesthesia should be used, because it allows early detection of signs of hypoglycemia.
- An intravenous solution of 5% dextrose should be administered, with hourly glucose monitoring.

SUGGESTED READING

1. Diamond MP, Moley KH, Pellicer A, Vaughn WK, DeCherney AH: Effects of streptozotocin- and alloxan-induced diabetes mellitus on mouse follicular and early embryo development. *J Reprod Fertil* 86:1–10, 1989
2. Diamond MP, Vaughn WK, Salyer SL, Cotton RB, Fields LM, Boehm FH: Antepartum fetal monitoring in insulin-dependent diabetic pregnancies. *Am J Obstet Gynecol* 153:528–35, 1985
3. Fog-Pedersen J, Molsted-Pedersen L, Moller S: Ultrasound studies on fetal growth. In *Carbohydrate Metabolism in Pregnancy and the Newborn*. Vol. 4. Sutherland HW, Stowers JM, Pearson DWM, Eds. London, Springer-Verlag, 1989, p. 83–93
4. Hobbins JC: Ultrasonography in the management of the diabetic pregnancy. *Diabetes Mellitus in Pregnancy*. Reece EA, Coustan DR, Eds. New York, Churchill Livingstone, 1988, p. 347–62
5. Reece EA, Davis N, Mahoney MJ, Baumgarten A: Maternal serum alpha fetoprotein in diabetic pregnancy: correlation with glycemic control (Letter). *Lancet* 2:275, 1987

5. Infants of Diabetic Mothers

CYNTHIA E. STRAND, MD, and
RICHARD A. EHRENKRANZ, MD

Approximately 1 in 200 pregnancies is complicated by overt diabetes, and gestational diabetes develops in an additional 2–3% of pregnancies. Because diabetes in pregnancy is associated with significant perinatal mortality and morbidity, this is clearly an important clinical entity. Common neonatal and fetal problems associated with infants of diabetic mothers (IDMs) are listed in Table 5.1.

PATHOGENESIS

The etiology of fetal and neonatal complications related to maternal diabetes is not entirely clear and probably involves more than one mechanism. These mechanisms include 1) fetal hyperglycemia and eventually fetal hyperinsulinemia secondary to maternal hyperglycemia and 2) decreased placental blood flow secondary to maternal and placental vascular disease associated with severe long-standing diabetes (White classification R and F).

Because the fetal pancreas does not make insulin until after 100 days gestation and insulin receptors are not found in the fetus until 26–27 wk gestation, congenital anomalies are not associated with fetal hyperinsulinemia but rather factors such as hyperglycemia or genetic predisposition. Macrosomia, cardiomyopathy, and septal hypertrophy are believed to be secondary to fetal hyperinsulinemia with increases in glucose and amino acid transport to fetal tissues, lipogenesis, and glycogen production. After delivery, hypoglycemia

Dr. Strand is a Fellow in Prenatal Medicine and Dr. Ehrenkranz is Professor of Pediatrics and Obstetrics and Gynecology at Yale University School of Medicine, New Haven, CT.

Table 5.1. COMMON FETAL AND NEONATAL PROBLEMS ASSOCIATED WITH DIABETES IN PREGNANCY

- Congenital anomalies
- Stillbirth
- Late-gestational death
- Intrauterine growth retardation
- Prematurity
- Macrosomia
- Cardiomyopathy and/or septal hypertrophy
- Respiratory distress syndrome
- Polycythemia
- Hypoglycemia
- Hypocalcemia
- Hyperbilirubinemia
- Renal vein thrombosis

will develop if this hyperinsulinemia persists and the maternal-to-fetal transfer of glucose is not replaced by an alternate glucose source. Hyperglycemia and/or hyperinsulinemia is associated with decreased production of lung surfactant, which can manifest as respiratory distress syndrome (RDS) in preterm infants. Intrauterine growth retardation is related to vascular disease. The cause of problems such as polycythemia, hypocalcemia, hyperbilirubinemia, renal vein thrombosis, prematurity, stillbirths, and late gestational deaths are unknown. Although gestational diabetes is not associated with the full spectrum of these problems, it is associated with hypoglycemia.

NEONATAL PROBLEMS AND MANAGEMENT

A full maternal history is important, including White classification and intrapartum maternal blood glucose level and management (e.g., insulin infusion, glucose-containing intravenous fluids). Newborn examination should include evaluation for macrosomia, congenital anomalies, and stigmata of growth retardation and an accurate gestational-age assessment. Table 5.2 lists characteristics of infants who should be evaluated and treated in a special-care nursery.

Birth Injury/Asphyxia

Macrosomic infants are at risk for asphyxia and birth injury secondary to difficult delivery. For this reason, delivery should take place where trained personnel are available and preparations can be made to deal with a potentially distressed infant.

Hypoglycemia

An early problem that the IDM may encounter is hypoglycemia. Macrosomic and appropriately grown infants are at risk for this

Table 5.2. INDICATIONS FOR EVALUATION AND TREATMENT IN SPECIAL-CARE NURSERY

All infants of insulin-dependent diabetic mothers
Infants of gestational diabetic mothers with complicating factors
    Preterm <37 wk
    Birth weight <2 kg
    Risk factors for sepsis
    5-min Apgar score <6
    Jitteriness
    Weak suck
    Hypothermia
    Bradycardia
    Tachycardia
    Tachypnea
    Poor tone

derangement within 30 min of cord clamping. Hypoglycemia is secondary to hyperinsulinemia, which persists even after cessation of maternal glucose transfer. The definition of hypoglycemia in the neonate is controversial, and, although variously reported as ranging from 17–72 mg/dl (0.95–4.03 mM), many clinicians accept levels ≤40 mg/dl (≤2.24 mM). Normal newborn blood glucose appears to depend on such factors as gestational age, postnatal age, hematocrit, type of blood sample (plasma, whole blood, serum), and method of analysis (e.g., glucose oxidase reagent-strip methods, glucose analyzers). The rapid reagent-strip methods are commonly used but have high variance (± 5–15 mg/dl [± 0.28–0.84 mM]) and poor reproducibility especially at blood glucose levels <50 mg/dl (<2.80 mM). A rapid glucose oxidase reagent-strip method for screening should be followed up with a laboratory glucose determination. The flow diagram in Fig. 5.1 represents one approach to monitoring and responding to blood glucose values in IDMs.

Respiratory Distress

Respiratory symptoms may develop in the IDM and may be due to polycythemia, congestive heart failure, hypoglycemia, sepsis, asphyxia, meconium aspiration, transient tachypnea of the newborn, and RDS. The IDM is known to have delayed lung maturation and inhibition of surfactant production. RDS has been described in IDMs where the amniotic fluid lecithin-sphingomyelin ratio is mature (>2:1) and the phosphatidylglycerol is absent. Although it is important to determine the primary cause of the respiratory symptoms, treatment of respiratory distress remains largely supportive.

Congenital Malformations

Once the infant is stabilized, he/she should be closely examined for evidence of any malformation. Cardiac malformations, including septal hypertrophy and cardiomyopathy, are the most common.

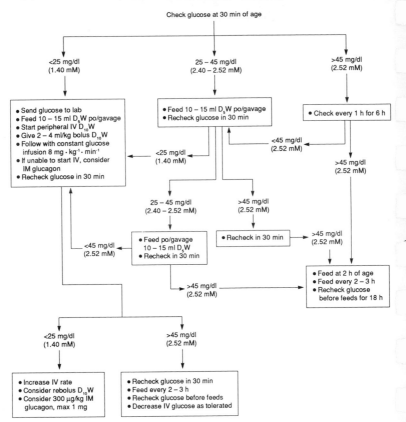

Figure 5.1. Management of hypoglycemia. D_5W, 5% dextrose solution; $D_{10}W$, 10% dextrose solution.

Caudal regression syndrome with hypoplasia of the sacrum and lower extremities occurs almost exclusively in IDMs. Gastrointestinal tract anomalies, particularly the small left colon syndrome, are also common.

Hypocalcemia

Hypocalcemia is defined by total serum calcium level of <7 mg/dl (<1.75 mM) or Ca^{2+} <3.5 mg/dl (<0.88 mM). As many as 50% of IDMs may have hypocalcemia. If the patient is asymptomatic, it is probably not necessary to monitor calcium levels or to treat with supplemental calcium. Symptoms such as jitteriness, irritability, seizures, hypotonia, or decreased myocardial contractility indicate that serum calcium level should be tested. In addition, serum calcium level should be tested in infants requiring intravenous glucose for hypoglycemia.

Treatment consists of 1–2 ml/kg 10% solution i.v. calcium gluconate administered initially as a slow infusion, with monitoring of heart rate. This should be followed by 100 mg/kg every 6 h until the hypocalcemia corrects or until total parenteral nutrition including calcium begins.

Polycythemia

Polycythemia is common in IDMs. Treatment consists of a reduction exchange transfusion to lower the hematocrit to 55%. The procedure should be done over 30 min. The volume to be exchanged is calculated by the formula

$$\text{exchange volume} = (\text{Hct-55/Hct}) \times \text{weight (kg)} \times 80 \text{ ml/kg}$$

where Hct is the starting hematocrit, and 80 ml/kg reflects the blood volume of a baby per kilogram of body weight.

Hyperbilirubinemia

Hyperbilirubinemia usually results from an exaggerated physiological jaundice, but pathological causes must be excluded. Treatment with phototherapy is almost always sufficient.

Renal Vein Thrombosis

When the symptoms of hematuria, signs of acute kidney failure, and a palpable renal mass are present, especially in the IDM, renal vein thrombosis is likely. Once suspected, a renal ultrasound with Doppler is indicated to confirm the diagnosis.

SUGGESTED READING

1. Conrad PD, Sparks JW, Osberg I, Abrams L, Hay WW Jr: Clinical application of a new glucose analyzer in the neonatal intensive care unit: comparison with other methods. *J Pediatr* 114:281–87, 1989
2. Cornblath M, Schwartz R, Aynsley-Green A, Lloyd JK: Hypoglycemia in infancy: the need for a rational definition. *Pediatrics* 85:834–37, 1990
3. Koh THHG, Eyre JA, Aynsley-Green A: Neonatal hypoglycemia: the controversy regarding definition. *Arch Dis Child* 63:1386–88, 1988
4. Oh W: The infant of the diabetic mother. In *Current Therapy in Neonatal-Perinatal Medicine II*. Nelson NM, Ed. Philadelphia, PA, Decker, 1990, p. 279–81
5. Warshaw JB: Infant of the diabetic mother. In *Principles and Practice of Pediatrics*. Oski F, DeAngelis C, Feigin R, Warshaw J, Eds. Philadelphia, PA, Lippincott, 1990, p. 429–31

6. Diabetic Ketoacidosis in Children

MARK A. SPERLING, MD

Children with diabetic ketoacidosis (DKA) differ from adults in requiring greater precision in the provision of fluids and electrolytes according to body weight and surface area; in a greater predilection to develop the complication of clinical cerebral edema, especially in children under age 5 yr; and in events commonly precipitating DKA.

DEFINITION

DKA is characterized by

1. Hyperglycemia with blood glucose usually >300 mg/dl (>17 mM)
2. Ketonemia with total ketones (β-hydroxybutyrate [βOHB] and acetoacetate) in serum >3 mM
3. Acidosis with blood pH <7.3 or serum bicarbonate ≤15 meq/L

Pure lactic acidosis (blood lactate >7 mM), salicylate ingestion, and nonketotic hyperglycemic coma should be distinguished from DKA.

PATHOPHYSIOLOGY

The metabolic derangements of DKA result from absolute or relative insulin deficiency amplified by the concerted action of the

Dr. Sperling is Professor of Pediatrics and Chairman of the Department of Pediatrics at the University of Pittsburgh School of Medicine, Pittsburgh, PA.

counterregulatory hormones catecholamine, glucagon, cortisol, and growth hormone, all of which are elevated in DKA.

Insulin deficiency is absolute if DKA is the initial presentation of newly diagnosed type I (insulin-dependent) diabetes or when the patient has inadvertently or deliberately omitted insulin; counterregulatory hormones are secondarily elevated with evolving stress. Insulin deficiency is relative if a major stress such as sepsis, trauma, or vomiting induces counterregulatory hormones that antagonize the effects of insulin or prevent its mobilization from subcutaneous depot sites due to dehydration. Stress and counterregulatory hormone secretion are the primary events.

Normally insulin is secreted with feeding, and the high insulin state is associated with anabolism, whereas the fasting low-insulin state is associated with catabolism. The increased counterregulatory hormones compound and accelerate the catabolic state. Acting in concert, they

1. Increase glucose production by glycogenolysis and gluconeogenesis (catecholamines, glucagon)
2. Impair glucose utilization by antagonizing the effects of insulin (catecholamines, cortisol, growth hormone)
3. Mobilize fatty acids by lipolysis (catecholamines, glucagon, growth hormone)
4. Induce ketogenesis with accumulation of the organic acids βOHB and acetoacetic acid (glucagon)

Excessive production and diminished utilization of these metabolites lead to hyperglycemia and polyuria due to osmotic diuresis when the renal threshold of ~180 mg/dl (~10 mM) is exceeded. Osmotic diuresis is associated with significant electrolyte losses compounded by vomiting and/or diarrhea (Table 6.1). Patients are commonly ≥10% dehydrated and manifest the signs and symptoms of dehydration, except for ongoing "good urine output" due to polyuria. Accumulating organic acids lead to metabolic acidosis with some lactic acidosis from poor perfusion and/or sepsis.

Table 6.1. FLUID AND ELECTROLYTE REQUIREMENTS IN DIABETIC KETOACIDOSIS

Fluid and Electrolyte	Maintenance Requirements	Losses
Water	1500 ml/m^2	100 ml/kg (60−100)
Sodium	45 meq/m^2	6 meq/kg (5−13)
Potassium	35 meq/m^2	5 meq/kg (4−6)
Chloride	30 meq/m^2	4 meq/kg (3−9)
Phosphate	10 mM/m^2	3 meq/kg (2−5)

Maintenance is expressed in surface area to permit uniformity because fluid requirements change as weight increases. Losses are expressed per unit of body weight because the losses remain relatively constant as a function of total body weight. Ranges are in parentheses.

CLINICAL MANIFESTATIONS

Clinical manifestations of ketoacidosis include

1. Deep-sighing respiration in an attempt to blow off carbon dioxide
2. Abdominal pain mimicking pancreatitis or an acute surgical abdomen
3. Possible elevation of nonspecific serum amylase
4. Elevated leukocyte count to 15,000–20,000/mm^3
5. Sepsis, pneumonia, urinary tract infection, or acute gastroenteritis identified in ~80% of patients
6. Fever
7. Progressive obtundation and loss of consciousness related to the degree of evolving hyperosmolality. Serum osmolality can be calculated as mosM = 2(Na + K) meq/L + glucose (mg/dl)/18.

CAVEATS

1. The degree of sodium loss may be overestimated due to the presence of hyperlipidemia and hyperglycemia. For each increase in glucose of 100 mg/dl (5.5 mM), serum sodium may be decreased by ~2 meq/L.
2. Serum potassium may be normal, but total-body potassium is commonly depleted. During acidosis, intracellular potassium moves to the extracellular compartment and may be lost in urine or vomitus. Hyperkalemia in DKA is therefore uncommon, unless renal shutdown has occurred. In contrast, hypokalemia may develop rapidly after treatment is initiated because the provision of insulin in the presence of hyperglycemia and the correction of acidosis promote the return of potassium to the intracellular compartment. Hypokalemia may be life threatening in its predilection for cardiac arrhythmias; therefore, provision of potassium and monitoring of its plasma concentration is of paramount importance in treating DKA.
3. Ketone bodies may cause spurious elevation in creatinine values in some assays. Also, only acetoacetic acid but not βOHB is measured by the commonly used semiquantitative and qualitative strip tests that depend on the sodium nitroprusside reaction. The concentration of βOHB is 4- to 10-fold higher than that of acetoacetic acid at initial presentation. With correction of acidosis, the βOHB is oxidized back to acetoacetate and is now measured. Hence, physicians should not be misled by the persistence of a strong ketone reaction as long as the patient manifests evidence of clinical and biochemical improvement in acidosis.
4. Ketoacidosis takes longer to correct than hyperglycemia. Therefore, insulin therapy should not be discontinued if ke-

toacidosis has not cleared even if glucose concentrations are approaching 300 mg/dl (17 mM).

5. The provision of excessive chloride is almost inevitable and usually presents no problem; the provision of some of the potassium deficits as potassium phosphate has certain theoretical and possibly practical benefits.

MANAGEMENT

Principles of DKA management in children is as follows (Tables 6.2–6.5).

1. Provision of fluid and electrolytes to correct dehydration, maintenance requirements, and ongoing losses. Fluid repair should extend over 36 h rather than 24 h to achieve a slower correction of serum hyperosmolality to avoid a rapid shift of water from the extracellular to the intracellular compartment, which is implicated in the development of cerebral edema. Similarly, the initial hydrating fluid should be normal saline, and the glucose concentration should be maintained at ~200–300 mg/dl (~11–17 mM) for the initial 36–48 h. The initial rate of fall in glucose concentration should, if possible, be limited to ~100–150 mg $\cdot$ dl^{-1} $\cdot$ h^{-1} (~5–8 mM/h).

2. Potassium replacement should begin slowly (after ~1 h intravenous treatment) if urine flow is established. Rate of potassium replacement should not exceed 6 meq $\cdot$ kg^{-1} $\cdot$ day^{-1}, unless plasma concentrations remain abnormally low (<3.5 meq/L) due to inordinate urinary or other losses. Some potassium can be given as potassium phosphate, thereby limiting the inevitable excess provision of chloride.

3. Bicarbonate therapy is not recommended unless the blood pH is <7.2. Bicarbonate (HCO_3^-), after combining with H^+, dissociates to CO_2 + H_2O. Whereas the HCO_3^- diffuses poorly across the blood-brain barrier, CO_2 diffuses freely into cerebrospinal fluid. Hence, inappropriate use of HCO_3^- may worsen cerebral acidosis

Table 6.2. FLUID AND ELECTROLYTE LOSSES BASED ON ASSUMED 10% DEHYDRATION IN CHILD WITH DIABETIC KETOACIDOSIS

Fluid and Electrolyte	Approximate Accumulated Losses With 10% Dehydration	Approximate Requirements for Maintenance (36 h)	Working Total (36 h)
Water (ml)	3000	2250	5500
Sodium (meq)	180	65	250
Potassium (meq)	150	50	200
Chloride (meq)	120	45	165
Phosphate (mM)	90	15	100

Body weight 30 kg; surface area 1.0 m².

Table 6.3. REPLACEMENT PROCEDURE FOR DIABETIC KETOACIDOSIS WITH 10% DEHYDRATION

Approximate Duration	Fluid (Composition)	Sodium (mM)	Potassium (mM)	Chloride (mM)	Phosphate (meq)
1st h	500 ml of 0.9% NaCl (normal saline)	75		75	
2nd h	500 ml of 0.45% NaCl (0.5 normal saline) plus 20 meq of KCl	35	20	55	
h 3–12 (200 ml/h for 10 h)	2000 ml of 0.45% saline with 30 meq/L of potassium phosphate	150	60	150	40
Total initial 12 h	3000 ml	260	80	280	40
Next 24 h 100 ml/h	0.2 normal saline in 5% glucose with 40 meq/L of potassium phosphate	75	100	75	60
Total (over 36 h)	5400 ml	335	180	355	100

Weight 30 kg; surface area 1.0 m^2. All replacement values should be halved if dehydration is estimated to be 5%. Maintenance requirements remain the same.

while serum acidosis improves. Also, the use of HCO_3^- may overcorrect acidosis, and the resultant alkalosis favors intracellular movement of potassium, thereby predisposing further to the development of hypokalemia. Bicarbonate should not be given as a bolus because it may precipitate cardiac arrhythmias.

4. Insulin is absolutely essential to fully correct the metabolic derangements of DKA, although fluid treatment alone has some corrective effects. After an initial bolus dose (0.15 U/kg), a continuous low-dose insulin infusion at $0.1 \ U \cdot kg^{-1} \cdot h^{-1}$ has become the recommended method of insulin delivery.

COMPLICATIONS

Electrolyte Changes

Inappropriate levels of serum electrolytes, particularly hyperkalemia and hypokalemia, hypophosphatemia, and hypocalcemia from too vigorous use of phosphate replacement can be avoided by scrupulous monitoring and appropriate adjustment of the electrolyte composition. If acidosis does not resolve, check the composition of the insulin mixture to ensure that an error in dilution has not occurred. If no error is identified and the acidosis does not resolve despite appropriate fluids and insulin, consider the coexistence of severe sepsis causing lactic acidosis and that certain bacteria possess insulin-degrading enzyme activity.

Table 6.4. **ADDITIONAL GUIDELINES FOR MANAGEMENT OF DIABETIC KETOACIDOSIS**

- A diabetic flowchart with laboratory data appropriately recorded must be maintained in the patient's chart.
- Insulin therapy by continuous low-dose intravenous method
  - Priming dose 0.15 U/kg i.v. regular insulin.
  - Continuous infusion $0.1 \ U \cdot kg^{-1} \cdot h^{-1}$ i.v. regular insulin.
- Directions for making insulin infusion
  Add 50 U regular insulin to 500 ml of physiological saline. Flush 50 ml through the tubing to saturate insulin binding sites. For a 30-kg patient, infuse at rate of 30 ml/h. When blood glucose concentration reaches 300 mg/dl (17 mM), continue the insulin infusion, and add glucose 5–10% to the infusate to maintain glucose concentration of 200–300 mg/dl (11.1–16.7 mM) until acidosis is corrected.
- Bicarbonate therapy*
  - For pH >7.2, no therapy necessary.
  - For pH 7.1–7.2, 40 mM/m² HCO_3^- over 2 h, then reevaluate.
  - For pH <7.1, 80 mM/m² HCO_3^- over 2 h, then reevaluate.
- New diabetic patients <2 yr of age with diabetic ketoacidosis and 10% dehydration or any diabetic with pH <7.0, blood glucose >1000 mg/dl (55 mM), or comatose should be managed in an intensive-care unit or equivalent.

*For more detailed discussion, see chapt. 10.

Table 6.5. STEPS IN MANAGEMENT OF DIABETIC KETOACIDOSIS

---

1. Confirm diagnosis
   Obtain: Blood glucose
            Serum electrolytes
            Acid-base status—pH, HCO_3^-, P_{CO_2}
   Consider: Urine microscopy/culture
            Chest X ray
            Blood culture
            Throat culture
   Intensive-care setting necessary: pH <7.00
                                    Age <2 yr
                                    Unconscious
                                    Blood glucose >1000 mg/dl
                                    (55 mM)
2. Begin intravenous fluids—20 ml/kg 0.9% (normal) saline (NaCl) over 1 h
3. Reassess patient—What precipitated this episode?   Noncompliance
                                                      Infection
                                                      Trauma
4. Follow protocol—Begin insulin with a bolus dose of 0.15 U/kg i.v. regular insulin followed by infusion of $0.1 \ U \cdot kg^{-1} \cdot h^{-1}$ i.v. regular insulin
5. Measure glucose every 2 h; electrolytes/acid-base every 2–4 h for first 24 h
6. Continue treatment with insulin even if glucose approaches 300 mg/dl (17 mM) as long as acidosis persists. Consider adding 5–10% glucose to intravenous infusion or occasionally reducing insulin to $0.05 \ U \cdot kg^{-1} \cdot h^{-1}$
7. If acidosis is not resolving (or improving) despite fluids and insulin of $0.1 \ U \cdot kg^{-1} \cdot h^{-1}$, consider severe sepsis causing lactic acidosis and/or insulin degradation
8. In children <10 yr old (especially <5 yr old),
   anticipate possible clinical cerebral edema
   after 4–6 h of treatment: Headache
                                    Change in consciousness level/response
                                    Unequal dilated pupils
                                    Delirium
                                    Incontinence
                                    Vomiting
                                    Bradycardia
9. If cerebral edema is clinically apparent: Reduce intravenous infusion rate
                                                  Give mannitol 1 g/kg i.v. ($10–120 \ g/m^2$)
                                                  Repeat in 2–4 h

---

Cerebral Edema

The major complication of DKA management in children is clinical cerebral edema. The etiology of this potentially devastating sequela is incompletely understood. Computed tomography of the head suggests that most patients with DKA have some evidence of raised intracranial pressure due to narrow ventricles during therapy, which then widen when the patient recovers. Only a few of these patients manifest clinical cerebral edema, which is more common in children <5 yr of age and includes the symptoms outlined in Table 6.5. Usually these are patients with new-onset diabetes whose clinical manifestations occur several hours after the institution of therapy and after clinical and biochemical indices have suggested improvement. The symptoms and signs of raised intracranial pressure, e.g., headache, deterioration in conscious state, bradycardia, papilloedema, development of fixed dilated pupils and occasionally polyuria secondary to diabetes insipidus, should alert the physician to the existence of this potentially fatal complication. Although the use of magnetic resonance imaging indicates that some children have cerebral thrombosis or infarction in addition to cerebral edema, early intervention with intravenous mannitol, reduction of the intravenous infusion rate and the institution of hyperventilation are indicated. The dose of mannitol is $10-20$ g/m^2 i.v., repeated after $2-4$ h if necessary. When instituted promptly (before coma), these measures can be lifesaving and may avoid neurological sequelae. Some authorities believe that the risks of cerebral edema can be reduced by limiting the rate of fluid administration to <4.0 L $\cdot$ m^{-2} $\cdot$ day^{-1}, avoiding the use of hypotonic solutions and avoiding the excessive use of bicarbonate. In the case of severe cerebral edema, the use of high-dose dexamethasone therapy should be considered.

The most efficient way to decrease the incidence of cerebral edema is by the prevention of DKA through the early diagnosis of diabetes mellitus and avoidance of recurrent episodes of DKA by effective patient/family education and support. Recurrent episodes of DKA in a child, particularly an adolescent, should be viewed as management failure on the part of the parents or a plea by the child to be removed from an environment that the child considers intolerable.

SUGGESTED READING

1. Foster DW, McGarry JD: The metabolic derangements and treatment of diabetic ketoacidosis. *N Engl J Med* 309:159–69, 1983
2. Harris GD, Fiordalisi I, Harris WL, Mosovich LL, Finberg L: Minimizing the risk of brain herniation during treatment of diabetic ketoacidemia: a retrospective and prospective study. *J Pediatr* 117:22–31, 1990
3. Krane EJ, Rockoff MA, Wallman JK, Wolfsdorf JI: Subclinical brain swelling in children during treatment of diabetic ketoacidosis. *N Engl J Med* 312:1147–51, 1985
4. Rosenbloom AL: Intracerebral crises during treatment of diabetic ketoacidosis. *Diabetes Care* 13:22–33, 1990
5. Sperling MA: Diabetic ketoacidosis. *Pediatr Clin North Am* 31:591–610, 1984

7. Type I Diabetes in Children

TIMOTHY W. JONES, MD, SUSAN D. BOULWARE, MD, and
WILLIAM V. TAMBORLANE, MD

The adequacy of diabetes care received during school-age years may
be the most important factor determining whether patients develop
the late degenerative complications of diabetes. On the other hand,
the rapid physiological and psychosocial changes that occur during
childhood and adolescence make these patients the most difficult
to manage.

INITIATION OF TREATMENT

Almost all children with newly diagnosed type I (insulin-dependent)
diabetes should be admitted to the hospital for the initiation of
treatment. The diagnosis of type I diabetes in a child is a major
shock and crisis for the family that requires time for adjustment
and healing. The hospital provides a reasonably safe place for this
process to begin. Three to 5 days of hospitalization are usually
necessary to accomplish basic diabetes education and initiation of
treatment.

INSULIN THERAPY

The aim of insulin replacement in the treatment of type I diabetes
is to simulate as closely as practically possible the fluctuations in
plasma insulin levels that are normally seen in nondiabetic individ-

*Dr. Jones is a visiting professor, Dr. Boulware is Assistant Professor of
Pediatrics, and Dr. Tamborlane is Professor of Pediatrics at the Yale University School of Medicine, New Haven, CT.*

uals (see chapt. 20). However, in the face of the severe insulin deficiency that characterizes type I diabetes in youth and practical considerations of acceptability and compliance, the ability to simulate normal insulin profiles is particularly limited in young patients. As the most generally acceptable compromise, newly diagnosed children should be started on 2 injections/day of a mixture of human intermediate-acting (NPH) and short-acting (regular) insulin at a total dose of ~0.5 U · kg^{-1} · day. Two thirds of the total is given in the morning before breakfast and one third as a predinner dose. As in the past with animal (beef and pork) insulins, the starting prebreakfast dose is usually divided in a 2:1 ratio of intermediate- to short-acting insulin, whereas the predinner dose is divided in a 1:1 ratio. However, due to the more rapid onset and shorter duration of action of human NPH, relatively more intermediate- and less short-acting insulin will ultimately be needed. This can be accomplished in the initial dosage-adjustment period by preferentially increasing the doses of intermediate-acting insulin until adequate control of the prebreakfast and predinner plasma glucose levels are achieved. Extra short-acting insulin should then be added, if needed, for control of prelunch and bedtime glucose levels.

Early in the course of the disease, many children go through a "honeymoon" or partial remission phase. This is usually heralded by recurrent biochemical or symptomatic hypoglycemia despite reductions in insulin dosage. At this stage, the evening dose of intermediate-acting insulin should be reduced or omitted if nocturnal hypoglycemia is a problem, because residual endogenous insulin secretion is usually sufficient to regulate the fasting blood glucose level. Most patients still require their morning mixture and predinner short-acting insulin. Recent evidence supports the concept of aggressive insulin therapy during the early stages of the disease. Such treatment may play an important role in helping to preserve residual β-cell function months or even years after diagnosis, which will, in turn, facilitate achievement of good diabetes control.

The primary goals of treatment of type I diabetes in children and adolescents have not changed substantially over the years. The treatment regimen should still be adjusted to minimize symptoms of hypoglycemia and hyperglycemia and promote normal growth and development. With intensive education, independence and self-management can be maximized to reduce the adverse psychosocial effects of this chronic disease. On the other hand, increasing effort is directed toward maintaining blood glucose profiles as close to normal as possible. Steadily increasing doses of insulin are required to meet these aims for several reasons:

- Weight and calorie intake increase with age.
- Residual endogenous insulin secretion declines after the honeymoon period so that most children and adolescents are totally insulin deficient after having had type I diabetes for 2–3 yr.
- Hormonal and physiological changes of puberty may themselves induce a state of relative insulin resistance.

As a result, the average daily insulin dose in children with long-standing diabetes is ~1 U/kg body wt, and doses of ≥1.5 U/kg may be required by well-controlled adolescents. These changes in the treatment program are best accomplished by frequent small alterations made by the parents or patients themselves with review by the medical staff on at least a 3- to 4-mo basis. More frequent telephone contact can also be helpful.

Day-to-day adjustments of insulin doses are of two types. In patients on 2 injections/day, small adjustments in the prebreakfast and predinner doses of short-acting insulin can be made if the blood glucose value is outside the target range. Patients and parents should be taught to look for repetitive patterns of hyperglycemia or hypoglycemia that indicate an adjustment in the usual dose is needed. Dosage changes of 5–10% at a time are usually recommended.

INTENSIFIED INSULIN THERAPY IN CHILDREN AND ADOLESCENTS

More aggressive insulin treatment with ≥3 injections/day or continuous subcutaneous insulin infusion (CSII) with a portable pump can provide means to more closely simulate normal insulin profiles and avoid some of the problems with the standard 2-shot schedule. A major problem with twice-daily injections is that the peak of the predinner intermediate-acting insulin may coincide with the time of minimal insulin requirement (i.e., 0200–0400). Subsequently, insulin levels fall off when basal requirements are increasing (i.e., 0400–0800). Thus, the tendency for blood glucose levels to rise before breakfast (dawn phenomenon) may be exaggerated by the release of anti-insulin hormones in response to a fall in glucose in the middle of the night (Somogyi phenomenon). A 3-injection schedule—mixed short- and intermediate-acting insulin at breakfast, short-acting insulin only at dinner, and intermediate-acting insulin at bedtime—may effectively compensate for these problems. Alternatively, a long-acting insulin (e.g., ultralente) can replace basal insulin and short-acting insulin given with each meal (see chapt. 20). Adherence and compliance issues have been the major obstacles that have limited the use of complex multiple-dose regimens in children. Use of convenience devices such as insulin pens and jet injectors may be helpful.

CSII has also been used sparingly in young patients with type I diabetes. There are several problems specific to CSII therapy, particularly in children. The most obvious disadvantage is the presence of the pump itself, because children are particularly sensitive to being different. Also, because only short-acting insulin is used with CSII, any interruption of the flow can lead to decompensation. The solution to this problem lies in meticulous care of the infusion system and frequent blood glucose measurements. The added responsibility of caring for the device, in addition to the disease, may be a problem for young patients.

of caring for the device, in addition to the disease, may be a problem for young patients.

Intensified insulin therapy takes a tremendous effort on the part of patients and their parents, and a great deal of support is required from the medical team. Only a small fraction of children and adolescents are either interested in or able to maintain this degree of intensity over the long run. On the other hand, such treatments should not be denied to youngsters with diabetes just because of their age. Indeed, if successful, the results of intensive therapy are especially gratifying in this age-group.

MONITORING GLUCOSE CONTROL

Self-Monitoring of Blood Glucose (SMBG)

SMBG represents one of the most important advances in diabetes management. To be helpful, SMBG must be performed accurately and frequently, and the results must be interpreted correctly. The parent or child must be taught what a normal blood glucose value is, what the target values are to be, the degree to which levels should be expected to vary, and what the relationship is between blood glucose and diet, insulin, and exercise.

Newly diagnosed patients are requested to perform at least four blood tests daily (before each meal and at bedtime), but it is difficult to sustain this level of activity over time. On the other hand, improved compliance with this aspect of management might be expected if the data are used by patients and parents for ongoing adjustments of insulin dosages. Waning enthusiasm for performing blood testing may result in falsification of SMBG data. This is more of a problem in children and adolescents than in adults with diabetes, and it is not readily correctable.

Glycosylated Hemoglobin

Glycosylated hemoglobin levels should be measured regularly (every 2–6 mo) because they provide an index of glucose control over the preceding 4- to 8-wk period. Measurement of glycosylated hemoglobin complements SMBG by providing a relatively simple way to independently and objectively assess diabetes control. Discrepancies between SMBG and glycosylated hemoglobin results are more commonly due to problems with the former than with the latter. HbA_{1c} levels in the normal range are rarely observed in conventionally treated children and adolescents except during the honeymoon period. Even in adults with type I diabetes enrolled in intensive treatment programs, HbA_{1c} values usually hover around or are modestly above the upper limit of normal. In adolescents receiving conventional treatment, HbA_{1c} levels are typically ≥50% higher than the upper limit of the normal range, i.e., values that correspond to mean plasma glucose levels of >250 mg/dl (>14 mM). Whereas these data suggest there is usually room for improvement, they also provide a realistic basis for comparison when evaluating control of young patients with type I diabetes.

DIET

Dietary guidance for children with type I diabetes requires careful instruction and frequent reinforcement. Involvement of a nutritionist who is knowledgeable about and comfortable working with children is strongly recommended (see chapt. 15). The American Diabetes Association diet is a good basis for dietary counseling. In addition to incorporating sound nutritional principles concerning the fat, fiber, and carbohydrate (complex rather than simple sugars) content, the importance of consistency in meal size and regularity in the timing of meals is emphasized. Paradoxically, the success of the nutritional program may ultimately depend on the degree to which the meal planning is individualized and tailored to well-established eating patterns in the family. Moreover, flexibility can be enhanced if blood glucose–monitoring results are used to evaluate the impact of deviations from the prescribed diet.

EXERCISE

Regular exercise and active participation in organized sports has positive implications concerning the psychosocial and physical well-being of young patients (see chapt. 16). Aerobic endurance exercise is preferred over weight lifting and other activities that involve straining and increase systemic blood pressure. Patients should be advised that different types of exercise may have different effects on blood glucose levels. For example, sports that involve short bursts of intensive exercise (e.g., hockey) may increase rather than decrease blood glucose levels. On the other hand, long-distance running and other prolonged activities are more likely to lower blood glucose levels.

At some centers, patients are discouraged from exercising if they are hyperglycemic (e.g., blood glucose >240 mg/dl [>14 mM]). However, if such a prohibition was enforced in young patients, virtually no teenager would be allowed to exercise. Therefore, exercise should be encouraged unless the patient is not feeling well and is ketotic.

ROUTINE OUTPATIENT CARE

Adolescents with type I diabetes should be routinely referred to a diabetes center that uses a multidisciplinary team knowledgeable and experienced in the management of young patients. This team should ideally consist of pediatric diabetologists, nurse educators, nutritionists, social workers, psychologists, exercise physiologists, and referral resources for eye, neurological, renal, and other problems.

During the first few weeks after diagnosis, patients and parents should maintain close follow-up with the treatment team. This is a critical period for the child and parent to learn the principles of adjusting insulin dosage and overall diabetes self-management. The parent or older child should be in daily telephone contact with the clinician. Clinical well-being, monitoring results, and the effect of changes in diet and exercise should be reviewed. The patient's thoughts about changes in the insulin regimen should be sought before making recommendations. The timing of phone calls should be prearranged and ideally made to the same clinician each day. Usually within 1–2 wk, the children (and parents) will feel more confident and should be able to make their own insulin adjustments.

Subsequently, regular follow-up on a 2- to 4-mo basis is recommended for each patient. The main purpose of these visits is to ensure that the patient is achieving the primary treatment goals of normal growth in the absence of significant symptomatic complaints related to hyperglycemia or hypoglycemia. In addition to serial measurements of height and weight, particular attention should be paid to monitoring of blood pressure and examinations of the optic fundus, thyroid, and subcutaneous injection sites. Limited mobility of the joints of the fingers in association with waxy thickening of the skin can indicate increased susceptibility to the microvascular complications of type I diabetes. Signs and symptoms referable to diabetes complications are sought. Such surveillance is complemented by use of the laboratory to measure lipids and circulating thyroid hormone levels, renal-function studies (including microalbuminuria), and retinal fundus photography. Routine outpatient visits provide an opportunity to review glucose monitoring and to adjust the treatment regimen. Follow-up advice and support should be given by the nutritionist, nurse educator, and behavioral scientist.

HYPOGLYCEMIA

The nonphysiological nature of conventional insulin replacement and relatively large insulin doses required by adolescents, defective glucagon responses, irregularities in diet and exercise, unreliability of blood glucose monitoring, and other problems contribute to the vulnerability of young patients to severe reductions in plasma glucose. On the other hand, brisk epinephrine responses are commonly observed in children with poorly controlled diabetes even when plasma glucose falls into the normal range, which can confuse the clinical assessment of hypoglycemic symptoms and emphasizes the need for accurate blood glucose testing.

Treatment of a mild to moderate reaction consists of at least 10 g of carbohydrate (40 cal), e.g., orange juice, regular soda, or glucose tablets. Candy bars or special treats are not recommended because the child may begin to feign reactions to get these things.

Proper insulin and dietary adjustments should be made to prevent further hypoglycemia. Parents must be taught how to inject glucagon for treatment of more severe reactions. They can also administer a quick glucose solution (e.g., honey or Insta-glucose) to the lips and cheeks.

SICK-DAY RULES

Children with intercurrent illnesses such as infections or vomiting should be closely monitored for elevations in blood glucose levels and ketonuria. On sick days, the blood glucose should be checked every 2 h if it is $\geq$240 mg/dl ($\geq$14 mM), and the urine should be checked for ketones every 3–4 h. Supplemental doses of short-acting insulin (0.1–0.3 U/kg) should be given every 2–4 h for elevations in glucose and ketones. Adequate fluid intake is essential to prevent dehydration. Fluids such as flat soda, clear soups, popsicles, and gelatin water are recommended to provide some electrolyte and carbohydrate replacement. If vomiting is persistent and ketones remain moderately to greatly increased after several supplemental insulin doses, arrangements should be made for parenteral hydration. Recurrent episodes of ketonuria and vomiting are usually the result of missed insulin doses or overall poor metabolic control.

SUGGESTED READING

1. Amiel SA, Tamborlane WV: New treatment methods in diabetes mellitus. In *Current Concepts in Pediatric Endocrinology*. Brook OGD, Styne DM, Eds. New York, Elsevier, 1987, p. 126–54
2. DCCT Research Group: The Diabetes Control and Complications Trial: results of the feasibility study (phase II). *Diabetes Care* 10:1–19, 1987
3. Shah SC, Malone JI, Simpson NE: A randomized trial of intensive insulin therapy in newly diagnosed insulin-dependent diabetes mellitus. *N Engl J Med* 320:550–54, 1989
4. Sperling MA: Outpatient management of diabetes mellitus. *Pediatr Clin North Am* 34:917–33, 1987

8. Psychosocial Adjustment in Children With Type I Diabetes

BARBARA J. ANDERSON, PhD, JOSEPH I. WOLFSDORF, MD, and ALAN M. JACOBSON, MD

Daily treatment of children with diabetes impacts and intrudes on everyday behavior in the family, alters family routines, and affects relationships among family members. How the family handles these intrusions determines the effectiveness with which childhood diabetes is managed. This chapter addresses these issues from a developmental perspective by examining the changing tasks of different-aged children and their families.

CRISIS AT DIAGNOSIS

The diagnosis of diabetes in a child or adolescent hurls the parent from a secure and known reality into a frightening and foreign world. At diagnosis, they grieve the loss of their healthy child and cope with such normal distress reactions as shock, disbelief and denial, fear, anxiety, anger, and extreme blame or guilt. However, parents must acquire an understanding of and behavioral skills to manage the illness at home and to assist the child in achieving acceptable blood glucose control.

Parents should receive the emotional support required to begin coping with the emotional distress and not be overwhelmed by unrealistic expectations from a well-meaning diabetes-treatment team (Table 8.1). Parents must find a sense of balance after the diagnosis

Dr. Anderson is Assistant Professor of Psychiatry, Dr. Wolfsdorf is Chief of Pediatrics, and Dr. Jacobson is Assistant Professor of Psychiatry at the Joslin Diabetes Center, Boston, MA.

Table 8.1. RECOMMENDATIONS FOR DIABETES-TREATMENT TEAM AT DIAGNOSIS

- Limit guidelines to basic skills
- Keep to a minimum the number of medical staff providing information and treatment
- Include both parents, in some fashion, in the diabetes-education program
- Encourage, in single-parent families, another adult (e.g., grandparent or neighbor) to support the parent

---

and should be encouraged to progress at their own pace with emotional support offered by a staff member or another parent.

DIABETES AND CHILD DEVELOPMENT

Diabetes presents family members with the task of being sensitive to the balance between the child's need for independence and mastery of self-care activities and the need for family support and involvement. The struggle to balance independence and dependence in relationships between the child and family members presents a long-term problem and raises different issues for families at different stages of child and adolescent development. Focusing on normal developmental tasks at each stage of the child's growth and development provides the most effective structure to address this concern.

INFANTS AND TODDLERS WITH DIABETES (0–3 YR OLD)

At this earliest stage of child development, the parent is the only appropriate patient with respect to diabetes management. Researchers have identified several problems facing parents with diabetic infants and toddlers (Table 8.2).

Children diagnosed before age 5 yr may be at risk for specific subtle cognitive deficits caused by severe hypoglycemic episodes. This relates to difficulties in administering and adjusting the small insulin doses needed by most infants and toddlers as well as the proverbal child's inability to recognize and communicate symptoms of hypoglycemia.

At this stage of development, two important aspects of care are *1*) how treatment responsibilities are shared between parents and *2*) the prevention of severe hypoglycemic episodes. The primary developmental task during infancy is to achieve a stable, trusting relationship between infant and primary-care provider.

The central task of the child from age 1 to 3 yr is to establish an initial sense of mastery over the world. Toddlers do not have the cognitive skills to understand why cooperation with the intrusive, sometimes painful procedures of the diabetic regimen is needed.

Table 8.2. CHALLENGES FACING PARENTS AND/OR CHILDREN WITH DIABETES

Parents of infants and toddlers (0–3 yr old)
- Monitoring diabetes control and avoiding hypoglycemia
- Establishing a meal schedule despite the child's normally irregular eating patterns
- Coping with the very young child's inability to understand the need for injections
- Managing the conflicts with older siblings that result from unequal sharing of parental attention

Preschoolers and early elementary schoolchildren (4–7 yr old)
- Mastering separation from the family and adapting to the expectations of teachers
- Blaming self for having diabetes; regarding injections and restrictions as punishments
- Educating school personnel, coaches, and scout leaders about diabetes (parents)

Later elementary schoolchildren (8–11 yr old)
- Engaging in a wide range of activities with peers
- Understanding long-term benefits of diabetes care
- Becoming involved in diabetes self-care tasks (selecting snacks, selecting and cleaning injection sites, and identifying symptoms of low blood glucose)

Early adolescence (12–15 yr old)
- Integrating physical changes into their self-image
- Acknowledging that the young teenager is on the threshold of becoming an adult (parents)
- Assuming increased responsibility for diabetes management in the face of physiological changes caused by puberty on insulin resistance and sensitivity
- Fitting in with the peer group
- Maintaining good glycemic control while concerned about possible weight gain

Later adolescence (16–19 yr old)
- Making decisions regarding post–high school plans
- Living more independently of parents
- Strengthening relationships with fewer friends
- Assuming more independent responsibility for health and health care

Thus, injections or fingersticks for blood glucose monitoring may become battlegrounds when the toddler resists and may require significant emotional stamina by the parent.

PRESCHOOLERS AND EARLY ELEMENTARY SCHOOLCHILDREN WITH DIABETES (4–7 YR OLD)

Nursery school or kindergarten may represent the first arena in which both parents and children face the social consequences of diabetes, including the need to educate others about the disease (Table 8.2). Thus, separation problems that often appear in children this age may be heightened in the child with diabetes.

The 4- to 7-yr-old with diabetes often applies cause-effect thinking and may blame himself/herself for having the disease or see injections and restrictions as punishments. Diabetic youngsters at this age benefit from informal contact and group interactions (diabetes camps) with other diabetic children.

At this stage of development, parents continue to be the primary recipients of diabetes education and to interact with the health-care team. However, the child's increasing motor coordination and cognitive skills enable him/her to become a more involved partner in diabetes self-care tasks. Children can select appropriate snacks, select and clean injection sites, and begin to identify symptoms of low blood glucose. The goal is for elementary school–aged children to be positively drawn into their own care without premature and unrealistic expectations for independence while parental control and supervision continue.

LATER ELEMENTARY SCHOOLCHILDREN (8–11 YR OLD)

The preadolescent child forms close friendships with children of the same sex, strives to gain approval from this peer group, and seriously begins to evaluate himself/herself by comparing abilities to those of peers. Diabetic children, in the process of making these social comparisons, should develop a strong positive self-image. In fact, preadolescent diabetic children with adjustment problems may often be overlooked because they are not overtly rebellious and hostile but rather are overdependent on family members and withdrawn from peers. Participation and positive self-image are key concepts at this age, and health-care providers should emphasize to parents the importance of a wide range of activities with peers.

Parents should focus diabetes education on realistic blood glucose goals and safety guidelines for prevention of hypoglycemia. That is, parent and child should be ready to increase monitoring of blood glucose and plan ahead for additional snacks with extra activity.

It is important to continue emphasizing the long-term benefits of continued diabetes care. Children this age can test blood glucose levels and give injections on occasion without supervision. Health-care providers should negotiate more directly with the child concerning issues and problems with diabetes rather than talking solely to the parents.

EARLY ADOLESCENCE (12–15 YR OLD)

During early adolescence, the change in balance of responsibility between the diabetic child and the family for diabetes management tasks continues. Dramatic changes occur in five areas:

- Physical development
- Family dynamics

- School experiences
- Cognitive development
- Social networks

It is common for families to change their expectations of the young adolescent and frequently "turn over" responsibility for diabetes management. However, physiological changes of puberty, which are associated with insulin resistance in both nondiabetic and diabetic adolescents, can complicate this transition. Reduced sensitivity to insulin probably contributes significantly to the difficulty experienced by many diabetic adolescents in achieving optimal glycemic control.

If the diabetes-care regimen makes a teen stand out from the peer group, conflicts can arise. Some diabetic teenagers may stop their self-care and try to prove they are "normal." Others may use diabetes as an excuse to withdraw. Many who never before hid their diabetes may now refuse to talk about it with friends.

Young teenagers have an increasing cognitive ability to analyze themselves and the world around them and do not accept authority but rather examine, criticize, and question. This growing ability leads many diabetic teenagers to a new sensitivity about their disease; e.g., they may vent their anger about having diabetes. Parents and health-care professionals frequently overestimate the teenager's conceptual understanding of diabetes. Parents also can overestimate the adolescent's ability to follow through with diabetes care tasks without immediate positive reinforcement and support, mistakenly assuming that long-term good health will provide motivation for adherence to the diabetes-treatment plan.

Diabetes can further threaten the young teenager's self-confidence. Fluctuating blood glucose levels that defy control contribute to younger teenagers feeling uneasy in their bodies. Insulin reactions, injections, and blood glucose monitoring can further undermine the child's ability to feel attractive or normal. Concerns about body image must be taken seriously by parents and health-care providers. For example, a problem seen frequently in young adolescent girls who are distressed about weight gain is a dramatic increase in blood glucose levels. When adolescent girls are worried about their weight, and parents and the health-care team focus exclusively on good control, many patients begin to secretly reduce their insulin and thereby purge calories and lose weight. This self-destructive behavior is similar to bulimia nervosa, and this diabetes-specific eating disorder often causes repeated hospitalizations for diabetic ketoacidosis in adolescent girls.

Because puberty causes such physiological barriers to controlling blood glucose, and because of the psychological and social vulnerabilities of this age, parents should continue involvement in and supervision of insulin administration and blood glucose testing throughout early adolescence. Negotiation of continued support and supervision is critical even if the young adolescent initially rejects it. Likewise, parents should recruit participation from the child even if the notion is rejected initially. Negative family interactions surrounding diabetes management contribute to compliance and metabolic control problems in adolescents with diabetes.

Families should also be encouraged to change their pattern of relationships with diabetes health-care providers. Young teenagers often have issues, e.g., concerns about sexuality, that they do not feel comfortable discussing in front of parents. Thus, health-care providers should begin seeing parents and young teenagers individually and sequentially.

Both young adolescents and their parents may benefit from contact with other families coping with similar struggles. Diabetes camps often provide an important forum for peer identification, and peer-group educational and support programs may be helpful for both children and parents.

LATER ADOLESCENCE (16–19 YR OLD)

As growth and change decrease and stabilize, so do conflicts over diabetes self-care. The central developmental tasks of the older adolescent are outlined in Table 8.2.

Some older diabetic teenagers who feel overwhelmed with the pressures of high school and the need to plan for the future ignore their self-care. When peer relationships are insecure or school work seems beyond their abilities, some teenagers may use their diabetes to avoid the conflicts at school. Some older teenagers with poor metabolic control reflect a chronic unmet need for more family support for self-care tasks. Poor control in a teenager can be a reflection of chaos and dysfunction at home. In these instances, more (not less) parental involvement may be needed. Family counseling can help parents and teenagers negotiate adjustments.

Conflicts over friendships are the primary cause of alienation between parents and teenagers. This is especially true when issues of alcohol and drugs, safety (driving), and sexual activity are raised. Older teenage girls (and their parents) should be educated about the importance of good metabolic control before conception and about the difficulties of managing a diabetic pregnancy.

During this stage of development, growth and the upheaval of puberty slows, and insulin needs stabilize. Many older adolescent

Table 8.3. FAMILIES BENEFITING FROM ADDITIONAL PSYCHOSOCIAL SUPPORT

- All families at the time of diagnosis
- Single-parent families
- Minority ethnic-group membership
- Families in which another member has a serious chronic physical or mental illness, including a learning disability
- Families with infants and toddlers with type I diabetes

Table 8.4. RISK FACTORS RELATED TO INDIVIDUAL CHILDREN

Children and their families should be referred for counseling if any one of the following is present:
1. Failure to master the tasks of normal child or adolescent development
2. Identification of the child/adolescent as a "problem" by the legal system or school (extended school absences, school failure)
3. Serious depression, anxiety, learning disability, or other severe mental disorder
4. Inability to show age-appropriate cooperation with the tasks of diabetes care
5. More than one diabetes-related hospitalization for unexplained causes during a 1-yr period
6. Weight loss and chronic hyperglycemia (elevated HbA_{1c}), especially in adolescent girls

girls continue to be concerned about weight gain caused by insulin dose increases and a meal plan that provides significantly more calories than needed to meet the requirements of accelerated growth. Patients should be evaluated for insulin manipulation whenever poor metabolic control remains unexplained in an adolescent girl concerned about her weight. More gradual separation from medical providers is not a sign of psychological problems or overdependence. Expectations are that the older adolescent can manage diabetes independently; however, each family situation must be assessed individually.

REFERRAL TO MENTAL-HEALTH PROFESSIONAL

Several types of families should be considered high risk and may benefit from additional psychosocial support resources and more frequent appointments with the health-care team (Table 8.3). Similarly, several warning signals are used to identify a child (Table 8.4) or family (Table 8.5) for whom mental-health intervention is required.

Table 8.5. RISK FACTORS RELATED TO ENTIRE FAMILY

Family therapy is recommended if any one of the following problems is present:
1. Prolonged intense conflict between parent and child over division of responsibilities for diabetes-care tasks
2. Life crisis, such as divorce or death of family member, which causes severe grief reactions within family
3. Suspicion of child sexual/physical/emotional abuse or neglect, which should also be reported immediately to state legal authorities

SUGGESTED READING

1. Amiel SA, Sherwin RS, Simonson DC, Lauritano AA, Tamborlane WV: Impaired insulin action in puberty: a contributing factor to poor glycemic control in adolescents with diabetes. *N Engl J Med* 315:215–19, 1986
2. Anderson BJ: Diabetes and adaptations in family systems. In *Neuropsychological and Behavioral Aspects of Diabetes*. Holmes C, Ed. New York, Springer-Verlag, 1990, p. 85–101
3. LaGreca AM, Schwartz LT, Satin W: Eating patterns in young women with IDDM: another look. *Diabetes Care* 10:659–60, 1987
4. Rovet JF, Ehrlich RM, Hoppe M: Intellectual deficits associated with early onset of insulin-dependent diabetes mellitus in children. *Diabetes Care* 10:510–15, 1987
5. Wolfsdorf JL, Anderson BA, Pasquarello C: Treatment of the child with diabetes. In *Joslin Diabetes Manual*. 13th ed. Weir G, Kahn R, Eds. Philadelphia, PA, Lea & Febiger. In press

9. Psychosocial Aspects in Adults

LAWSON R. WULSIN, MD, and ALAN M. JACOBSON, MD

ORIGIN OF PSYCHOSOCIAL COMPLICATIONS

Diabetes itself does not cause psychiatric illness or changes in personality. That is, the prevalence of psychiatric illness is no greater in the diabetic population than in other chronic illness groups. However, particular subgroups of the diabetic population appear to be at risk for developing psychosocial complications. Women with type I (insulin-dependent) diabetes mellitus seem to have a higher prevalence of eating disorders, such as anorexia nervosa and bulimia, and those with long-standing diabetes and major medical complications have a higher prevalence of symptoms of depression and anxiety.

Older patients with type II diabetes may have associated alterations in cognitive or intellectual functioning, but the pathophysiology of these cognitive changes is not well understood.

Stress

Stress is one of many factors that may interfere with glycemic control. Two pathways, one behavioral and one humoral, mediate the effect of stress on glucose levels. Stress may cause the person to change key behaviors that upset self-care habits, e.g., increased alcohol intake or decreased exercise. Alternatively, stress hormones, e.g., catecholamines and cortisol, directly alter glucose levels in response to stress.

Dr. Wulsin is Assistant Professor of Psychiatry at the University of Cincinnati, Cincinnati, OH. Dr. Jacobson is Assistant Professor of Psychiatry at the Joslin Diabetes Center, Boston, MA.

Table 9.1. **BARRIERS TO SELF-CARE**

Patient attitudes and beliefs that affect self-care
- Anticipating early cure
- Believing that self-care regimen is too difficult
- Believing that treatment is unlikely to improve or control health problems

Psychosocial factors affecting self-care
- Stressful events in patient's life
- Development of new complication
- Availability and quality of social support for patient
- Psychiatric problems unrelated to patient's diabetes
- Health-care provider's approach to medical care

Barriers to Self-Care

Psychological and social factors can profoundly influence a patient's success in adhering to the prescribed self-care regimen (Table 9.1). Several medical problems can be reliable indicators of psychosocial barriers (Table 9.2).

Detection of Psychosocial Factors

The framework that favors early detection of complicating psychosocial factors is an effective working relationship with the patient. Periodically, examine the patient's experience by asking open-ended questions (Table 9.3):

- Ask patients to describe any stressful events or situations.
- Determine whether patients have adequate social and family support.
- Ask about problems concerning mood, anxiety, and sense of well-being.
- Ask young women who might be at risk for eating disorders whether they have skipped insulin doses, dieted excessively, eaten in binges, or vomited.
- Engage the patient, and at times the family, in monitoring behaviors or events as well as glucose levels.

Inquiries along these lines collect practical information that guide interventions and build the collaborative alliance. Over time, this alliance may lead to better glycemic control by helping the patient address such self-care barriers as low motivation, preconceived judg-

Table 9.2. **MEDICAL PROBLEMS INDICATING PSYCHOSOCIAL BARRIERS TO DIABETES CONTROL**

- Recurrent hypoglycemia
- Frequent episodes of ketoacidosis
- Very high glycosylated hemoglobin levels
- Brittle diabetes

Table 9.3. OPEN-ENDED QUESTIONS FOR PATIENTS WITH SELF-CARE PROBLEMS

Practitioners should ask about
- Importance of glycemic control
- Feasibility of adhering to prescribed diet
- Importance of self-monitoring of blood glucose
- Patient's susceptibility to developing complications
- Efficacy of treating complications
- Reasonableness of practitioner's recommendations and expectations

ments about treatment, and fears about diabetes. Even if this approach does not exact better glycemic control, it will help the patient feel more accepted and keep open lines of communication until he/she is more prepared to effect change.

THERAPY

Table 9.4 summarizes the major principles of effective glycemic control when psychosocial factors impair that control. The first six steps are behavioral and focus on accomplishing a goal; the latter two steps recognize the importance of maintaining a strong long-term working relationship.

A systematic approach to glycemic control following these principles may require a considerable initial investment of time and energy from the patient and clinician. The physician or nurse clinician should coordinate the effort, delegating responsibilities to the appropriate people and communicating the current plans to all involved. Nurses and physician assistants can be helpful in carrying out the plan once it has been developed.

This systematic coordinated approach is designed to reduce the number of diabetic crises and the emotional turmoil from failed

Table 9.4. GUIDELINES FOR IMPROVING ADHERENCE TO DIABETES REGIMENS

1. Give specific instructions, written and oral, about who will do what, tailored to the patient's specific needs and situation.
2. Train the patient and family in the skills necessary for the regimen and monitoring.
3. Monitor self-care behaviors in several ways by several people.
4. Increase the frequency of self-care behaviors with reminders.
5. Reinforce or reward steps toward adherence to the regimen.
6. Begin with small tasks and achievable goals; shape behaviors with successive revisions of the plan or contract as short-term goals are met.
7. Meet the patient at the level of effort the patient is prepared to make.
8. Avoid chastising patients when they fail to achieve a goal; instead, revise the goal or the approach.

From Wulsin and Jacobson (4).

Table 9.5. PATIENTS REQUIRING REFERRAL TO MENTAL-HEALTH SPECIALIST

- Patients who have had two or more episodes of severe hypoglycemia or diabetic ketoacidosis without obvious causes in 1 yr
- Patients whom you find frustrating

efforts at glycemic control while improving the working relationships among the patient, family, and clinicians. The approach justifies the time and effort required when past patterns of poor control have caused increasing stress on the patient's resources or when stress and other behavioral factors have interfered with glycemic control.

Problems with glycemic control may require thorough inquiry into several factors in addition to the occurrence of a stressful event or situation. Effective management strategies make use of a thorough assessment to develop a systematic treatment plan following principles that enhance adherence to medical regimens. The effectiveness of this approach depends on the doctor's ability to negotiate specific steps of the plan with the patient and to delegate responsibility to the appropriate people.

REFERRAL TO SPECIALIST

The practitioner will need to identify, for possible referral, mental-health professionals who are knowledgeable about diabetes and who can serve as collaborators in treating the patient (Table 9.5). Encourage patients to attend group sessions for patients and families.

Remember that diabetes is a chronic illness. Even if treatment activities fail to bring change in the short term, remaining involved with the patient and family and providing an accepting atmosphere may lead to increased motivation for change in the future.

SUGGESTED READING

1. Bradley C: Psychological aspects of diabetes. In *The Diabetes Annual.* Vol 1. Alberti KGMM, Krall LP, Eds. New York, Elsevier, 1985
2. Feste C: *The Physician Within.* Minneapolis, MN, Diabetes Center, 1987
3. Jacobson AM, Hauser ST: Behavioral and psychological aspects of diabetes. In *Diabetes Mellitus: Theory and Practice.* Ellenberg M, Rifkin H, Eds. New York, Med. Exam., 1983, p. 1037–52
4. Wulsin LR, Jacobson AM: Management of stress and glycemic control in diabetes. *Intern Med Specialist* 9:100–16, 1988

10. Diabetic Ketoacidosis and Hyperglycemic Hyperosmolar Coma in Adults

SAUL GENUTH, MD

DIABETIC KETOACIDOSIS (DKA)

DKA occurs in 2–5% of type I (Insulin-dependent) diabetic patients per year, and death due to failure of or delay in diagnosis, complications associated with treatment such as hypokalemia, or precipitating comorbid conditions such as sepsis still occurs in 1–10% of patients depending on treatment circumstances and locale. The pathophysiology of DKA is presented in chapter 6.

Diagnosis

Any person presenting with

- Coma
- Shock
- Dehydration
- Respiratory distress
- Any other evidence of major illness

should have an immediate screening of blood or urine glucose and urine ketones. If this simple rule is followed, new-onset cases of diabetes that present in DKA should never be missed.

Any known diabetic patient with nausea or vomiting, abdominal pain, CNS depression, shortness of breath, fever, localized signs of

---

Dr. Genuth is Professor of Medicine at Case Western Reserve University, Cleveland, OH.

infection, or unexplained blood glucose >250 mg/dl (>14 mM) is a candidate for DKA. Urine ketones (ketosticks or acetest tablets) should be checked at once. A negative, trace, or small reaction virtually excludes DKA (with the rare exception of the patient in uremia or with a high "reduced state" in his/her liver from alcohol intoxication or lactic acidosis). A moderate or large urine ketone reaction raises the possibility of existing or impending DKA. If vomiting cannot be controlled and fluid intake ensured at home and/or if urinary ketones do not promptly diminish with extra insulin, the patient must be examined. Clinical evidence of dehydration and acidosis suggests DKA:

- Decreased skin turgor or eyeball pressure
- Dry mucous membranes
- Hypotension
- Tachycardia
- Tachypnea
- Kussmaul respirations

Laboratory confirmation is obtained by the values shown in Table 10.1, with some exceptions. The plasma bicarbonate concentration may be misleadingly higher than expected or even normal if the patient has coexisting chronic respiratory acidosis from pulmonary disease. Conversely, the blood pH may be misleadingly higher than expected or even normal if there is a concurrent metabolic alkalosis due to diuretic ingestion or excessive mineralocorticoid action. Occasionally, plasma glucose may be <250 mg/dl (<14 mM) in a diabetic patient who has ingested large amounts of alcohol. Measured plasma sodium averages 130 meq/L, but when corrected for the plasma glucose level, it is usually in the normal range.

Corrected sodium =

$$\text{measured sodium} + 1.6 \times \frac{\text{plasma glucose (mg/dl)} - 100}{100}$$

or

$$\text{measured sodium} + 1.6 \times \frac{\text{plasma glucose (mM)} - 5.5}{5.5}$$

Plasma potassium averages 5.2 meq/L but can be <3.5 or >6 meq/L on occasion. Plasma blood urea nitrogen (BUN) and creatinine tend to be slightly elevated due to reduced renal blood flow.

Body fluid losses can be estimated by subtracting the admission weight from a recently known dry weight. Hypotension suggests at least 10% dehydration. A precipitating infection is not excluded by a normal body temperature and should be assiduously sought. Meningeal signs call for computed axial tomography scan or magnetic resonance imaging of the head followed by a lumbar puncture. Necrotic lesions in the nasal turbinates suggest mucormycosis. Rec-

Table 10.1. TYPICAL LABORATORY FINDINGS IN DIABETIC KETOACIDOSIS

	Average	Range
Plasma glucose	600 mg/dl	200–2000 mg/dl
	(33 mM)	(11–110 mM)
Plasma ketones (positive)	1:16	1:2–1:64
Plasma HCO_3^- (meq/L)	10	4–15
Blood pH	7.15	6.80–7.30
P_{CO_2} (mmHg)	20	14–30
Plasma anion gap	23	16–30
($Na^+ - [Cl^- + HCO_3^-]$)(meq/L)		

tal and pelvic examinations should not be deferred because appendicitis, pelvic inflammatory disease, diverticulitis, cholecystitis, etc., may be the cause of the patient's abdominal pain. The urine sediment should be checked for evidence of urinary tract infection or gram-negative sepsis. Pulmonary infection should be routinely excluded by a chest X ray, and an acute silent myocardial infarction in older adults or in patients with type I diabetes for >15 yr should be excluded by electrocardiogram (ECG).

Treatment

An intensive-care unit is the preferred setting for treatment of DKA. When this is not available, an attending physician or resident must personally monitor the patient's progress at intervals of no less than 1–2 h until the acidosis is broken and the patient is "out of the woods." An appropriate monitoring scheme is shown in Table 10.2.

The essential components of metabolic therapy are insulin administration, fluid replacement, and potassium repletion (Table 10.3). Bicarbonate, phosphate, and magnesium administration are not routinely required but may be needed or advantageous in certain situations.

Insulin. Short-acting (regular) insulin should always be used. Intermediate-acting (NPH and lente) insulins are not suitable and should only be used as a temporizing measure if DKA occurs in isolated circumstances where short-acting insulin is unavailable. Whenever possible, short-acting insulin should be administered as a continuous intravenous infusion in a starting dose of 10 U or 0.1 $U \cdot kg^{-1} \cdot h^{-1}$ via pump. If this is not feasible, 10 U/h short-acting insulin i.m. or s.c. is a satisfactory substitute. An initial intravenous bolus of 10 U, although not essential, guarantees an immediate therapeutic level of insulin while the rest of the treatment regimen is being prepared. Lower doses than these should not be used at the outset, and higher initial doses offer no advantage.

In response to insulin, plasma glucose should fall at an average rate of 75 $mg \cdot dl^{-1} \cdot h^{-1}$. If no response has occurred by 4 h, an unusual degree of insulin resistance may be present. The dose of

Table 10.2. MONITORING PATIENTS IN DKA

1. Weight: admission and every 6−12 h
2. Fluid intake and output: every 1−2 h (Foley catheter if incontinent)
3. Blood pressure, pulse, respirations, mental status: every 1−2 h
   Temperature: every 8 h
4. Blood (fingerstick) or plasma (laboratory) glucose: every 1−2 h
5. Plasma K^+: every 2−4 h
6. Plasma Na^+, chloride, HCO_3, and serum ketones: every 4 h
7. Arterial blood pH, Pco_2, Po_2: admission; repeat as needed until arterial pH >7.0−7.1
8. Plasma phosphate, Mg^{2+}, Ca^{2+}: admission; if low, repeat every 4 h; otherwise, every 8−12 h
9. Urine for ketones: every voiding
10. ECG: admission; repeat if follow-up plasma K^+ abnormal or unavailable
11. Complete blood count, blood urea nitrogen, creatinine, urinalysis, appropriate cultures, chest X ray: admission

All of the above should be carried out until the patient is stable, glucose levels are maintained at 150−250 mg/dl (8−14 mM), and acidosis is largely reversed. An intensive-care setting is preferred.

short-acting insulin should then be raised to 20−100 U/h i.v., with the higher doses being given for more extreme hyperglycemia and sicker patients. The dose should be further doubled every 2 h until plasma glucose definitely declines. The effectiveness of insulin therapy should also be demonstrated within 4−8 h by an increase in plasma bicarbonate, a decrease in the plasma anion gap, and a decrease in plasma ketones. It is not necessary to monitor arterial pH routinely, but it should be rechecked if there is evidence of inadequate response to insulin, if sodium bicarbonate has been administered (see below), or if coexisting pulmonary disease complicates the acid-base picture. Consultation with a diabetologist is strongly recommended if there is insulin unresponsiveness, insulin allergy, an admission pH of <7.0, or coma.

Table 10.3. ESSENTIAL COMPONENTS IN TREATMENT OF DKA

Insulin
- 10 U short-acting (regular) insulin/h by continuous i.v. infusion
- Increase 2- to 10-fold if no response by 4 h
- Decrease to 1−2 U/h when acidosis is corrected

Fluids
- 2−3 L 0.9% saline over first 3 h
- Subsequently, 0.45% saline at 150−300 ml/h
- Add 5% glucose when plasma glucose reaches 250 mg/dl (14 mM)

K^+
- 10−20 meq/h when plasma K^+ <6.0, ECG normal, urine flow documented
- 40−80 meq/h when plasma K^+ <3.5 or if bicarbonate is given

Once plasma glucose has reacted 250 mg/dl (14 mM), glucose should be added to the replacement fluids. This permits continued administration of insulin to abolish ketosis completely while protecting the patient from hypoglycemia. The insulin dose may be reduced when plasma bicarbonate has risen to 18 meq/L, the anion gap has decreased to 15 meq/L, plasma ketones and urine ketones have virtually disappeared, or arterial pH has risen to 7.30. Two units per hour intravenously is usually a satisfactory insulin dosage— along with 5% glucose at 100–150 ml/h (5–7.5 g glucose/h)—with which to clear any residual ketosis and to maintain plasma glucose at 150–250 mg/dl (8–14 mM).

Once the patient is judged capable of reliable oral intake, the insulin infusion should be stopped. For practical reasons, this is best done the morning after admission. Before stopping the insulin infusion, it is vital to administer 4–10 U short-acting insulin s.c. It is a common mistake not to do so on the grounds that plasma glucose is satisfactory at that point. However, ketosis often recurs if subcutaneous insulin is not administered until prominent hyperglycemia returns. In patients with previously known diabetes and no precipitating stress, their usual morning dose of intermediate- or long-acting insulin can also be given with the short-acting insulin. In new-onset patients, 20 U of intermediate-acting insulin is a reasonable addition to the short-acting insulin, if desired.

Fluids. The initial goal of fluid therapy is to restore circulating volume and protect against cerebral, coronary, or renal hypoperfusion. In this phase, isotonic fluid is needed. Generally 0.9% saline is used, although Ringer's lactate without glucose is also satisfactory. One liter should be administered in the first 30–60 min, followed by a 2nd L in the ensuing hour. In patients who are initially hypotensive or with estimated 10% dehydration, a rapid 3rd L of isotonic fluid is advisable. Frank shock may call for a colloidal volume expander such as plasma.

The second objective of fluid therapy is to replace total-body and intracellular losses and is achieved more slowly. Because total sodium and water losses are approximately in half-isotonic proportions, 0.45% saline is logical. Once plasma glucose reaches 250 mg/dl (14 mM), 5% glucose in 0.45% saline, 0.2% saline, or water should be administered. This choice is guided by the plasma sodium level, which should rise as plasma glucose falls, and by the patient's cardiac status. Measured or even corrected plasma sodium levels reaching 150 meq/L or a history of congestive heart failure indicates the need for more hypotonic fluids. The optimal rate of fluid replacement after circulatory volume has been initially stabilized cannot be stated categorically because it will vary with the original degree of dehydration, with renal or cardiac function, and with time into treatment. The range of rates is 150–500 ml/h. This should be tapered until an overall positive balance of 6 L on average is achieved. In the average case, fluid repletion is completed in 12–24 h. In mild cases of DKA, handled in an emergency-room setting, 6–8 h may suffice.

It is vital to document that a cumulative positive balance is occurring by comparing fluid intake with output every 1–2 h. Urine flow can remain 100–300 ml/h until plasma glucose has declined to 250 mg/dl (14 mM). In addition, there may be continuing gastrointestinal fluid losses or excessive ventilatory losses due to fever. Plasma sodium should be checked to ensure that it is gradually increasing as plasma glucose falls. If this is not happening, there may be excessive administration of free water, which may increase the risk of clinically significant cerebral edema.

Potassium. Nothing in the treatment of DKA requires more care and finesse than potassium replacement. Deaths have resulted from hypokalemia and, more rarely, from hyperkalemia. The average deficit of potassium is ~ 5 meq/kg body wt. If the patient has lain undiagnosed in coma from DKA or has delayed seeking treatment for 24 h, the deficit can reach 500–1000 meq. Despite the body potassium losses, plasma potassium on admission is usually normal or increased. Values <4.0 meq/L always indicate unusually large losses and require frequent subsequent plasma potassium measurement. The objective of therapy is simple:

Maintain plasma potassium >3.5 meq/L at all times.

This should prevent hypokalemic death from cardiac arrhythmia or from respiratory arrest until DKA is reversed. Total potassium repletion by the intravenous route is not necessary; it is completed later when oral intake is resumed.

Plasma potassium begins to decline as soon as insulin starts to act. Therefore, potassium should be administered from the outset unless the initial plasma level is >6.0 meq/L or oligoanuria is demonstrated by bladder catheterization. If plasma potassium cannot be rapidly ascertained, a normal pretreatment ECG will exclude life-threatening hyperkalemia. Potassium should be administered continuously at a beginning rate of 10–30 meq/h (not necessarily equivalent to 10–30 meq/L). The lower the initial plasma potassium, the higher the rate should be. If hypokalemia is present at the outset or if bicarbonate is given, 40–80 meq/h may be needed initially.

Potassium chloride is preferred to start with. Later, some potassium may be given as the phosphate to reduce the chloride load. Each 1 mM of potassium phosphate provides ~1.5 meq of potassium. Serial ECGs can help track potassium status: flattened or inverted T waves and the appearance of U waves indicate hypokalemia; tall symmetrical T waves, widened QRS complex, and loss of P waves indicate hyperkalemia. However, discrepancies and misinterpretations can occur so that it is always best to measure plasma potassium directly (Table 10.2).

Bicarbonate. Treatment with bicarbonate is not essential to and does not increase the rate of recovery from hyperglycemia or hyperketonemia. The acidosis of DKA will be corrected in due time by insulin inhibition of ketogenesis. Therefore the routine administration of alkali in all cases is not recommended. Furthermore, giving bicarbonate has the demonstrated disadvantage of significantly increasing the risk of hypokalemia and the theoretical disadvantages of decreasing tissue oxygen delivery and CNS pH.

However, in some instances, metabolic acidosis per se may be so severe or directly deleterious that it warrants emergency amelioration (Table 10.4). When buffering reserve is dangerously low, as indicated by pH <7.0 or plasma bicarbonate <5.0 meq/L, a slight increase in acid production or decrease in ventilation can result in lethal acidosis. Rarely, hyperkalemia is severe enough on admission to require immediate reversal by bicarbonate. If acidosis blunts vasoconstrictor responsiveness to catecholamines, dangerous hypotension can persist despite vigorous fluid replacement. Severe acidosis can also compromise cardiac output, leading to pulmonary edema and lactic acidosis, or it can impair ventilation, superimposing respiratory acidosis. Rarely, non−anion-gap hyperchloremic acidosis of sufficient severity to warrant alkali treatment develops late in the course of DKA.

If it is decided that any of these circumstances requires directly attacking the acidosis, sodium bicarbonate should be administered promptly to a defined end point. Doses of 50–100 meq in 250–1000 ml 0.45% saline can be administered in 30–60 min. Arterial pH should be rechecked after each 50–100 meq administered, and bicarbonate treatment should be continued until the pH has reached at least 7.10. To prevent hypokalemia, an extra 10 meq of potassium chloride should accompany each dose of bicarbonate unless hyperkalemia was the original indication for alkali treatment.

Phosphate and Magnesium. Although plasma levels of phosphate and magnesium are usually normal or elevated on admission, body stores of both are somewhat depleted by DKA. This becomes evident as insulin administration regularly produces hypophosphatemia, often to levels <1.5 mg/dl, and a less dramatic fall in plasma magnesium. However, clinical consequences of these changes are seldom observed, and prospective studies of routine phosphate supplementation have shown no particular benefit. Still, some physicians deem it wise to correct, or at least attenuate, hypophosphatemia by administering potassium phosphate in doses of 1–2 mM phosphate/kg body wt i.v. over 6–12 h. If rhabdomyolysis, CNS deterioration, cardiac dysfunction, or hemolysis parallel the initial fall in plasma phosphate, then phosphate therapy as described is definitely indicated. Plasma calcium should then be monitored care-

Table 10.4. INDICATIONS FOR CONSIDERING BICARBONATE THERAPY

- pH <7.0 or HCO_3^- <5.0 meq/L
- Hyperkalemia (K^+ >6.5 meq/L)
- Hypotension unresponsive to fluid replacement
- Severe left-ventricular failure
- Respiratory depression
- Late hyperchloremic acidosis

fully because hypocalcemia and even tetany have occurred with phosphate therapy. Magnesium is indicated when ventricular arrhythmias occur that are not accounted for by hypokalemia. Doses of 10–20 meq i.v. of magnesium should be given over 30–60 min as emergency therapy in the form of 2.5–5.0 ml of 50% magnesium sulfate diluted in 100 ml of fluid. The need for additional doses is determined by ECG monitoring.

HYPERGLYCEMIC HYPEROSMOLAR COMA (HHC)

HHC should probably not be considered a specific syndrome but rather one end of the spectrum of severe metabolic decompensation in diabetes. In the pure case, HHC is differentiated from DKA by the absence of significant ketosis and by the presence of higher average levels of plasma glucose and osmolality. By definition, plasma glucose should be >600 mg/dl (>33 mM), and osmolality should be >320 mosM in HHC. By these osmolar criteria, ~50% of all cases of extreme diabetic decompensation are HHC. However, in 35% of these, acidosis (pH <7.30) is also present. This may be due to accompanying lactic acidosis or uremia but also occasionally indicates significant accumulation of ketoacids. The distinction between pure and mixed cases of HHC is of little practical importance because the main elements of therapy are similar in both.

HHC is responsible for ~1/1000 hospital admissions. It occurs predominantly in adults over age 50 yr and almost exclusively in patients with type II (non-insulin-dependent) diabetes, 35% of whom are previously undiagnosed. In one survey, 40% of patients had accompanying infection, 38% had been on diuretics, and 28% were living in nursing homes. Mortality rates in various series range from 12–42%. Death is associated with age >70 yr, nursing-home residency, higher plasma osmolality, and higher plasma sodium but not with higher plasma glucose or anion gap. This emphasizes the key pathogenetic features of HHC. Ketosis is relatively suppressed, perhaps by more available endogenous insulin and by hyperosmolarity itself, compared with DKA. However, losses of total-body water, especially relative to total-body sodium, are greater than in DKA. This is probably due to a combination of age and dementia-related diminished thirst, decreased kidney function, and the absence of ketosis-associated vomiting as a warning sign of decompensation. In turn, the greater degree of dehydration causes more prerenal reduction in glomerular filtration rate and secondarily raises plasma glucose to even higher levels than usually seen in DKA.

HHC is more insidious in nature, and patients typically come to medical attention later and sicker. Precipitating conditions can include otherwise silent myocardial infarction, pancreatitis, sepsis, stroke, and an array of drugs (glucocorticoids, diuretics, phenytoin, β-blockers, and Ca^{2+}-channel blockers). CNS findings range from confusion to complete coma, but in contrast to DKA, patients can also present with generalized or focal seizures, myoclonic jerking, and reversible hemiparesis.

Diagnosis

HHC should be suspected in any elderly person with or without diabetes who exhibits acute or subacute deterioration of CNS function and is severely dehydrated. Blood pressure is low or lower than expected if the patient is known to have hypertension. Either hyperthermia or hypothermia may be present. A fingerstick blood glucose above the readable range of any test strip suggests HHC. Average plasma values on admission are

- Glucose, 1000 mg/dl (55 mM)
- Osmolality, 360 mosM
- Sodium, 140 meq/L
- BUN, 65 mg/dl (23 mM)
- Creatinine, 3.0 mg/dl (265 μM)
- Potassium, 4.9 meq/L
- Anion gap, 23 meq/L

Arterial pH is usually >7.30 but may be decreased by accompanying metabolic acidosis.

Management

Fluids. The most critical element in the management of HHC is the choice of replacement fluid and its rate of administration. As noted above, both the total losses of fluid and the proportion represented by free water are usually greater in HHC than in DKA. The average admission plasma sodium is 10 meq/L higher in HHC, despite a greater degree of hyperglycemia. Furthermore, the degree of CNS abnormality in HHC correlates best with the level of hyperosmolarity, which reflects intracellular dehydration. Therefore, rehydrating brain cells is of great therapeutic importance. On the other hand, overhydrating brain cells can also impair their function. This may be a risk during treatment of HHC, because animal studies suggest that brain cells respond to hypotonic dehydration by generating intracellular osmoles of unknown identity. The benefit of this response is to diminish the amount of water that must leave brain cells to maintain osmolar equilibrium in the face of rising plasma osmolarity. However, if these intracellular osmoles persist as plasma glucose is being rapidly reduced with treatment, they can stimulate overcorrection of CNS dehydration because they attract extra water back into the brain cells.

Such considerations may explain why many patients with HHC do not completely recover their baseline CNS function until some time after plasma glucose is decreased to <300 mg/dl (<17 mM). In some instances, it is because of continued hyperosmolarity, as revealed by a very high plasma sodium (Fig. 10.1). This can result

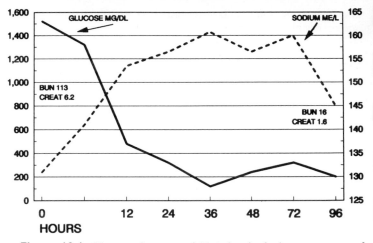

Figure 10.1. Plasma glucose and Na⁺ levels during treatment of hyperosmolar coma. BUN, blood urea nitrogen; creat, creatinine.

from inadequate free-water replacement and may be aggravated by persistent renal losses of free water as kidneys recover from functional impairment due to severe prior dehydration. In other instances, slow CNS recovery may occur because of too rapid correction of hyperosmolarity, as would be indicated by development of a low plasma sodium level as plasma glucose declines.

As in DKA, the initial objective of fluid therapy is to immediately raise the circulating volume. Hence, 1 L of 0.9% saline should be administered in the first 30 min. If the patient remains hypotensive, a 2nd L of 0.9% saline should be given in the next 30–60 min. Thereafter, all fluids should ordinarily be hypotonic. The ensuing 2–3 L should be 0.45% sodium chloride infused at ~500 ml/h. This rate may be slowed thereafter, but ultimately as much as 12 L positive fluid balance may be required over 24–36 h to restore normal body fluid content. When plasma glucose has declined to 250–300 mg/dl (14–17 mM), 5% glucose should be added to 0.45% sodium chloride. If plasma sodium exceeds 150 meq/L at this point, 5% glucose in 0.2% sodium chloride or in water is indicated. The rate of fluid administration must be guided by body weight, urine output, kidney function, and presence or absence of pulmonary congestion and jugular venous distention. In patients with prior congestive heart failure or renal insufficiency or in those with acute kidney failure secondary to HHC, catheter monitoring of central venous pressure is also indicated. Most important, the patient's neurological status must be observed frequently. Failure to show any improvement may indicate inadequate rates of fluid replacement or of reduction in plasma osmolarity. Regression after initial improvement may indicate too rapid a reduction in plasma osmolarity. A slow but steady improvement in CNS function is the best evidence that fluid management is satisfactory.

Other Therapy. Insulin should be infused at an initial rate of 10 U/ h i.v. as in DKA. Although fluid repletion itself has a major impact on hyperglycemia, it should not be relied on as the sole therapy of HHC. On the other hand, rapidly lowering plasma glucose by giving insulin without adequate fluids is also dangerous, because water will shift into cells and temporarily lower circulating volume and perfusion of vital organs. Once plasma glucose has reached 250–300 mg/dl (14–17 mM), the insulin infusion can be reduced to 1–2 U/ h. This should be adjusted to maintain plasma glucose around the recommended level until rehydration has been accomplished. Subcutaneous insulin should be started after recovery from HHC, as it is in DKA. However, because patients with HHC almost always have type II diabetes, they may be subsequently tried on sulfonyl-urea drugs or diet alone if they prove sensitive to insulin.

Potassium repletion is also necessary in HHC. Although potassium losses are less well established in HHC, they are probably lower than in DKA because of less acidosis and vomiting. Because initial oliguria is more common in HHC, potassium may not be needed at the outset, and the rates of administration should be more cautious, e.g., 10–20 meq/h. Bicarbonate is not needed unless there is severe lactic acidosis (see chapt. 11). Phosphate and magnesium can be given as in DKA and for similar reasons. Overall monitoring of the patient should be conducted essentially as outlined in Table 10.2.

COMPLICATIONS OF DKA AND HHC

Persistent Vomiting

Nasogastric suction is helpful to prevent aspiration pneumonia. Stomach contents often test positive for occult blood, but significant blood loss requiring investigation or transfusion is unusual.

Infection

Appropriate antibiotics for pulmonary, urinary tract, abdominal, soft tissue, or CNS infection should be given intravenously to ensure that they reach the bloodstream promptly. Amphotericin is specifically indicated for mucormycosis. In febrile patients who appear very ill or are hypotensive, obtain blood cultures and treat with an antibiotic regimen that covers the common gram-positive and gram-negative organisms as well as pseudomonas and anaerobes.

Acute Kidney Failure

Severe volume depletion and/or papillary necrosis may lead to secondary kidney failure. Anuria on admission or persistent oliguria despite rehydration calls for nephrological consultation.

Acute Respiratory Distress Syndrome

Tachypnea, after acidosis is corrected, calls for repeat chest X ray. A "shock-lung" or "white-out" picture requires positive-pressure oxygen, central venous pressure monitoring, and more cautious fluid replacement.

Disseminated Intravascular Coagulation (DIC)

The picture of multiple thromboses and/or bleeding, accompanied by thrombocytopenia, low fibrinogen levels, prolonged prothrombin time and partial thromboplastin time, and the presence of circulating fibrin products is characteristic of DIC. Therapy with heparin is usually indicated. In elderly patients without DIC but with a history of venous thrombosis, pulmonary embolism, or congestive heart failure, prophylactic low-dose heparin (5000 U s.c. every 12 h) should be considered.

PREVENTION OF DKA AND HHC

Clear instructions should be given always to test blood glucose and urine ketones when symptoms of diabetic decompensation or intercurrent illness appear. The physician or nurse should be called at once for vomiting, when blood glucose is >500 mg/dl (>28 mM), or when blood glucose is >250 mg/dl (>14 mM) and urine ketones are moderate or large. In turn, the physician and/or nurse should maintain constant (every 2–4 h) telephone or office contact with the patient either until extra insulin, fluids, antiemetics, etc., have aborted development of DKA or HHC or until a decision to hospitalize the patient is made. If extra insulin is given at bedtime because of acute hyperglycemia and/or ketosis, the patient must set an alarm and check blood glucose and urine ketones 4 h later. If these remain dangerously high, the physician must be called again. A routine instruction to "call back in the morning" is not an adequate response to the threat of DKA or HHC.

SUGGESTED READING

1. Adroque HJ, Wilson H, Boyd AE, Suki WN, Eknoyan G: Plasma acid-base patterns in diabetic ketoacidosis. *N Engl J Med* 307:1603–10, 1982
2. Carrol P, Matz R: Uncontrolled diabetes mellitus in adults: experience in treatment of diabetic ketoacidosis and hyperosmolar nonketotic coma with low-dose insulin and a uniform treatment regimen. *Diabetes Care* 6:579–85, 1983
3. Fisher JN, Kitabchi AE: A randomized study of phosphate therapy in the treatment of diabetic ketoacidosis. *J Clin Endocrinol Metab* 57:117–80, 1983
4. Foster DW, McGarry JD: The metabolic derangements and treatment of diabetic ketoacidosis. *N Engl J Med* 309:159–69, 1983

5. Genuth SM: Diabetic ketoacidosis. In *Clinical Diabetes: Modern Management*. Podolsky S, Ed. New York, Appleton-Century-Crofts, 1980, p. 173–207
6. Keller U: Diabetic ketoacidosis: current views on pathogenesis and treatment. *Diabetologia* 29:71–77, 1986
7. Lever E, Jaspan JB: Sodium bicarbonate therapy in severe diabetic ketoacidosis. *Am J Med* 75:263–68, 1983
8. Matz R: Hyperosmolar nonacidotic uncontrolled diabetes: not a rare event. *Clin Diabetes* 6:25, 1988
9. Soler NG, Bennet MA, Dixon K, Fitzgerald M, Malins J: Potassium balance during treatment of diabetic ketoacidosis with special reference to the use of bicarbonate. *Lancet* 2:665–67, 1972
10. Wachtel TJ, Silliman RA, Lamberton P: Prognostic factors in the diabetic hyperosmolar state. *J Am Geriatr Soc* 35:737–41, 1987

11. Lactic Acidosis

SCOTT E. BUCHALTER, MD, and
ROBERT A. KREISBERG, MD

Lactic acidosis (LA) is usually due to inadequate oxygen delivery or utilization in patients with serious underlying diseases but can also occur in disorders without obvious tissue hypoperfusion. LA is the most common form of metabolic acidosis in hospitalized patients. Regardless of cause, the accumulation of lactic acid indicates that the balance between lactate production and utilization has been disturbed.

CLASSIFICATION OF LACTIC ACIDOSIS

A modest elevation in blood lactate concentration (usually <5.0 meq/L) can occur without changes in blood pH and may represent an increased "set point" for lactate, such as occurs with some hypermetabolic states. In contrast, true LA, in which an elevated blood lactate (usually ≥ 5.0 meq/L) is associated with significant hemodynamic and metabolic decompensation, usually has a lowered blood pH. The most widely used classification divides LA into two broad categories: type A, associated with disorders in which there is reduced O_2 delivery (Do_2), and type B, which is not associated with reduced Do_2 (Table 11.1).

Type A LA

Type A LA is much more common than type B LA and forms the basis for most of the understanding of LA biochemistry. Type A

Dr. Buchalter is Assistant Professor of Medicine and Dr. Kreisberg is Professor of Medicine and Vice-Chairman of the Department of Medicine at the University of Alabama at Birmingham School of Medicine, Birmingham, AL.

Table 11.1. SOME CAUSES OF LACTIC ACIDOSIS

Type A (clinical evidence of inadequate O_2 delivery)
  Shock (septic, cardiogenic, hypovolemic)
  Severe hypoxemia or anemia
  CO poisoning
Type B (no clinical evidence of inadequate O_2 delivery)
  B_1 (associated with underlying disease)
    Diabetes mellitus
    Malignancy
    Liver disease
    Sepsis
  B_2 (due to drugs/toxins)
    Biguanides
    Ethanol/methanol
    Ethylene/propylene glycol
    Acetaminophen
    Salicylates
    Cyanide
    Nitroprusside
  B_3 (due to congenital defects in gluconeogenesis or pyruvate oxidation)
    Deficiency of:
      Glucose-6-phosphatase
      Pyruvate carboxylase
      Fructose-1,6-diphosphatase
      Pyruvate dehydrogenase
      Oxidative phosphorylation

LA occurs when DO_2 is inadequate to meet the metabolic demands of tissues, resulting in anaerobic glycolysis. Systemic shock and regional hypoperfusion, hypoxemia, anemia severe enough to reduce DO_2, and CO intoxication are examples of LA related to decreased DO_2. Vigorous exercise, seizures, and severe asthma are examples of type A LA where tissue O_2 demand outstrips supply. With type A, the hemodynamic abnormalities of mismatched supply and demand precede and lead to the LA.

Type B LA

Type B LA develops in settings in which there is no clinical evidence for reduced DO_2 to tissues. It has been further divided into subcategories related to underlying disease (type B_1), drugs or toxins (type B_2), and inborn errors of metabolism (type B_3). Although some cases of type B LA may have occult tissue hypoperfusion, many occur without evidence for primary DO_2 problems. There are several causes of type B LA.

Diabetes Mellitus. Lactate metabolism is abnormal in diabetes. LA occurring in the setting of diabetes, even with diabetic ketoacidosis, is rare. When it does occur in association with diabetes, it is usually the result of reduced DO_2 and/or tissue hypoxia related to severe volume contraction, myocardial dysfunction, or sepsis. Therefore, when LA is present in patients with diabetes, underlying causes for LA related to reduced DO_2 should be found.

Liver Disease. An association between liver disease and altered lactate metabolism is expected because of the central role of the liver in lactate homeostasis. LA is frequent in patients with serious liver disease, and acidemia may be masked because of coexistent metabolic and respiratory alkaloses. Basal blood lactate concentrations appear to be normal in these patients, but clearance of infused lactate may be prolonged by ~20%. Thus, while basal lactate production and utilization are matched, any condition that increases production of lactate may result in hyperlactatemia and LA due to impaired hepatic clearance. Shunting of lactate around the liver via collateralization (e.g., in cirrhotics) may play a role in reducing lactate utilization by the liver.

Malignancy. LA is associated with malignant disease, most commonly with uncontrolled leukemia (usually lymphocytic, rarely myelocytic) and less commonly with solid tumors (most often with associated hepatic or bone marrow metastasis). The mechanism is not completely understood, although the LA in malignancy has most often been attributed to overproduction. Underutilization (e.g., reduced clearance) has also been proposed as a mechanism for tumor-associated LA, often with almost complete replacement of the liver with malignant cells. Both overproduction and underutilization probably occur in LA associated with malignancy. Again, inadequate tissue Do_2 (e.g., sepsis, volume depletion, or cardiac dysfunction) is still the most common cause of LA in cancer patients and must be evaluated and treated aggressively.

Sepsis. Sepsis is common and often associated with hyperlactatemia and/or LA. Both type A and type B LA can occur in sepsis. Type A LA clearly occurs in the setting of septic shock, because of a marked vasodilation of systemic vessels, varying degrees of myocardial depression, and most often, a reduction of intravascular volume. This acute shock state, identified clinically by a marked reduction in systemic vascular resistance, severe hypotension, and systemic signs of reduced Do_2, is easily diagnosed. As in any other form of shock with acidemia, confirming the presence of an elevated blood lactate is unnecessary diagnostically, at least initially, because therapy would be immediately directed toward improving Do_2 and tissue perfusion. Depending on myocardial dysfunction and depression, volume status, and degree of initial volume resuscitation, patients with sepsis have a normal or high cardiac output and therefore normal Do_2 with significant LA. Depending on the underlying pathophysiology, this type B LA is probably related to occult tissue hypoperfusion or, in contrast, to an isolated or coexistent cellular metabolic defect, which alters lactate metabolism and produces hyperlactatemia and acidosis independent of tissue hypoperfusion.

DIAGNOSIS OF LACTIC ACIDOSIS

The measurement of lactate in the setting of obvious clinical shock with acidemia may be unnecessary to aid in diagnosis. However, in the absence of clinical signs of hypoperfusion, or when an unexplained anion-gap acidosis exists, particularly in a critically ill patient, an elevated blood lactate concentration may allow for the diagnosis of LA and indicates that a search for occult tissue hypoperfusion be undertaken.

A blood lactate concentration of >5 meq/L and a pH of <7.35 constitute the criteria for defining LA in which false-positive and false-negative diagnoses would be minimized. LA frequently occurs in association with disorders in which dynamic acid-base disturbances are common, e.g., the metabolic alkalosis of liver disease or hyperventilation related to early sepsis or mechanical ventilation. The initial pH may be normal or near normal, thus masking a significant acidemia.

TREATMENT

The cornerstone of therapy for LA is treatment of the underlying and predisposing disorders (Table 11.2). Although such therapy is essential for survival, a poor outcome relates to both the seriousness of the associated primary disorder and the inability to specifically treat LA.

Optimization of Do$_2$

In addition to therapy of the underlying disorder, another treatment approach is optimization of Do$_2$. Beyond clinically obvious shock, which should be dealt with swiftly and aggressively, many critically ill patients enter a clinical and biochemical gray zone. These patients may have mild to moderate hyperlactatemia (2–5 meq/L) with or without an associated acidosis. Because noninvasive assessment of Do$_2$ and Vo$_2$ in these patients is relatively inaccurate and maintenance of Do$_2$ and consumption at supranormal levels reduces subsequent multiple organ-system failure and improves survival, the use of hemodynamic monitoring and a trial to determine whether an occult perfusion defect and supply dependency exists is important for further therapeutic decisions in these patients with hyperlactatemia.

Table 11.2. TREATMENT OF LACTIC ACIDOSIS

1. Correct perfusion
2. Maximize tissue O$_2$ delivery
3. Treat any underlying sepsis
4. Judicious use of bicarbonate to raise pH to 7.2 and serum bicarbonate to 12 meq/L
5. Dichloroacetate, an experimental drug, may be helpful in refractory cases

Acidosis has undesirable clinical effects, including

- Significant adverse effects on the cardiovascular system
- Reduced cardiac contractility, cardiac output, systemic blood pressure, and heart rate
- Decreased hepatic and renal blood flow
- Impaired responsiveness to endogenous and exogenous catecholamines
- Increased susceptibility to ventricular arrhythmias

These deleterious effects, which generally occur at pH <7.2, would further decrease tissue Do_2 and worsen the developing LA.

The use of bicarbonate as a buffering agent seems appropriate. Unfortunately, use of bicarbonate is not without potential adverse effects, and its use has undergone intense scrutiny recently. Because of the large quantities of bicarbonate usually required, hypernatremia, hyperosmolality, and volume overload can become significant problems, especially in the setting of already reduced flow, poor renal perfusion, and reduced renal secretion of sodium and water.

There may be adverse effects directly related to bicarbonate therapy that may be of considerable clinical importance and largely unmanageable. The administration of sodium bicarbonate increases production of CO_2, which rapidly diffuses into the myocardial cell, causing a decrease in intracellular pH and worsening myocardial function. The reduced contractility and cardiac output that occurs might be of great potential importance in settings where CO_2 removal is a problem (such as ventilatory failure or during resuscitation).

Furthermore, bicarbonate may have a detrimental effect on lactate production, probably related to the effect of pH on phosphofructokinase (PFK) activity, which increases dramatically as pH increases from 6.8 to 7.2. Thus, bicarbonate administration might increase PFK activity, stimulating lactate production and possibly nullifying any potential benefit.

Although adverse effects may exist when bicarbonate is administered to patients with LA, sodium bicarbonate should be administered in severely acidemic patients with cardiovascular compromise to correct the systemic pH to 7.2 and the serum bicarbonate to 12 meq/L, with careful attention to volume status and cardiac output. Bicarbonate should be administered as a continuous infusion, because bolus administration has caused a transient drop in systemic vascular resistance and blood pressure. The amount and route of infused bicarbonate requires clinical judgment and must be tailored to specific clinical conditions.

A new drug, dichloroacetate (DCA), may be useful in the treatment of LA. DCA has a beneficial effect on LA production and utilization in both type A and type B LA. DCA activates pyruvate dehydrogenase and improves oxidation of pyruvate and lactate utilization. It also has a positive inotropic effect, increases cardiac output, and produces peripheral vasodilation. DCA improves survival in some types of experimentally induced LA when compared with bicarbonate or saline therapy. Many patients with LA who fail to respond to bicarbonate will respond to DCA administration with a significant decrease in lactate levels and an improvement in acidosis. However, DCA is currently an investigational drug and not available for routine use. Nevertheless, no clear improvement in survival has been demonstrated in humans, which underscores the seriousness of the underlying disorders in these critically ill patients.

SUGGESTED READING

1. Buchalter SE, Crain MR, Kreisberg R: Regulation of lactate metabolism in vivo. *Diabetes Metab Rev* 5:379–91, 1989
2. Cohen RD, Woods HF: *Clinical and Biochemical Aspects of Lactic Acidosis*. Boston, MA, Blackwell, 1976
3. Kreisberg RA: Lactic acidosis: an update. *J Intensive Care Med* 2:76–84, 1987
4. Madias NE: Lactic acidosis. *Kidney Int* 29:752–74, 1986
5. Mizock BA: Lactic acidosis. *Disease-a-Month* 35:235–300, 1989
6. Narins RG, Cohen JJ: Bicarbonate therapy of organic acidosis: the case for its continued use. *Ann Intern Med* 106:615–18, 1987
7. Stacpoole PW: Lactic acidosis: the case against bicarbonate therapy. *Ann Intern Med* 105:276–79, 1986

12. Role of Diabetes Educator in Patient Management

RUTH FARKAS-HIRSCH, MS, RN, CDE, and
IRL B. HIRSCH, MD

This chapter focuses on clarification of the training and roles of the diabetes educator, suggestions for effective utilization of the educator, and methods for recruitment of or referral to an educator or program. Of fundamental importance is the knowledge that patient education is the cornerstone of diabetes management, and the educator/specialist is an integral part of the diabetes health-care team.

THE DIABETES TEAM

The benefits of a team approach to diabetes management have been well documented. The makeup of a team can vary considerably. A minimal number of health-care workers would typically consist of a physician and a nurse or nutritionist. A more comprehensive team could also include a social worker/psychologist, exercise physiologist, pharmacist, physicians' assistant, or certified nurse practitioner. Many physicians' offices employ a nurse educator, but only some can also provide nutritional or psychosocial support services. A clearly defined team is the "gold standard" for the current management of all diabetic patients.

- Diabetes educator—Anyone involved with the education of patients or professionals in the field of diabetes.
- Diabetes teaching nurse—A nurse who spends most of his/her time in diabetes education.

Ms. Farkas-Hirsch is a Diabetes Clinical Specialist and Dr. Hirsch is Assistant Clinical Professor of Medicine and Medical Director at the Diabetes Care Center, University of Washington School of Medicine, Seattle, WA.

- Diabetes nurse clinician—This title implies some type of specialized training, although much of it may be on-the-job training. Clinicians generally provide care, management, and instructional services; most have at least an undergraduate degree.
- Diabetes nurse specialist or diabetes clinical specialist—This is the most advanced level of practitioner, who may also be a nonnurse professional. These individuals have at least Master of Science degrees in a specialized area of study. They have the training, expertise, and autonomy to provide most clinical management responsibilities and patient and professional education.

All diabetes educators should have sufficient educational background and expertise to fulfill certain requirements. They need a thorough and current knowledge base of the principles of diabetes care and management and of principles of learning and teaching. Their roles usually demand flexibility because the type and age of patients and the clinical settings vary considerably. The health-care team works under the auspices and guidance of the physician. Diabetes educators can act as true "physician extenders" by offering valuable and continuous service and support that is difficult or impossible for physicians to provide. Studies have shown that patients can only recall about 50% of their doctor's specific recommendations immediately after an interview. After initial instruction, patients need continuing personal and telephone contact by the educator. Many handicapped or elderly patients require repeated instruction, and, in some cases, other family members must also be instructed.

Diabetes educators must use their own discretion in scheduling frequency and length of teaching sessions. For example, if the physician asks the educator to teach the patient self-monitoring of blood glucose (SMBG), the instruction must also include a review of basic information of diabetes mellitus, symptoms and treatment of hypoglycemia, actual monitoring technique, record keeping, rationale for SMBG, and the interaction of food, exercise, and insulin. It is unrealistic to request a 20-min session on SMBG without any of the accompanying vital information. Diabetes educators are aware of this and are obligated to provide more comprehensive instruction.

RECRUITMENT AND REFERRAL

The American Diabetes Association (ADA) published the "National Standards for Diabetes Patient Education," which can be extremely valuable in determining the level of patient training to be provided. It includes guidelines for a curriculum that should be made available to diabetic patients and the minimal standards for professional expertise and training. Structured inpatient or outpatient programs can apply for "recognition" by ADA if they meet these standards and the review criteria. Even the smallest office practice will find these guidelines helpful in planning any type of diabetes education services. Patients and families can and should be referred to these recognized programs for more comprehensive structured classes. ADA can also provide a directory of all ADA-recognized diabetes education programs.

The American Association of Diabetes Educators (AADE) published "Diabetes Education: A Core Curriculum for Health Professionals," which is a comprehensive outline of all aspects of knowledge required by the educator or specialist. This guide can be invaluable in assisting health professionals in the acquisition of a more specialized or advanced knowledge base.

Diabetes educators can now become Certified Diabetes Educators (those who pass an examination add CDE after their name and degree). AADE can provide the specific requirements for CDEs and supply a directory of CDEs. "CDE" implies certain minimal standards of knowledge, expertise, and skills in all aspects of diabetes education.

EXAMPLES OF EDUCATIONAL AND SUPPORT SERVICES

Under physician supervision, the nurse specialist/educator can provide the following individualized instructional and support services over several hours, days, or weeks. The topics are based on those included in the ADA-approved curriculum for diabetes education programs.

1. Educational assessment and development of an individualized curriculum and class schedule
2. Explanation of general aspects of diabetes mellitus, including classification, symptoms, diagnosis, and importance of medical management
3. Nutritional evaluation and development of a meal plan (usually performed by nutritionist); explanation of interaction of medication, food intake, and physical activity
4. Guidelines for exercise, including referrals to exercise physiologist, if appropriate; review of precautions related to hypoglycemia
5. Instruction in blood glucose and urine ketone monitoring, including selection of appropriate methods and supplies; review of importance of record keeping and rationale for monitoring
6. Instruction on insulin action (or oral agents), types of treatment regimens, selection of appropriate insulin regimen, injection technique, and types of injectors
7. Explanation of insulin adjustments (algorithms), including the setting of target blood glucose and glycosylated hemoglobin levels
8. Instruction on causes, symptoms, treatment, and prevention of hypoglycemia, hyperglycemia, and diabetic ketoacidosis; review of sick-day guidelines and emergency procedures including glucagon administration

9. Explanation of glycemic guidelines during pregnancy and specific aspects of antepartum management and risk factors
10. Discussion of chronic complications, including prevention, scheduling, and frequency of screening examinations and clinical management; review of importance of regular dental, foot, and skin care
11. Review of community resources, insurance reimbursement, health-care agencies, and benefits and responsibilities of care
12. Assistance in psychological adjustment to living with a chronic disease and importance of family support; referral to social worker or psychologist as needed
13. Instruction on and initiation of insulin-infusion pump therapy in conjunction with the physician's medical plan

ALTERNATE EDUCATIONAL RESOURCES

If the physician cannot recruit or use a diabetes educator or specialist for his/her office, then referral of the patient should be made to an ADA-recognized patient education program (Table 12.1).

Table 12.1. REASONS TO REFER PATIENT TO DIABETES EDUCATOR, NURSE SPECIALIST, OR ADA-APPROVED PROGRAM

- Improved individualized and comprehensive patient instruction and follow-up
- Improved retention of knowledge and skills by the patient and his/her family
- Continuity of care and facilitation of communication within a multidisciplinary team
- Encourages referrals to other educational specialists or programs, as appropriate
- Information on sources of insurance and reimbursement, diabetes supplies, and community agencies
- Allows more time for the physicians to provide other services
- Promotes autonomy and self-care in the patient with a chronic disease
- Provides ongoing emotional support for the patient and family

SUGGESTED READING

1. Anderson RM, Funnell MM: The role of the physician in patient education. *Pract Diabetol* 9:10–12, 1990
2. Anderson RM, Lockwood D, Dedrick RF, Hiss RG: The diabetes care and education provided by nurses working in physicians' offices. *Diabetes Educ* 14:532–36, 1988
3. Flavin K, White NH: The intensive therapy team. *Diabetes Educ* 15:249–52, 1989
4. Guthrie DW: Diabetes patient education: nurse specialist approach. *Diabetes Educ* 12:131–34, 1986
5. Pichert JW: Strategies for effective patient teaching. *Pract Diabetol* 6:1–4, 1987

13. Monitoring Diabetes Mellitus

DAVID M. NATHAN, MD

Monitoring metabolic status in diabetes mellitus is critical to patient safety and a necessary element of self-management. The past decade of clinical research resulted in major advances in monitoring, including the development and refinement of methods for self-monitoring of blood glucose (SMBG) and for measurement of chronic glycemia with glycosylated protein assays. In the absence of definitive data that support a specific glucose target, beyond that necessary to eliminate symptoms of hyperglycemia and hypoglycemia, recommendations for monitoring are problematic. Nevertheless, the demonstrated import of tight control in pregnant diabetic women and those planning pregnancy, the need to avoid hypoglycemia in all insulin- and oral-agent–treated patients, and other practical considerations with regard to self-management dictate the need for monitoring guidelines. The relative lability of blood glucose profiles in type I (insulin-dependent) compared with type II (non-insulin-dependent) diabetes requires more complex treatment and monitoring schedules.

MEASUREMENT OF GLUCOSE

The measurement of glucose levels, either laboratory based or patient performed, represents the most common means of assessing metabolic control in diabetes. Modern enzymatic (hexokinase or glucose oxidase) methods provide rapid reliable and accurate measurements. Serum and plasma levels are ~10–15% higher than

Dr. Nathan is Director of the Diabetes Research Center and the Diabetes Clinic at Massachusetts General Hospital and Associate Professor of Medicine at the Harvard Medical School, Boston, MA.

simultaneous whole-blood levels. Glucose oxidase–impregnated strips, read with either a color chart or meter, provide patients with the opportunity to self-monitor. A list of products available for SMBG can be found in the American Diabetes Association's *Physician's Guide to Insulin-Dependent (Type I) Diabetes: Diagnosis and Treatment* (p. 42).

Urine glucose measurements are not generally recommended. They are an indirect semiquantitative reflection of blood glucose levels. Urine tests are "blind" to blood glucose levels below the renal threshold (generally 180–220 mg/dl [10–12.2 μM] in nonpregnant adults); they are incapable of distinguishing between blood glucose values in the normal to hypoglycemic range. Moreover, urine glucose concentration represents an average of blood glucose levels over the time that the urine collects.

Type I Diabetes

Type I diabetes is characterized by frequent, major fluctuations in blood glucose levels. Blood glucose monitoring is the method of choice for type I diabetes. Although intermittent office- or laboratory-based glucose assays may be useful in specific instances, labile glucose profiles in type I diabetes make sporadic measurements difficult to interpret. Isolated measurements may not be representative of values at other times or on other days. In addition, isolated measurements correlate poorly with the average level of glycemic control. Therefore, sporadic office-based glucose measurements are of limited value.

The logical method of monitoring type I diabetes is SMBG. Table 13.1 describes the more commonly used regimens. The frequency of SMBG is predicated on the intensity and goals of the treatment regimen. Intensive treatment regimens (continuous subcutaneous insulin infusion with pumps or ≥3 daily injections) with glucose goals that approximate the nondiabetic range are associated with an increased risk for severe hypoglycemia. To adjust insulin doses and to prevent hypoglycemia, frequent blood glucose monitoring is required. On the other hand, patients treated with minimal treatment regimens, designed to prevent symptomatic hyperglycemia and ketosis with 1 or 2 daily insulin injections, require less frequent monitoring. Here, the goal is to prevent hypoglycemia and to adjust insulin on sick days.

Type II Diabetes

Blood glucose profiles are more stable in type II than in type I diabetes. Fasting levels tend to be similar from day to day and generally correlate closely with average glycemia. The arguments that SMBG can help motivate obese type II diabetic patients to lose weight or can aid in controlling hyperglycemia have not been proved by clinical studies. Thus, SMBG has not been demonstrated to be useful or necessary in the management of diet-treated type II dia-

Table 13.1. **SELF-MONITORING OF BLOOD GLUCOSE IN TYPE I DIABETES***

Level of Treatment	Goals of Therapy	Expected HbA$_{1c}$ (%)	Time of Testing				
			Prebreakfast	Prelunch	Predinner	Prebedtime	Other†
Minimal 1–2 injections insulin/day; Frequent insulin adjustments are not made	Avoid symptomatic hyperglycemia and hypoglycemia	9–11	x	— or —	x		x
Average 2 injections mixed-split insulin/day; Insulin adjustments made on more regular basis	Avoid symptomatic hyperglycemia and hypoglycemia	7–9	x		x — or —	x	x
Intensive 3 or 4 injections insulin/day or insulin pump; Frequent adjustments of insulin made	Achieve near-normal glycemia	<7	x	x	x	x	x

*Insulin-treated type II diabetic patients usually require minimal monitoring, consistent with their simple insulin-injection regimen.
†More frequent tests performed on sick days or when ketonuria is present, with changes in exercise or meal patterns, on travel days, or when hypoglycemia is suspected or imminent. Intensively treated patients should perform a test at 0300 on a weekly basis.

betic patients. Intermittent measurements (laboratory or office) of fasting blood glucose or daily urine measurements may suffice in stable non–insulin-treated type II patients (Table 13.2).

Type II diabetic patients treated with oral agents or insulin face the risk of hypoglycemia. Although the frequency of hypoglycemia may be less than in type I diabetes, the clinical sequelae may be more severe, given the greater prevalence of coronary and cerebral vascular disease in this older population. Type II diabetes insulin-treatment regimens are less intensive than type I diabetes treatment regimens and, because of the relative stability of glucose profiles, may not require frequent change. Therefore, SMBG frequency can be similar to the frequency recommended for "minimal" or, if >1 daily injection is used, "average" type I diabetes treatment regimens (Table 13.1). However, some type II diabetic patients require intensive insulin treatment and must be monitored accordingly.

MEASUREMENT OF CHRONIC GLYCEMIA

Recognition that minor hemoglobin fractions, representing glycosylated adducts, increase in diabetic patients proportional to the

Table 13.2. **MONITORING OF TYPE II DIABETES TREATED WITH DIET OR ORAL HYPOGLYCEMIC AGENT**

Treatment Regimen	Method of Monitoring	Comments
Diet	Intermittent fasting blood or plasma glucose (laboratory or office)	Relatively stable blood glucose profiles; makes timed samples meaningful.
	SMBG	May be useful to help patient understand impact of diet, exercise, and life stresses on glycemia. Useful during periods of stress and infection. Frequency usually 1 or 2×/wk (prebreakfast or prebedtime) if used.
Oral agent	Intermittent fasting blood or plasma glucose (laboratory or office)	May suffice; useful to confirm accuracy of SMBG.
	SMBG	May be useful in adjusting dose and detecting hypoglycemia. Usual frequency 1×/day (prebreakfast or prebedtime). For stable program, may only be necessary 1 or 2×/wk.

SMBG, self-monitoring of blood glucose.

average blood glucose over the preceding 2–3 mo led to the implementation of the glycosylated hemoglobin assay (HbA$_{1c}$, HbA$_1$, or fast hemoglobin depending on the assay method used) as an accurate objective measure of chronic glycemia in diabetes. The characteristics of this assay are listed in Table 13.3.

HbA$_{1c}$ measured every 3 mo helps physicians identify type I patients with poor metabolic control, lower their average glycemic level, and prevent hospitalizations for metabolic instability. Note that the assay does not provide any measure of acute glucose levels; once HbA$_{1c}$ measurement has identified patients who require adjustments in regimen, measures of glucose levels, such as SMBG, are required to direct the change in therapy.

The role of HbA$_{1c}$ assay as the most accurate single assay for glycemic status indicates its use in all diabetic patients. Whether knowing average glycemia will influence treatment and improve long-term outcome in type II diabetes is under investigation. Although HbA$_{1c}$ may theoretically be a more physiological measure of chronic glycemia than nonphysiological stress tests, e.g., the oral glucose tolerance test, glycosylated hemoglobin assays are not sufficiently standardized to be acceptable for screening.

MEASUREMENT OF URINE KETONES

Type I diabetic patients are ketosis prone, whereas type II diabetic patients are generally ketosis resistant. Urine ketones, measured with dipsticks or tablets, should be tested routinely during sick days in all diabetic patients (even type II diabetic patients can become ketotic in the setting of severe illness). Because ketoacidosis may be associated with gastrointestinal symptoms indistinguishable from gastroenteritis, patients and physicians should be particularly attentive to such symptoms and test ketones if they occur. In addition, type I diabetic patients should test urine ketones once or twice daily if their SMBG indicates blood glucose levels consistently >300 mg/dl (>16.7 mM).

Table 13.3. GLYCOSYLATED HEMOGLOBIN ASSAY

- Measures average level of glucose over preceding 2–3 mo
- Provides objective index not provided by other measures
- Different assay methods measure different fractions; must check nondiabetic range for each assay
- Interfering factors (sickle-cell hemoglobin and other hemoglobinopathies) may affect measurement, depending on method
- May be used to validate accuracy of SMBG; discrepancy between SMBG levels and HbA$_{1c}$ suggests inaccurate SMBG results
- Optimal frequency not certain, but 3–4 assays/yr can influence management and complement SMBG in type I diabetes; in stable type II diabetes, 2 assays/yr should suffice

SMBG, self-monitoring of blood glucose.

SUGGESTED READING

1. Allen BT, DeLong ER, Feussner JR: Impact of glucose self-monitoring on non–insulin-treated patients with type II diabetes mellitus: randomized controlled trial comparing blood and urine testing. *Diabetes Care* 13:1044–50, 1990

2. American Diabetes Association: Consensus statement on self-monitoring of blood glucose. *Diabetes Care* 10:95–99, 1987

3. Larsen ML, Horder M, Mogensen EF: Effect of long-term monitoring of glycosylated hemoglobin levels in insulin-dependent diabetes mellitus. *N Engl J Med* 323:1021–25, 1990

4. Nathan DM, Singer DE, Hurxthal K, Goodson JD: The clinical information value of the glycosylated hemoglobin assay. *N Engl J Med* 310:341–46, 1984

5. Singer DE, Nathan DM, Coley CM, Samet JH: Tests of glycemia in diabetes mellitus. *Ann Intern Med* 110:125–37, 1989

14. Nutritional Management

ANNE DALY, MS, RD, CDE, and RONALD A. ARKY, MD

Nutritional management is a cornerstone of treatment for diabetes. Current nutritional recommendations of the American Diabetes Association are similar to those for healthy individuals without diabetes as developed by the National Research Council, the American Heart Association, and the American Cancer Society. For some patients, it can be the only intervention needed to control metabolic abnormalities associated with the disease. A resurgence of interest in nutritional management of diabetes mellitus has been prompted by new and emerging information. However, questions exist regarding the optimal carbohydrate, protein, and fat intake; use of fiber; role of glycemic index; liberalization of sucrose; value of ω-3 fatty acids; and alternative meal planning approaches to the exchange system. Greater variety in insulin regimens and self-monitoring of blood glucose (SMBG) allows increased individualization and flexibility of meal planning. Together, these changes may result in better adherence and improved blood glucose control.

ROLE OF HEALTH-CARE PROVIDER

The physician should take an active role in the definition of the patient's meal plan and integrate that plan with the patient's medication and physical activity pattern. Referral to a registered dietitian (RD) for nutrition education and the development of a practical and flexible meal plan is strongly recommended.

Ms. Daly is Program Director at the Springfield Diabetes and Endocrinology Center, Springfield, IL. Dr. Arky is Charles S. Davidson Professor of Medicine at Harvard Medical School, Boston, and Chairman of the Department of Medicine at Mount Auburn Hospital, Cambridge, MA.

The dietitian will consider the age and nutritional status of the patient, the presence of complications, and cultural, ethnic, and socioeconomic factors to develop an individualized meal plan. The final meal program is then shared with all health professionals caring for the patient. These health professionals should understand initial educational objectives related to nutrition. This may require considerable time but should be viewed as an important aspect of diabetes care. All diabetic patients should receive an individualized diet with education, with an intense follow-up program.

Supporting dietary adherence of the patient is the responsibility of all treatment team members. This can be accomplished by involving the patient and family; being supportive, nonjudgmental, positive, and helpful; using terms and language the patient understands; considering the patient's life-style; reinforcing instructions of other team members; providing feedback on progress; and arranging for adequate follow-up.

RATIONALE

For type I (insulin-dependent) diabetic individuals at desired weight, the meal plan is not intended as a restricted-calorie diet but rather as a guideline for consistency in food intake. Calorie intake and insulin administration should be adjusted so that adequate calories are consumed to cover periods of peak insulin action. As metabolic control improves, fewer calories will be lost through glycosuria, and calorie consumption should be reduced and/or activity increased accordingly.

In overweight people with diabetes, insulin resistance is enhanced. Weight loss decreases insulin resistance and results in decreased hepatic glucose production and increased peripheral glucose uptake. Significant calorie restriction can lower plasma glucose even before notable weight loss is achieved. Decreased calorie intake and reduction of dietary fat composition are necessary to promote weight loss. Also, spreading calories evenly throughout the day allows adequate time for postprandial glucose concentration to return to preprandial levels. In addition, SMBG aids the RD to plan food distribution and helps evaluate meal composition.

THERAPY

Considerations

Immediately after diagnosis of diabetes, patients (or parents, if appropriate) should meet with an RD or nutrition counselor to discuss basic dietary principles. Physicians and dietitians must consider several age-related factors when developing the overall meal plan (Tables 14.1 and 14.2).

Table 14.1. PRINCIPLES OF MEAL PLANNING (TYPE I DIABETES)

Ages 2–13 yr
- Adequate calorie intake to ensure normal growth and development
  - Assess growth every 3–4 mo
  - Protein intake 1.0–1.5 g/kg ideal body weight
- Limit foods/beverages with concentrated sucrose (soda)
  - Evaluate glycemic effects of specific foods with self-monitoring of blood glucose
  - Prevent severe hypoglycemia
- Encourage families to eat meals together
- Coordinate meals with insulin action
  - Knowledge of effects of exercise on insulin action
  - Never omit insulin when sick

Teenagers, adolescents, young adults
- Coordinate meals with insulin action
  - Eat regularly; avoid missing meals
  - Self-monitor glucose; know glycemic effects of specific foods, snacks, and meals
  - Make food adjustments for exercise and physical activity
- Avoid high-fat diets
  - Maintain ideal weight; avoid excessive weight gain
  - Fat content ≤30% of total calories; refrain from fast foods
  - Measure cholesterol and triglyceride yearly
  - Emphasize complex carbohydrate and soluble fibers
- Alcohol in moderation only
  - If taken, consume with food to avoid hypoglycemia
  - 1–2 equivalents once or twice weekly
- Be flexible; consider social demands and peer pressure of adolescence

Elderly
- Avoid hypoglycemia
  - Food intake to cover insulin
  - Eat regularly
- Avoid excessive weight gain
- Balanced diet
  - Fat to comprise 30% of total calories
  - Most calories from carbohydrate and protein

Table 14.2. PRINCIPLES OF MEAL PLANNING (TYPE II DIABETES)

Young, middle-aged, or elderly
- Calorie restriction and exercise are therapeutic cornerstones
- If overweight, reduce total calories and prescribe exercise
  - Maintain balanced nutrition, control portion sizes
  - Fat restriction is important; first step, ≤30% calories from fats
- Restrict foods/beverages with concentrated sucrose
  - Encourage sugar-free beverages
  - Measure fasting triglycerides

Nutrition Goals

The goal of nutritional management for diabetes is to maintain reasonable weight and control blood glucose and lipid levels without compromising overall nutrition or health. The current nutritional recommendations for people with diabetes are given in Table 14.3. Nutrition intervention varies according to the type of diabetes, the

Table 14.3. TARGET NUTRITIONAL GOALS FOR PEOPLE WITH DIABETES

Calories
- Sufficient to achieve and maintain reasonable body weight

Carbohydrate
- May be 55–60% of total calories
- Liberalized individualized emphasis on unrefined carbohydrate with fiber
- Modest amounts of sucrose and other refined sugars may be acceptable contingent on metabolic control and body weight

Protein
- Usual intake of protein is double amount needed
- Exact ideal percentage of total calories is unknown; however, usual intake is 12–20% of total calories
- RDA is 0.8 g/kg body wt for adults; it is modified for children, pregnant and lactating women, elderly, and those with special medical conditions

Fat
- Ideally <30% of total calories; however, this needs to be individualizod*
- Polyunsaturated fats, 6–8%
- Saturated fats, 10%
- Monounsaturated fats, remaining percentage
- Cholesterol <300 mg/day

Fiber
- Up to 40 g/day
- 25 g/1000 kcal for low-calorie intakes

Alternative sweeteners
- Use of various nutritive and nonnutritive sweeteners is acceptable

Sodium
- ≤3000 mg/day
- Modified for special medical conditions

Alcohol
- ≤1–2 equivalents 1–2×/wk
- 1 equivalent = 1.5 oz distilled liquor, 40-oz glass of wine, 12-oz glass of beer

Vitamins/minerals
- No evidence that diabetes influences need

---

*Controversy has developed over whether restriction of dietary fat to 30% is advisable for all patients with type II diabetes because of susceptibility to develop or worsen hypertriglyceridemia. This is not a problem when total calories are also restricted, but when diets are isocaloric, carbohydrate must also be increased. In some patients, it may be prudent to monitor serum triglycerides. RDA, recommended daily allowance.

drugs prescribed, and the patient's readiness to make dietary changes (Table 14.4).

Changing dietary habits is best done gradually, beginning with a patient's current food habits. Actual food records, rather than a dietary recall, are useful to identify priority areas for dietary change. A skilled dietitian will identify the procedures most likely to be successful in accomplishing dietary goals. Because changing food habits is a process requiring professional assistance, it is best to manipulate diet first and adjust medication accordingly.

Consistency of food intake and synchronizing the timing of insulin's action with the timing and composition of meals is of primary importance for patients with type I diabetes. However, most people with diabetes (90–95%) have type II (non-insulin-dependent) diabetes, and 60–80% of these are obese. Consequently, reaching and maintaining a reasonable weight is the primary management goal in type II diabetes.

Although an adequate trial of dietary treatment alone should first be attempted, some patients will need addition of oral hypoglycemic agents or insulin if a weight reduction diet is not effective. However, with weight reduction, some patients may be able to reduce or discontinue their medications. Even modest weight loss (10–20 lb) can improve insulin efficiency and produce a substantial reduction in serum glucose levels.

Table 14.4. PRIORITIES FOR MEAL-PLANNING STRATEGIES

Strategy	Type I Diabetes	Obese	Nonobese	Impaired Glucose Tolerance	Gestational Diabetes Mellitus
Timing of meals	High	Moderate	Moderate	Low	High
Consistency of day-to-day intake	High	Moderate	Moderate	Low	High
Fat modification	High	High	High	High	Moderate
Sucrose limitation	Moderate	Moderate	Moderate	Moderate	Moderate
Exercise snack	High	Low	Low	Low	Moderate
Calorie restriction	Low	High	Low	Moderate	Low
Other nutrition variables	Moderate	Moderate	Moderate	Moderate	Moderate

Patients with type II diabetes who are on insulin may need to follow type I diabetes strategies for timing and consistency more closely. If overweight, weight reduction is encouraged. Weight gain should follow weight grid for pregnancy. Reprinted from *Handbook of Diabetes Nutritional Management*, p. 50, with permission of Aspen Publishers, Inc., © 1987 (5).

Calorie Prescriptions

The first step in determining a diet prescription is to evaluate body weight in relation to height and body frame. Although various methods are available to determine desirable body weight (DBW), Table 14.5 presents a simple method that is consistent with the 1959 Metropolitan Life Insurance Company height-weight tables.

Calories should be prescribed to achieve and maintain DBW. Baseline calorie needs depend on height, weight, need for weight loss or gain, and usual activity/exercise patterns. During childhood, adolescence, and pregnancy and lactation, the body requires additional calories. Guidelines for initial calculation of calorie requirements through all phases of the life cycle are listed in Table 14.6.

The calorie prescription should also consider weight history and desired level of metabolic control. For children, it is necessary to monitor growth on a weight-height grid to ensure nutritional adequacy and reach and maintain DBW.

Calculating Calories for Weight Loss

One pound of body fat contains ~3500 kcal. Eating 500–1000 cal/day less than usual intake or less than maintenance calorie needs should result in a weight loss of 1–2 lb/wk. The minimum recommended calorie level is 1200 cal for women and 1500 cal for men to ensure the diet is nutritionally adequate in vitamins and minerals. Some individuals may require special efforts such as very-low-calorie diets or supervised supplemented fasting to achieve weight loss. To assist with weight loss, exercise (average of 250–300 kcal expended/day) is recommended.

Distribution of Meals and Snacks

Distribution of meals and snacks depends on life-style and activity patterns. With increasing use of more flexible insulin regimens, it is usually not necessary to divide the meal plan into specific intake fractions throughout the day. With consistent food intake from day to day, insulin therapy can usually be adjusted to the patient's usual food intake. For patients with type II diabetes, smaller meals spaced throughout the day may be a good nutrition intervention, because

Table 14.5. ESTIMATION OF DESIRABLE BODY WEIGHT

Build	Women	Men
Small	−10%	−10%
Medium	100 lb for 1st 5 ft of height; 5 lb/inch for each inch >5 ft	106 lb for 1st 5 ft of height; 6 lb/inch for each inch >5 ft
Large	+10%	+10%

Consult growth grids for desirable body weight of children.

Table 14.6. GUIDELINES FOR CALCULATING
CALORIE REQUIREMENT

Age	Calorie Requirements
0–12 yr	1000 cal for 1st yr + 100 cal/yr over age 1 yr
12–15 yr	
Female	1500–2000 cal + 100 cal/yr over age 12 yr
Male	2000–2500 cal + 200 cal/yr over age 12 yr
15–20 yr	
Female	13–15 cal/lb (29–33 kcal/kg) DBW
Male	15–18 cal/lb (33–40 kcal/kg) DBW
Adults	
Physically active	14–16 cal/lb (31–35 kcal/kg) DBW
Moderately active	12–14 cal/lb (26–31 kcal/kg) DBW
Sedentary	10–12 cal/lb (22–26 kcal/kg) DBW
Sedentary >55 yr, obese and/or inactive	10 cal/lb (22 kcal/kg) DBW
Pregnancy	
1st trimester*	12–16 cal/lb (26–35 kcal/kg) DBW
2nd and 3rd trimesters	13–17 cal/lb (29–37 kcal/kg) DBW
Lactation	15–17 cal/lb (33–37 kcal/kg) DBW

DBW, desired body weight.
*2- to 4-lb weight gain; calories may be reduced slightly if obese, with early excessive weight gain, or with sedentary life-style.

less insulin may be required to achieve blood glucose control. Another approach to improve glycemic control is to space meals 5–6 h apart to allow insulin time to lower blood glucose.

Meal-Planning Approaches

An individualized flexible meal plan is crucial to the success or failure of a nutrition-care plan. Various meal-planning approaches or strategies are available to the dietitian to effectively teach a patient. The type of approach used should depend on the patient's learning needs and abilities, nutritional needs, and personal needs and life-style. Some examples of meal-planning approaches commonly used are

- Basic nutrition guidelines
- Healthy food choices
- Exchange lists
- Calorie counting
- Carbohydrate counting
- Fat counting
- Sample menus

The exchange system remains the most widely used approach by dietitians, especially those working in hospital settings. Exchanges are convenient to standardize food delivery in an institutional setting. They teach food portions and help patients identify questions before discharge. In outpatient settings, however, dietitians are increasingly using the exchange system in combination with other meal planning approaches.

SUGGESTED READING

1. American Diabetes Association: Position statement: nutritional recommendations and principles for individuals with diabetes mellitus: 1986. *Diabetes Care* 10:126–32, 1987
2. Diabetes Care & Education Practice Group: Introducing Meal Planning and Meal Planning Approaches in Diabetes Management. In *Meal Planning Approaches in the Nutrition Management of the Person With Diabetes*. Chicago, IL, Am. Diet. Assoc., 1987, p. 9–15
3. *Nutrition Guide for Professionals: Diabetes Education and Meal Planning*. Alexandria, VA, Am. Diabetes Assoc., 1988, p. 29
4. *Physician's Guide to Insulin-Dependent (Type I) Diabetes: Diagnosis and Treatment*. Sperling MA, Ed. Alexandria, VA, Am. Diabetes Assoc., 1988, p. 47
5. Powers MA: Diabetes nutritional management. In *Handbook of Diabetes Nutritional Management*. Powers MA, Ed. Rockville, MD, Aspen, 1987, p. 50

15. Accessing Nutrition Care

MARGARET A. POWERS, MS, RD, CDE

Nutrition care is a continuous and integral component of complete diabetes management. It should be viewed as ongoing therapy that involves changing behaviors and determining an optimal food intake pattern (Tables 15.1 and 15.2).

Table 15.1. WHEN TO CONSULT WITH REGISTERED DIETITIAN

First contact
  1. When diabetes is first diagnosed or considered. This includes people with impaired glucose tolerance, obesity with a family history of diabetes, and android obesity
  2. When first seeing a patient with prediagnosed diabetes

Routine care
  1. For continued development of a goal-directed meal plan
  2. For continued education and counseling
  3. Before initiation of diabetes medication, if possible, to determine
      • Whether diet manipulation or activity adjustment will prevent the use of drugs
      • Usual eating behaviors so the best drug regimen can be selected

Additional indicators for intervention
  1. When the patient anticipates or has a life-style change such as a job change, marriage, or pregnancy
  2. When the patient expresses frustration about food choices
  3. When the patient feels unmotivated to adhere to what he/she feels is the best eating pattern
  4. When the patient wants to improve glycemic control
  5. If there are unexplainable excursions in blood glucose levels
  6. When weight control is a concern

Ms. Powers is President of Powers and Associates Health Promotion and Communications, St. Paul, MN.

Table 15.2. TIME FRAMES FOR NUTRITION INTERVENTION

Initial workup/assessment
   1−2 h, 1−2 appointments
Education/counseling
   Biweekly or monthly sessions for 2−4 mo, 15−45 min each
   Daily/weekly phone calls with self-monitored blood glucose records
Follow-up
   As needed
   With life-style and life-cycle changes
   Minimum follow-up for children every 3−6 mo, for adults every 6−12
     mo

WHO SHOULD PROVIDE NUTRITION CARE

Complete nutrition counseling is best done by a qualified nutrition professional with appropriate training and experience (e.g., an RD). The questions in Table 15.3 are guidelines for selecting a dietitian to work with and are similar to those that might be used to evaluate other medical consultants. Inpatient hospital stays are no longer considered the ideal educational setting for changing life-style behaviors (Tables 15.4 and 15.5).

Table 15.3. INTERVIEW QUESTIONS WHEN SELECTING REGISTERED DIETITIAN (RD)

Qualifications
   1. Is the nutrition counselor registered by the American Dietetic Association's Commission on Dietetic Registration, the qualification for an RD?
   2. What specific qualifications does the RD have to manage the nutrition care of your patients with diabetes? Answers should include experience with diabetes patient care and with nutrition counseling in individual and group settings.
Treatment philosophy
   1. Does the RD uses various meal-planning approaches rather than trying to fit each patient into one method of planning food intake?
   2. Does the RD use self-monitored blood glucose (SMBG) records to determine the most appropriate arrangement of food intake and/or to make recommendations about medication adjustments?
Patient relationship
   1. Have the RD describe what types of phone calls he/she might expect from patients. For example, the patient is asked to review the labels on several specific food products and calls the dietitian to discuss them. You want to determine whether the dietitian is amenable to these types of calls, which indicates a responsive and creative educator.
   2. Does the RD use support resources such as community exercise programs, cooking classes, and library books?

Table 15.4. HOW TO ACCESS NUTRITION CARE

- Word of mouth
  Ask peers who they use for nutrition care.
- Local hospital
  Find out whether nutrition outpatient services are available.
- Advertise to employ a registered dietitian
- Yellow pages
  Because not all states require licensure, telephone listings for nutrition or nutritionist should be checked to ensure that the individual is competent in the area of diabetes nutrition care.
- State licensing board
  Some states have licensure for dietitians.
- Local health programs
  Local public-health departments, community or neighborhood health centers, may provide nutrition services that encompass basic diabetes care.

WHAT TO EXPECT

The physician should expect follow-up correspondence from the RD regarding the diet history, instruction, follow-up plans, and other pertinent information that will influence diabetes care.

Specific needs and expectations should be discussed with the RD. Include the RD in team meetings or discussions to enhance an understanding of each other's approach to diabetes management more quickly and efficiently.

Table 15.5. PROFESSIONAL ORGANIZATIONS THAT SUPPORT NUTRITION CARE

- The American Dietetic Association, 216 West Jackson Boulevard, Suite 800, Chicago, IL 60606-6995; (312)899-0040, extension 4853. Ask the National Center for Nutrition and Dietetics for the list of dietitians in your area.

- American Diabetes Association, 1660 Duke Street, Alexandria, VA 22314; (800)ADA-DISC.
  Ask for the address and phone number of your state affiliate or local chapter or locate in your local phone book. They can help guide you in locating dietitians with a specialty in diabetes.

- American Association of Diabetes Educators, 500 North Michigan Avenue, Suite 1400, Chicago, IL 60611; (312)661-1700.
  A directory is available that includes dietitians who have a special interest in diabetes care.

16. Exercise

EDWARD S. HORTON, MD

Regular physical exercise has been recommended as an important component of the treatment of all people with diabetes. However, exercise potentiates the action of insulin, resulting in lower insulin requirements and an increased risk of hypoglycemic reactions during and after exercise. Also, in patients with type I (insulin-dependent) diabetes, exercise may cause a further rise in blood glucose and the rapid development of ketosis. Even in well-controlled patients, vigorous exercise may result in sustained hyperglycemia. Because of these problems with regulation of blood glucose and ketones during or after exercise, many type I diabetic patients have found it difficult to participate in sports or other recreational activities or, for that matter, to manage exercise as part of their daily lives. This has led to the opinion that exercise should not be recommended for all patients with type I diabetes but that efforts should be focused on making it possible for those who want to exercise to be able to do so as safely as possible. The availability of self-monitoring of blood glucose and the increased use of multiple-dose insulin regimens has led to the development of strategies for the management of exercise in type I diabetic patients, making it possible for them to participate safely in a wide range of physical activities and thus to lead a normal or near-normal life-style. In type II (non-insulin-dependent) diabetic patients, on the other hand, regular activity is an important component of treatment and should be prescribed along with appropriate diet and oral hypoglycemic agents as part of a comprehensive treatment program. This requires a careful assessment of the expected benefits and associated risks of exercise in individual

Dr. Horton is Professor of Medicine at the Medical Center Hospital of Vermont, Burlington, VT.

patients, the development of a well-planned exercise program, and appropriate monitoring to avoid complications.

BENEFITS

The benefits of exercise for patients with diabetes are listed in Table 16.1. Moderate sustained exercise in patients with either type I or type II diabetes may be used to help regulate glucose on a day-to-day basis and may be the mechanism by which regular physical exercise assists in achieving improved long-term metabolic control. Physical training results in lower fasting and postprandial insulin concentrations and increased insulin sensitivity. In patients with type I diabetes, increased insulin sensitivity results in lowered insulin requirements. In patients with type II diabetes, the improvement in insulin sensitivity resulting from regular physical exercise may be of major importance in improving long-term glycemic control.

Another benefit of regular exercise is a reduction of cardiovascular risk factors through improvement of the lipid profile and reduction of hypertension in diabetic patients. Physical training is associated with a significant decrease in serum triglycerides, particularly very-low-density lipoproteins, and an increase in high-density lipoprotein 2 cholesterol. There is also usually a slight reduction in low-density lipoprotein cholesterol levels with exercise. This improvement in the lipid profile requires a fairly high intensity of physical training. It is observed with running $\geq 9-12$ miles/wk and increases progressively up to distances of ~ 40 miles/wk. Lower levels of physical activity have little, if any, effect on serum lipids. The effect of physical training to improve mild to moderate hypertension is independent of weight loss or a change in body compo-

Table 16.1. BENEFITS OF EXERCISE FOR PATIENTS WITH DIABETES

1. Lower blood glucose concentrations during and after exercise
2. Lower basal and postprandial insulin concentrations
3. Improved insulin sensitivity
4. Lower glycosylated hemoglobin levels
5. Improved lipid profile
   - Decreased triglycerides
   - Slightly decreased LDL cholesterol
   - Increased high-density lipoprotein 2 cholesterol
6. Improvement in mild-to-moderate hypertension
7. Increased energy expenditure
   - Adjunct to diet for weight reduction
   - Increased fat loss
   - Preservation of lean body mass
8. Cardiovascular conditioning
9. Increased strength and flexibility
10. Improved sense of well-being and quality of life

sition. Decreases in both systolic and diastolic blood pressures of 5–10 mmHg are common and are often correlated with decreases in serum insulin and triglyceride concentrations.

In addition to improvement in cardiovascular risk factors, physical exercise may be an effective adjunct to diet for weight reduction. This is usually seen when exercise is combined with moderate calorie restriction. When patients are treated with very-low-calorie diets (600–800 kcal/day), exercise may not have a significant effect on the amount or composition of weight loss beyond that of the diet alone.

Finally, exercise improves cardiovascular function (decreased resting heart rate, increased stroke volume, and decreased cardiac work), increases fitness and physical working capacity, and improves sense of well-being and quality of life.

RISKS

There are several risks for patients with diabetes (Table 16.2). In type I diabetic patients, late-onset postexercise hypoglycemia can occur 6–15 h after completion of the exercise and may persist for up to 24 h after prolonged strenuous exercise. In contrast to hypoglycemia, vigorous exercise may result in a rapid increase in blood glucose, which can persist for several hours after the exercise is

Table 16.2. **RISKS OF EXERCISE FOR PATIENTS WITH DIABETES**

1. Hypoglycemia, if treated with insulin or oral agents
   - Exercise-induced hypoglycemia
   - Late-onset postexercise hypoglycemia
2. Hyperglycemia after very strenuous exercise
3. Hyperglycemia and ketosis in insulin-deficient patients
4. Precipitation or exacerbation of cardiovascular disease
   - Angina pectoris
   - Myocardial infarction
   - Arrhythmias
   - Sudden death
5. Worsening of long-term complications of diabetes
   - Proliferative retinopathy
     - Vitreous hemorrhage
     - Retinal detachment
   - Nephropathy
     - Increased proteinuria
   - Peripheral neuropathy
     - Soft tissue and joint injuries
   - Autonomic neuropathy
     - Decreased cardiovascular response to exercise
     - Decreased maximum aerobic capacity
     - Impaired response to dehydration
     - Postural hypotension

discontinued. Even moderate-intensity exercise may result in hyperglycemia and the rapid development of ketosis or ketoacidosis in type I diabetic patients.

Careful screening for underlying cardiac disease is important for all patients with diabetes before starting an exercise program. In addition, degenerative joint disease is more common in obese individuals and may be exacerbated by weight-bearing exercises.

Several complications of diabetes may be aggravated by exercise, and all patients should be screened before they start an exercise program. The most important of these is proliferative retinopathy, in which exercise may result in retinal or vitreous hemorrhage. Exercises that increase blood pressure, e.g., heavy lifting or exercise associated with Valsalva-like maneuvers, are particularly dangerous and should be avoided by patients with proliferative retinopathy. Exercise resulting in jarring or rapid head motion may precipitate hemorrhage or retinal detachment. Physical exercise is also associated with increased proteinuria in patients with diabetic nephropathy, probably due to changes in renal hemodynamics. It is not known whether this has any long-term deleterious effect on renal function, but it may cause concern in patients with diabetic nephropathy.

Patients with peripheral neuropathy have an increased risk of soft tissue and joint injuries and, if autonomic neuropathy is present, the capacity for high-intensity exercise is impaired due to a decrease in maximum heart rate and aerobic capacity. In addition, patients with autonomic neuropathy may have impaired responses to dehydration and develop postural hypotension after exercise. With proper selection of the type, intensity, and duration of exercise, most of these complications can be avoided.

GUIDELINES FOR EXERCISE

Screening

Before starting an exercise program, all patients should have a complete history and physical examination, with particular attention to identifying any long-term complications of diabetes. An exercise-stress ECG is recommended for all patients >35 yr of age. This test will help identify silent ischemic heart disease and may identify patients who have an exaggerated hypertensive response to exercise and/or may develop postexercise orthostatic hypotension. A careful ophthalmological examination to identify proliferative retinopathy, renal function tests including screening for microalbuminuria, and a neurological examination to determine peripheral and/or autonomic neuropathy should be performed. If abnormalities are found, exercises should be selected that will not pose significant risks for worsening complications. In general, young active patients with diabetes of brief duration and no evidence of long-term complications do not require formal exercise prescriptions, although they need specific recommendations regarding strategies for managing exercise and avoiding injuries.

Selection of Types of Exercise

If there are no contraindications, the types of exercise a patient performs can be a matter of personal preference. In general, moderate-intensity aerobic exercises that can be sustained for ≥30 min are preferred, although intermittent high-intensity and resistance exercises, e.g., weight lifting, can also be managed successfully.

Some types of exercise may be less desirable for people with diabetes. For example, high-resistance exercises, e.g., weight lifting, are less desirable because of the high incidence of orthopedic and vascular side effects. Exercises that traumatize the feet, e.g., running and jogging, should be limited in patients with peripheral neuropathy, and body-contact sports should be avoided by patients with proliferative retinopathy.

Exercise Sessions

Each exercise session should begin with a warm-up of low-intensity aerobic exercise and stretching for 5–10 min to prevent musculoskeletal injuries. The higher-intensity portion of the exercise session should last 20–45 min, except in highly trained individuals in whom longer workouts are possible. Exercises should be of moderate intensity (50–75% of the individual's maximum aerobic capacity), if the complications of diabetes permit and blood-pressure response is not excessive. In general, exercise intensity should be limited so that systolic blood pressure does not exceed 180 mmHg. The intensity of exercise can be estimated from the heart-rate response, i.e., the resting pulse rate determined before arising in the morning and the maximum heart rate determined during exercise. Fifty percent of a subject's maximal effort can be estimated by the formula 0.5 (maximum heart rate − resting heart rate) + resting heart rate. When the true maximal heart rate is unknown, it can be estimated by the formula 220 − patient's age. However, this is less accurate than a direct determination of the maximum heart rate under controlled conditions and may significantly overestimate the maximum heart rate in patients with autonomic neuropathy. Once the heart-rate response to exercise is determined for an individual patient, exercise intensity can be conveniently monitored by teaching the patient to measure his/her own pulse periodically during exercise and recording the results. The end of each exercise session should consist of a cool-down for at least 5–10 min to reduce the risk of postexercise cardiac and musculoskeletal complications. This is best done at an intensity of ~30% of maximum aerobic capacity and should include activities such as walking, stretching, and slow rhythmic exercises.

Frequency of Exercise

Patients should exercise ≥ 3 days/wk or on an every-other-day sched-ule to achieve cardiovascular conditioning and improved insulin sensitivity and glycemic control. If exercise is being used as an adjunct to diet for weight reduction, exercise should be done ≥ 5 days/wk.

Special Precautions

Feet should be inspected daily and always after exercise for cuts, blisters, and infections. Exercise should be avoided in extreme hot or cold environments and during periods of poor metabolic control. Special guidelines for patients taking insulin are described below.

Compliance

Several things can be done to improve the patient's motivation and participation on a regular basis. These include choosing activities the patient enjoys, providing a variety in types and settings for exercise, performing exercise at a convenient time and location, encouraging participation in group activities, involving the patient's family and associates for reinforcement, and measuring progress to provide positive feedback. Most important is to start slowly, build up gradually, and not set excessive or unrealistic goals.

Instruction and Monitoring

For patients who have not participated regularly in exercise in the past or who have significant complications of diabetes or other impediments to exercise, supervised exercise programs may be ben-eficial. Often, cardiac rehabilitation programs will be of assistance in supervising exercise programs for people with diabetes, partic-ularly if the patients are at high risk for cardiovascular disease. There are an increasing number of diabetes treatment centers that offer supervised exercise programs for patients with either type I or type II diabetes. Many patients, however, do not need formal supervision once an initial assessment has been completed and an appropriate exercise plan has been established.

MANAGEMENT IN TYPE I DIABETIC PATIENTS

Whereas changes in blood glucose are small in nondiabetic individ-uals during exercise, several factors may complicate glucose regu-lation during and after exercise in type I diabetic patients. Plasma insulin concentrations do not decrease normally during exercise, thus upsetting the balance between peripheral glucose utilization and hepatic glucose production. With insulin treatment, plasma insulin concentrations stay the same or may even increase if exercise is undertaken within 1 h of an insulin injection. Enhanced insulin absorption during exercise is most likely to occur when the insulin injection is given immediately before or within a few minutes of the onset of exercise. The longer the interval between injection and onset of exercise, the less significant this effect will be and the less important it is to choose the site of injection to avoid an exercising area.

The sustained insulin levels during exercise increase peripheral glucose uptake and stimulate glucose oxidation by exercising muscle. In addition, insulin inhibits hepatic glucose production. The hepatic glucose production rate cannot match the rate of peripheral glucose utilization, and blood glucose concentration falls. During mild to moderate exercise of short duration, this may be a beneficial effect of exercise, but during more prolonged exercise, hypoglycemia may result. On the other hand, if exercise is vigorous, sympathetic nervous stimulation of hepatic glucose production may result in a rapid and sustained rise in blood glucose concentrations. If there is also insulin deficiency, hepatic ketone production is stimulated, and ketosis or ketoacidosis may occur.

A checklist of factors to consider before the onset of exercise is provided in Table 16.3. Obviously, it is not possible to predict all

Table 16.3. PREEXERCISE CHECKLIST FOR TYPE I DIABETIC PATIENTS

1. Consider the exercise plan
   - What is the duration and intensity of the planned exercise?
   - Is the exercise habitual or unusual?
   - How does the exercise relate to the level of physical conditioning?
   - What is the estimated calorie expenditure?
2. Consider the insulin regimen
   - What is the usual insulin-dosage schedule? Should it be decreased?
   - What is the interval between injection of insulin and the onset of exercise?
   - Should the site of injection be changed to avoid exercising areas?
3. Consider the plan for food intake
   - What is the interval between the last meal and the onset of exercise?
   - Should a preexercise snack be eaten?
   - Should carbohydrate feedings be taken during exercise?
   - Will extra food be required after exercise?
4. Check blood glucose
   - If <100 mg/dl (<5.5 mM), eat a preexercise snack.
   - If 100–250 mg/dl (5.5–14 mM), it should be all right to exercise.*
   - If >250 mg/dl (>14 mM), check urine ketones.
5. Check urine ketones (if glucose is >250 mg/dl [>14 mM])
   - If negative, all right to exercise.
   - If positive, take insulin; do not exercise until ketones are negative.

*See Table 16.4.

situations, because exercise is often spontaneous or intermittent and varies greatly in intensity and duration.

By considering the exercise plan and making adjustments in insulin dosage and food intake, type I diabetic patients can avoid severe hypoglycemia or hyperglycemia. If exercise is of moderate intensity and long duration, blood glucose levels will fall, whereas vigorous exercise of short duration will often cause blood glucose to rise. Attention should be paid to the amount, timing, and site of insulin administration. Food intake before, during, and after exercise should be considered. It is also important to measure blood glucose before starting exercise and, if necessary, during and after exercise. With this information, the strategies outlined in Table 16.4 can be used to avoid either hypoglycemia or hyperglycemia.

Usually a snack containing 20–25 g carbohydrate every 30 min is sufficient to provide enough glucose to maintain normal blood levels during prolonged exercise. Carbohydrate requirements will depend on factors such as the intensity and duration of exercise, the level of physical conditioning, the antecedent diet, and the circulating insulin levels.

If the exercise is planned, the insulin-dosage schedule may be altered to decrease the likelihood of hypoglycemia. Individuals who take a single dose of intermediate-acting insulin may decrease the dose by 30–35% on the morning before exercise or may change to a split-dose regimen, taking 65% of the usual dose in the morning and 35% before the evening meal. Those who are taking a combination of intermediate- and short-acting insulin may decrease the short-acting insulin by 50% or omit it altogether before exercise; they also may decrease the intermediate-acting insulin before exercise and take supplemental doses of short-acting insulin later if needed. For those on multiple-dose therapy with short-acting insulin, the dose before exercise may be decreased by 30–50%, and postexercise doses may be adjusted based on glucose monitoring and experience with postexercise hypoglycemia. If insulin-infusion

Table 16.4. **STRATEGIES TO AVOID HYPOGLYCEMIA AND HYPERGLYCEMIA WITH EXERCISE**

1. Eat a meal 1–3 h before exercise.
2. Take supplemental carbohydrate feedings during exercise at least every 30 min if exercise is vigorous and of long duration.
3. Increase food intake for up to 24 h after exercise, depending on intensity and duration of exercise.
4. Take insulin at least 1 h before exercise. If <1 h before exercise, inject in a nonexercising area.
5. Decrease insulin dose before exercise.
6. Alter daily insulin schedule.
7. Monitor blood glucose before, during, and after exercise.
8. Delay exercise if blood glucose is >250 mg/dl (>14 mM) and ketones are present.
9. Learn individual glucose responses to different types of exercise.

devices are used, the basal infusion rate may be decreased during exercise and premeal boluses decreased or omitted.

EXERCISE PROGRAMS FOR TREATMENT OF TYPE II DIABETES

Exercise programs improve insulin sensitivity and lower average blood glucose concentrations. The increased energy expenditure associated with exercise, when combined with calorie restriction, may improve weight reduction. Thus, regular exercise is an important component of the treatment of type II diabetic patients.

On the other hand, type II diabetic patients are usually older, are frequently obese, and may have significant long-term complications, making the initiation of exercise programs difficult. In this group of patients, exercises with a decreased risk of injury that enhance motivation and participation should be selected. Increasing daily activities such as walking, climbing stairs, and other familiar activities is an excellent start.

Unlike patients treated with insulin, problems in glucose regulation do not occur, with the exception of occasional problems with hypoglycemia in patients taking sulfonylureas. In patients being treated with diet alone, supplemental feedings before, during, or after exercise are unnecessary except when exercise is unusually vigorous and of long duration.

In patients being treated with low-calorie diets, physical exercise is generally well tolerated and does not pose any additional risks if the diet is adequately supplemented with vitamins and minerals and adequate hydration is maintained. In patients treated with very-low-calorie diets (600–800 kcal/day), the diet should contain at least 35% of calories as carbohydrate to maintain normal muscle glycogen stores, which are needed to maintain high-intensity exercise. On the other hand, very-low-calorie diets severely restricted in carbohydrate are compatible with moderate-intensity exercise after an adaptation period of ≥2 wk. However, these offer little, if any, advantage over carbohydrate-containing diets.

An exercise program for obese patients with type II diabetes should start slowly, build up gradually, and include exercises that are familiar to the patient and least likely to cause injuries or worsening of long-term diabetes complications.

SUGGESTED READING

1. American Diabetes Association: Position statement: diabetes and exercise. *Diabetes Care* 13:804–805, 1990
2. American Diabetes Association: Technical review: exercise and NIDDM. *Diabetes Care* 13:785–89, 1990
3. Horton ES: Exercise and diabetes mellitus. *Med Clin North Am* 72:1301–21, 1988

17. Sulfonylurea Drugs

HAROLD E. LEBOVITZ, MD

Sulfonylurea drugs have been used for 40 years in the management of hyperglycemia in patients with type II (non-insulin-dependent) diabetes. The mechanism of action of sulfonylurea agents is complex. Acutely, they augment insulin secretion. After several months of therapy, however, plasma insulin levels return to pretreatment values, whereas plasma glucose levels remain improved. These findings have led to the suggestion that sulfonylurea drugs also exert extrapancreatic effects on glucose metabolism. Several metabolic effects of sulfonylureas have been clearly defined. They reduce the accelerated rates of hepatic glucose production in type II diabetes, partially reverse the postreceptor defect in insulin action and lead to an increase in the number of cellular insulin receptors, and increase the efficiency of insulin secretion. The relative importance of each of these actions in ameliorating hyperglycemia is unclear, but it is likely that pancreatic and extrapancreatic effects of these agents combine to produce the antidiabetic action of these drugs. Because type II diabetes is a disorder in which insulin secretion is decreased and insulin action is impaired, the sulfonylurea drugs are useful agents in controlling hyperglycemia in such patients.

Several features are essential in understanding the proper use of sulfonylurea drugs. They are ineffective in lowering blood glucose in patients who have a marked reduction or total loss of functioning β-cells, and hypoglycemia can be a serious consequence of their inappropriate use. For reasons that are still unknown, not all type II diabetic patients respond to the antidiabetic action of sulfonylureas (primary failure), and many patients who do respond very

---

Dr. Lebovitz is Professor of Medicine, Chief of Endocrinology and Metabolism/Diabetes, and Director of the Clinical Research Center at the State University of New York Health Science Center at Brooklyn, Brooklyn, NY.

well initially may lose this antidiabetic response after several years of treatment (secondary failure). Sulfonylurea drugs do not replace dietary management of type II diabetic patients, they complement it; i.e., they are unlikely to be effective if dietary management is ignored.

CHOICE OF SULFONYLUREA DRUG

All sulfonylurea drugs appear to exert their antidiabetic actions through the same mechanism of action. The clinical use of a particular sulfonylurea is based on the characteristics described in Table 17.1. Intrinsic antidiabetic activity varies considerably, with glyburide and glipizide being the most and tolbutamide being the least potent. The intrinsic potency of each sulfonylurea is important in determining the effective dose of the drug that is necessary. Clinical response in controlling hyperglycemia, however, is not significantly different among the various sulfonylureas at their effective doses except for tolbutamide, which is less effective in controlling the hyperglycemia of type II diabetes than the other drugs.

Type II diabetes is characterized by a relative decrease in meal-stimulated insulin secretion and a delay in insulin release. The delay in insulin release contributes to the excessive postprandial rise in blood glucose levels. The more rapid the onset of action of a sulfonylurea, the less delay in the rise in postprandial insulin secretion. Thus, the interval between administration of the drug and the meal should be considered.

Duration of action of a sulfonylurea drug is of considerable importance. A long-acting sulfonylurea is more likely to be associated with severe, prolonged, and sometimes fatal hypoglycemia in susceptible patients, i.e., those who are elderly (>70 yr of age), have poor nutrition, are likely to miss meals, or have concomitant hepatic, renal, or cardiovascular disease. Shorter-acting sulfonylureas are significantly safer in this population.

The mode of metabolism and excretion are also important in determining the frequency and severity of hypoglycemic reactions. Sulfonylureas that are metabolized to active metabolites are associated with more hypoglycemic reactions. Likewise, drugs or active metabolites primarily excreted by the kidney are more likely to

Table 17.1. **CHARACTERISTICS BY WHICH TO SELECT SPECIFIC SULFONYLUREA**

- Intrinsic antidiabetic potency
- Rapidity of onset of action
- Duration of action
- Mode of metabolism and excretion
- Beneficial and detrimental side effects

cause hypoglycemia in patients with renal dysfunction than drugs excreted via the biliary tract.

Side effects occur that are independent of antidiabetic action. Some, e.g., water retention and hyponatremia, appear to be unique to chlorpropamide. Others, e.g., alcohol-induced flushing, may occur with first-generation (low-intrinsic-potency) sulfonylureas such as chlorpropamide and tolbutamide but not with second-generation (high-intrinsic-potency) agents.

Characteristics of Specific Sulfonylurea Drugs

Table 17.2 lists the characteristics of the commonly used sulfonylurea drugs. The dose range is a function of the intrinsic potency, but the clinical effectiveness at the appropriate dose is the same for all sulfonylureas except tolbutamide. Onset and duration of action are determined by the unique pharmacokinetic properties of each agent. Most sulfonylureas are metabolized in the liver to active or inactive metabolites, except for chlorpropamide, which is excreted unchanged in significant quantities in the urine. Biliary excretion is significant with glyburide and to a lesser extent with glipizide. Major side effects other than hypoglycemia are most commonly seen with chlorpropamide.

HYPOGLYCEMIA

The most serious complication of sulfonylurea therapy is hypoglycemia. This is best avoided or minimized by the following procedures:

1. Start sulfonylurea therapy with the lowest possible dose and increase the dose incrementally every 4–7 days.
2. Patients susceptible to severe and prolonged hypoglycemia should be treated with shorter-acting sulfonylureas.
3. Sulfonylureas should be used cautiously in patients with renal dysfunction. Sulfonylureas with short duration of action, inactive metabolites, and biliary excretion are preferred.
4. Encourage patients not to skip meals after taking sulfonylurea drugs.
5. Be careful of drug interactions.

The treatment of mild hypoglycemia in sulfonylurea-treated patients is managed by giving food, careful monitoring, and a reduction in dosage or change in specific sulfonylurea. The treatment of severe sulfonylurea-induced hypoglycemia requires vigorous and prolonged treatment. Patients who present with gluconeuropenic symptoms and plasma glucose levels <50 mg/dl (<2.8 mM) should be given 50 ml of 50% glucose i.v. followed by continuous glucose (5 or 10%) and frequent monitoring of blood glucose. These patients must be monitored and treated for at least 24 h. With long-acting

Table 17.2. CHARACTERISTICS OF SPECIFIC SULFONYLUREA DRUGS

Drug	Dose Range (mg/day)	Peak Level* (h)	Half-Life (h)	Metabolites	Excretion
Tolbutamide	500–3000	3–4	4.5–6.5	Inactive	Kidney
Chlorpropamide	100–500	2–4	36	Active or unchanged	Kidney
Tolazamide	100–1000	3–4	7	Inactive	Kidney
Glipizide	2.5–40	1–3	2–4	Inactive	Kidney, ~20% in bile
Glyburide	1.25–20	~4	10	Inactive and weakly active	Kidney 50%, bile 50%

*After a single oral dose.

sulfonylureas, patients should be monitored for 72 h because recurrence of the hypoglycemia is common. The patients cannot be given 50% glucose intravenously and sent home. The reason for the severe hypoglycemia must be sought and appropriate therapeutic changes made.

INDICATIONS FOR SULFONYLUREA THERAPY

Ideal candidates for sulfonylurea therapy are type II diabetic patients who still have adequate β-cell function. Patients likely to show good glycemia responses to sulfonylureas

- Had onset of their hyperglycemia after age 30 yr
- Have had diagnosed hyperglycemia for <5 yr
- Are normal weight or obese
- Are willing to follow a reasonable dietary program
- Are not insulin dependent

Contraindications for sulfonylurea therapy are given in Table 17.3.

PROPER USE OF SULFONYLUREA DRUGS

Sulfonylurea drugs should be administered to type II diabetic patients who have been unable to adequately control their plasma glucose on a reasonable trial (4–6 wk) of appropriate diet therapy. When sulfonylurea therapy is added, dietary management must continue. Sulfonylurea therapy is unlikely to have significant beneficial effects in an individual who has a fasting plasma glucose level >250 mg/dl (>13.9 mM) while on a reasonable diet program.

Initiation of a newly diagnosed type II diabetic patient with hyperglycemia >300 mg/dl (>16.7 mM) on sulfonylurea therapy is inappropriate. If the hyperglycemia is acute and severe, the patient should be treated initially with insulin and placed on an appropriate diet. After adequate glycemic control is obtained (fasting plasma glucose <140 mg/dl [<7.8 mM]), sulfonylurea therapy may replace insulin therapy. The ideal goal of therapy is to maintain a fasting plasma glucose level of 115–140 mg/dl (6.4–7.8 mM).

Table 17.3. CONTRAINDICATIONS FOR SULFONYLUREA DRUG THERAPY

- Type I diabetes or pancreatic diabetes
- Pregnancy
- Major surgery
- Severe infections, stress, or trauma
- History of severe adverse reaction to sulfonylurea or similar compound (sulfa drug)
- Predisposition to severe hypoglycemia, e.g., patients with significant liver or kidney disease

Sulfonylurea therapy should be instituted with a low dose and increased at 4- to 7-day intervals. After adequate glycemic control is obtained and maintained for several weeks to months, discontinue sulfonylurea therapy to see whether diet therapy alone will maintain normoglycemic control. If not, the sulfonylurea therapy should be reinstituted.

Chronic sulfonylurea therapy should be continued only as long as it maintains the plasma glucose and glycosylated hemoglobin levels in the target ranges sought for that particular patient. When this is no longer achieved, a change in therapy is indicated.

EFFECT OF OTHER DRUGS ON SULFONYLUREA ACTIONS

Many commonly used drugs can potentiate sulfonylurea effects and precipitate hypoglycemia or antagonize sulfonylurea effects and worsen glycemic control. Table 17.4 lists some of the more important interactions. Alcohol and aspirin interactions may provoke prolonged and severe hypoglycemia. β-Blockers interfere with both the recognition and counterregulatory responses to hypoglycemia. Anticoagulants are competitive inhibitors of sulfonylurea metabolism, and when both classes of drugs are used, the doses of both may have to be appropriately reduced.

Any concomitant drug treatment in a patient on or to be started on sulfonylurea therapy must be evaluated for possible drug interactions. Because sulfonylureas with high intrinsic activity are given in smaller quantities and have somewhat different binding characteristics, they are likely to have fewer drug interactions than those with low intrinsic activity.

Table 17.4. **DRUG INTERACTIONS WITH SULFONYLUREAS**

Increase hypoglycemia
- Drugs that displace sulfonylurea from albumin-binding sites, e.g., aspirin, fibrates, trimethoprim
- Competitive inhibitors of sulfonylurea metabolism, e.g., alcohol, H_2 blockers, anticoagulants
- Inhibitors of urinary excretion of sulfonylureas, e.g., probenecid, allopurinol
- Concomitant use of drugs with hypoglycemic properties, e.g., alcohol, aspirin
- Antagonist of endogenous counterregulatory hormones, e.g., β-blockers, sympatholytic drugs

Worsen glycemic control
- Drugs that increase sulfonylurea metabolism, e.g., barbiturates, rifampin
- Agents that antagonize sulfonylurea action, e.g., β-blockers
- Inhibitors of insulin secretion or action, e.g., thiazides and loop diuretics, β-blockers, corticosteroids, estrogens, phenytoin

Table 17.5. **COMMON CAUSES OF SECONDARY SULFONYLUREA FAILURE**

Patient-related factors
- Overeating and weight gain
- Poor patient compliance
- Lack of physical activity
- Stress
- Intercurrent illnesses

Disease-related factors
- Decreasing β-cell function
- Increasing insulin resistance

Therapy-related factors
- Inadequate drug dosage
- Desensitization to chronic sulfonylurea exposure
- Impaired absorption of drug due to hyperglycemia
- Concomitant therapy with diabetogenic drugs

Modified from Groop et al. (2).

EXPECTED RESULTS

Initial treatment of type II diabetic patients with sulfonylureas results in one-third with excellent, one-third with good, and one-third with poor glycemic control. Of those with excellent or good glycemic control, the glycemic control appears comparable to that obtained with insulin therapy. Many type II diabetic patients who have excellent to good glycemic control initially tend to slowly lose their responses so that, at the end of 5 yr, only about half of them still have a favorable response. Whether this secondary failure is due to progression of the disease, loss of responsiveness to the drug, obesity, or some other unknown factor is unclear. The common causes of secondary failure are listed in Table 17.5. If possible, correction of some of these factors may restore sulfonylurea responsiveness.

Little is known about the effects of long-term (>5 yr) treatment of type II diabetic patients with either sulfonylureas or insulin. Because diabetic microvascular disease is a consequence of hyperglycemia and type II diabetic patients have the same microvascular complications as type I (insulin-dependent) diabetic patients, long-term glycemic control with sulfonylureas should provide symptomatic relief and have a beneficial effect on long-term morbidity and mortality.

SUGGESTED READING

1. A multicenter study: UK Prospective Diabetes Study. II. Reduction in HbA$_{1c}$ with basal insulin supplement, sulfonylurea, or biguanide therapy in maturity-onset diabetes. *Diabetes* 34:793–98, 1985
2. Groop LC, Pelkonen R, Koskimies S, Bottazzo GF, Doniach D: Secondary failure to treatment with oral antidiabetic agents in non-insulin-dependent diabetes. *Diabetes Care* 9:129–33, 1986

3. Lebovitz HE: Oral hypoglycemic agents. In *Diabetes Mellitus: Theory and Practice*. 4th ed. Rifkin H, Porte D Jr, Eds. New York, Elsevier, 1990, p. 554–74
4. Lebovitz HE: Non-insulin-dependent diabetes mellitus in current therapy. In *Endocrinology and Metabolism*. 4th ed. Bardin CW, Ed. Philadelphia, PA, Decker, 1991, p. 343–48
5. Management of type II diabetes. In *Physician's Guide to Non-Insulin-Dependent (Type II) Diabetes: Diagnosis and Treatment*. 2nd ed. Lebovitz HE, Ed. Alexandria, VA, Am. Diabetes Assoc., 1988, p. 37–46
6. Melander A, Bitzen P-O, Faber O, Groop L: Sulphonylurea antidiabetic drugs: an update of their clinical pharmacology and rational therapeutic use. *Drugs* 37:58–72, 1989

18. Metformin

HAROLD E. LEBOVITZ, MD

Biguanides are guanidine derivatives that have been used to treat hyperglycemia in patients with diabetes mellitus since the 1950s. Three biguanides were available initially for clinic usage: phenformin, metformin, and butformin. Phenformin, widely prescribed in the United States, and butformin have been removed from the market because of a significant incidence of associated lactic acidosis. Metformin, which was introduced in France in 1959, continues to be used worldwide and is undergoing clinical investigation in the U.S.

Metformin is an oral antidiabetic agent that has a different structure and different modes of action than sulfonylurea drugs. This drug is an effective and safe agent for the control of hyperglycemia in patients with diabetes mellitus.

MODE OF ACTION AND RATIONALE FOR USE

Considerable controversy exists concerning the mechanism of the antidiabetic action of metformin. Table 18.1 lists the mechanisms that have been proposed and supported by some studies but refuted by others. The important and consistent features of the mode of action of metformin are:

- Metformin does not stimulate insulin secretion.
- Treatment with metformin results in either no weight gain or a modest weight loss of several kilograms.

Dr. Lebovitz is Professor of Medicine, Chief of Endocrinology and Metabolism/Diabetes, and Director of the Clinical Research Center at the State University of New York Health Science Center at Brooklyn, Brooklyn, NY.

- Metformin does not cause hypoglycemia.
- Metformin lowers hyperglycemia in diabetic patients but does not lower blood glucose levels in nondiabetic individuals.

An important feature of metformin treatment in type II (non-insulin-dependent) diabetic patients is an associated decrease in plasma very-low-density lipoprotein triglyceride levels and an increase in serum high-density lipoprotein cholesterol levels.

TREATMENT

Metformin should be given orally in a dosage of 1.0–3.0 g/day in 2 or 3 divided doses. The administration of metformin is frequently associated with gastrointestinal symptoms, and therapy should be started with a single dose of 500 mg/day and increased at weekly intervals until the desired glycemic effect is obtained or the tolerable maximum dose is achieved.

Metformin is useful as an oral agent for the treatment of hyperglycemia in type II diabetic patients only after a reasonable trial (4–12 wk) of diet therapy. Metformin may be used as a primary pharmacological therapy or given in combination with a sulfonylurea or insulin.

Indications of Metformin Treatment

Whereas metformin is generally effective in decreasing hyperglycemia in type II diabetic patients, it is particularly useful in the treatment of obese type II diabetic patients whose hyperglycemia cannot be adequately controlled by diet alone. Metformin alone or combined with sulfonylureas may be effective in controlling hyperglycemia in patients who are primary or secondary failures with sulfonylureas alone.

Contraindications for Metformin Treatment

Metformin is ineffective as a primary treatment in type I (insulin-dependent) diabetic patients. Some studies suggest that metformin

Table 18.1. PROPOSED MECHANISMS FOR ANTIDIABETIC ACTION OF METFORMIN

- Increase insulin receptors on the cell surface of insulin-sensitive tissues
- Increase glucose-transport units in insulin-sensitive cells
- Increase muscle and adipose tissue glucose uptake
- Decrease hepatic glucose production
- Potentiate insulin action
- Decrease gastrointestinal absorption of glucose
- Cause anorexia

as an adjunct to insulin might decrease insulin requirements, but no data support any long-term beneficial effect from the combination of insulin and metformin.

Although lactic acidosis is a rare complication of metformin therapy, the drug should not be given to individuals with a propensity to develop lactic acidosis, e.g., those with kidney or liver disease, alcoholism, or cardiorespiratory insufficiency. Obviously, a drug such as metformin is contraindicated during pregnancy.

Side Effects of Treatment

The major side effects of metformin are gastrointestinal. These effects occur in ~10–30% of patients and include anorexia, nausea, abdominal discomfort, and diarrhea. The gastrointestinal side effects are worse initially and lessen during chronic therapy. The initial gastrointestinal side effects are lessened by initiating therapy with a low dose of metformin and increasing it gradually.

Precipitation of lactic acidosis is not a major problem with metformin therapy. The reason for the low risk of lactic acidosis in metformin treatment is that it does not bind to liver or plasma proteins, is not metabolized, and is excreted from the kidney through an active tubular secretion. In almost every reported case of lactic acidosis associated with metformin therapy, the patient had either renal, liver, or cardiorespiratory disease that should have been a contraindication to the use of the drug. Nonetheless, periodic monitoring of blood lactate levels in patients on metformin is advisable.

EXPECTED RESULTS

Several studies of metformin as a primary treatment for obese and nonobese type II diabetic patients who had failed on diet therapy alone concluded that metformin is as effective as sulfonylureas in reducing hyperglycemia. Approximately 80% of metformin-treated patients are reported to have improved glycemic control (blood glucose decreases of 25–30% from pretreatment levels). Some data suggest that metformin has a greater effect in lowering postprandial plasma glucose levels than fasting plasma glucose levels. Table 18.2 lists additive benefits of metformin therapy.

Table 18.2. ADVANTAGES OF METFORMIN THERAPY IN TYPE II DIABETIC PATIENTS

- Usually modest weight loss
- No hypoglycemia
- Decreased plasma very-low-density lipoprotein triglycerides
- Unchanged or slightly decreased plasma insulin levels

SUGGESTED READING

1. Klip A, Leiter LA: Cellular mechanism of action of metformin. *Diabetes Care* 13:696–704, 1990
2. Lucis OJ: The status of metformin in Canada. *Can Med Assoc J* 128:24–26, 1983
3. Vigneri R, Goldfine ID: Role of metformin in treatment of diabetes mellitus. *Diabetes Care* 10:118–22, 1987
4. Wu M-S, Johnston P, Sheu WH H, Hollenbeck CB, Jeng C-Y, Goldfine ID, Chen Y-DI, Reaven GM: Effect of metformin on carbohydrate and lipoprotein metabolism in NIDDM patients. *Diabetes Care* 13:1–8, 1990

19. α-Glucosidase Inhibitors in Treatment of Hyperglycemia

HAROLD E. LEBOVITZ, MD

In diabetic patients the ingestion and rapid absorption of carbohydrate causes significant postprandial hyperglycemia, whereas a lesser ingestion and slower absorption of carbohydrate leads to lesser postprandial hyperglycemia. Because dietary management has not been as successful as it could be due to difficulty with compliance, pharmacological agents have been developed that delay the digestion and absorption of sucrose and complex carbohydrates. The α-glucosidase inhibitors are in this class of drugs.

MECHANISM OF ACTION

α-Glucosidases are located in the brush border of enterocytes of the small intestine. They are responsible for the cleavage of sucrose, maltose, maltotriose, and other oligosaccharides into D-glucose, D-galactose, and D-fructose. Acarbose, which is the only approved α-glucosidase inhibitor, effectively inhibits human glucoamylase, sucrase, and maltase, which results in a marked diminution in the digestion of sucrose, starch, maltose, and complex carbohydrates. Carbohydrate digestion and absorption therefore occurs slowly and throughout the length of the small intestine rather than rapidly and primarily in the duodenum and upper jejunum. Carbohydrate that escapes digestion in the small intestine is metabolized to short-chain

Dr. Lebovitz is Professor of Medicine, Chief of Endocrinology and Metabolism/Diabetes, and Director of the Clinical Research Center at the State University of New York Health Science Center at Brooklyn, Brooklyn, NY.

fatty acids by bacteria in the large intestine. These are absorbed and metabolized.

α-Glucosidase inhibitors decrease the peak postprandial glucose rise in both type I (insulin-dependent) and type II (non-insulin-dependent) diabetic patients. They prolong absorption, so that the postprandial rise is more evenly distributed over a longer period.

Additionally, α-glucosidase inhibitors decrease meal-induced rises in gastric inhibitory polypeptide and other gastrointestinal peptides. The smaller rises in postprandial hyperglycemia result in smaller rises in plasma insulin postprandially.

CLINICAL USE OF ACARBOSE

Acarbose is an α-glucosidase inhibitor that has been approved for use in the treatment of patients with diabetes in several European and Central and South American countries. It should be administered orally $3\times$/day and chewed with the first mouthful of food. The initial recommended dose is 50 mg $3\times$/day. The dose may be increased after 2 wk to 100 mg $3\times$/day. Thereafter, if necessary, the dosage should be adjusted by stepwise increments at ~4-wk intervals until the desired glycemic goal or the maximum recommend dose is achieved. The preferred method of titrating the dose is to measure the 1-h postprandial plasma glucose. Side effects, which are primarily gastrointestinal, appear to increase with increasing dosages of acarbose.

Indications and contraindications for the use of acarbose are listed in Table 19.1. Acarbose has its greatest effect in lowering postprandial glycemic rises. About 35–50% of type II diabetic patients will have a modest decrease in fasting plasma glucose on chronic therapy. As primary therapy for these patients, it is most useful when fasting plasma glucose levels are ≤200 mg/dl (≤11.1 mM). As an adjunct to insulin or sulfonylurea therapy, it can be used to better control the postprandial glycemic rise. Acarbose may be useful for type I diabetic patients on insulin who have large excursions of glycemia after meals, because it can dampen these large excursions.

EXPECTED RESULTS

In patients who are on a diet consisting of ≥50% carbohydrate, acarbose is likely to have significant effects in reducing glycemia. As a primary therapy in obese or nonobese type II diabetic patients, acarbose has been shown to decrease fasting plasma glucose by ~15–25 mg/dl (~0.83–1.40 mM) and postprandial plasma glucose by ~50 mg/dl (~2.8 mM). The fall in HbA_{1c} is usually 0.5–1.0%. As an adjunct to sulfonylurea therapy, the postprandial glycemic rise decreases by ~30 mg/dl (~1.7 mM), and the HbA_{1c} falls ~0.5%.

Table 19.1. CLINICAL USE OF ACARBOSE

Indications
1. Primary therapy of mild to moderate hyperglycemia in patients with type II diabetes
2. Adjunct therapy with insulin or sulfonylureas in the treatment of patients with type II diabetes
3. Adjunct therapy with insulin in patients with type I diabetes to reduce insulin dosage and smooth out glycemic control

Contraindications
1. Primary therapy for patients with type I diabetes
2. Patients with significant gastrointestinal disorders
3. Patients who are pregnant or lactating

In insulin-treated patients, acarbose therapy results in a modest decrease in insulin dosage (10–30%) and gives a dampened postprandial glycemic excursion profile.

COMPLICATIONS AND SIDE EFFECTS OF TREATMENT

The major side effects of therapy with α-glucosidase inhibitors are gastrointestinal, i.e., abdominal fullness, borborygmi, increased intestinal flatulence, and occasional diarrhea. The side effects are both dose and substrate related. They generally decrease with chronic treatment.

Hypoglycemia does not occur with α-glucosidase inhibitors as primary therapy. If hypoglycemia occurs in insulin- or sulfonylurea-treated patients on acarbose, it must be treated with glucose and not sucrose or complex carbohydrates because glucose absorption is not affected by α-glucosidase treatment.

Concurrent administration of antacids, bile acid resins, intestinal adsorbents, or digestive enzyme preparations may reduce the effect of α-glucosidase inhibitors and should be used with great care.

SUGGESTED READING

1. Clissold SP, Edwards C: Acarbose. *Drugs* 35:214–43, 1988
2. Creutzfeldt W: *Proc. Int. Symp. Acarbose, 1st.* Amsterdam, Excerpta Med., 1982 (Int. Congr. Ser. 594)

20. Insulin Treatment

JAY S. SKYLER, MD

GENERAL CONSIDERATIONS

Types of Insulin

There are three major characteristics of insulin preparations: time course of action, degree of purity, and species of origin. The time course of action falls into three general categories: short acting or rapid onset, e.g., regular (soluble) insulin; intermediate acting, e.g., NPH (isophane) or lente (insulin zinc suspension) insulin; and long acting, e.g., ultralente (extended insulin zinc suspension) or protamine zinc insulin (PZI).

Purity of insulin preparations is reflected by the amount of non-insulin pancreatic proteins in the preparation. Proinsulin content is usually used to reflect purity. Insulins are defined as *purified* when they contain <10 ppm of proinsulin. This is true of all insulin preparations sold in the United States and is increasingly true in most other Western countries.

Insulin has been derived by extraction from bovine and porcine pancreas. Many commercial preparations contain mixtures of beef and pork insulin, and others are of single-species origin. Over the past decade, insulin of the same amino acid sequence as native human insulin has been commercially produced both by recombinant DNA technology and by enzymatic conversion of pork insulin to the human sequence. Human insulin preparations are less immunogenic than animal preparations.

Dr. Skyler is Professor of Medicine, Pediatrics, and Psychology at the University of Miami School of Medicine, Miami, FL.

Adverse Effects of Insulin Therapy

The major potential problem with insulin therapy is the risk of hypoglycemia. Other problems are cutaneous and immunologic reactions to insulin, leading to insulin allergy and insulin resistance (see chapt. 22).

THERAPY FOR TYPE I DIABETES

Insulin Secretion

Physiological insulin secretion is of two types: continuous basal insulin secretion and incremental prandial insulin secretion, controlling meal-related glucose excursions (Fig. 20.1). Basal insulin secretion restrains hepatic glucose production, keeping it in equilibrium with basal glucose utilization by brain and other tissues that are obligate glucose consumers. After meals, prandial insulin secretion stimulates glucose utilization and storage while inhibiting hepatic glucose output.

Flexible Insulin Programs

Contemporary insulin regimens for type I diabetes have multiple components that attempt to mimic the two normal types of endogenous physiological insulin secretion.

Prandial Insulin Therapy. Prandial incremental insulin secretion is best duplicated by giving preprandial injections of short-acting insulin (regular) before each meal. Each preprandial insulin dose is adjusted individually to provide meal insulinemia appropriate to the size of the meal. The use of preprandial insulin doses permits total flexibility in meal timing.

Regular insulin administered subcutaneously is rapid but not immediate in its onset of action. Therefore, it is best to give prandial injections at least 20–30 min before eating a given meal.

Basal Insulin Therapy. Basal insulinemia is given either as *1*) intermediate-acting insulin (NPH or lente) at bedtime and in a small morning dose or *2*) 1 or 2 injections/day of long-acting insulin (ul-

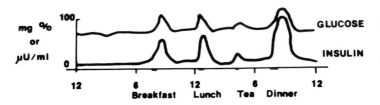

Figure 20.1. Twenty-four-hour plasma glucose and insulin profiles in hypothetical nondiabetic individual.

tralente), which is relatively peakless after steady state has been attained in most patients (Figs. 20.2 and 20.3).

The intermediate-acting insulins have their onset of action ~2 h after injection and produce peak insulin levels ~8–10 h after injection. Bedtime intermediate-acting insulin provides overnight basal insulinemia with peak serum insulin levels before breakfast, a time

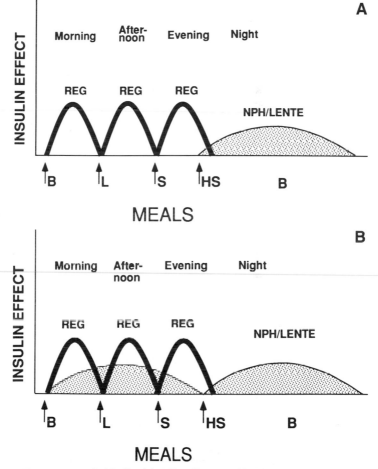

Figure 20.2. *A*: idealized insulin effect provided by multiple-dose regimen providing preprandial injections of short-acting insulin (REG) before meals and basal intermediate-acting insulin (NPH or LENTE) at bedtime. *B*: idealized insulin effect provided by multiple-dose regimen providing preprandial injections of short-acting insulin (REG) before meals, and basal regimen consisting of 2 daily injections of intermediate-acting insulin (NPH or LENTE). B, breakfast; L, lunch; S, supper; HS, bedtime snack. *Arrow*, time of insulin injection, 30 min before meals.

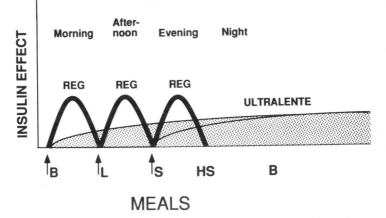

Figure 20.3. Idealized insulin effect provided by multiple-dose regimen providing preprandial injections of short-acting insulin (REG) before meals and basal long-acting insulin (ultralente). B, breakfast; L, lunch; S, supper; HS, bedtime snack. *Arrow*, time of insulin injection, 30 min before meals.

of relative insulin resistance known as the dawn phenomenon. Bedtime administration of intermediate-acting insulin also eliminates nocturnal peaks of insulin action, thus reducing the risk of nocturnal hypoglycemia. A small morning dose of intermediate-acting insulin provides daytime basal insulinemia.

Human ultralente insulin has a broad peak ~12–16 h after injection and sustains its action up to 24 h and sometimes beyond. In most patients, the peak of human ultralente insulin is sufficiently blunted at steady state to permit use of this preparation as a "peakless" basal insulin. As a consequence of waning insulin effect around 24 h, there may be a rise in fasting glucose if human ultralente insulin is administered in a single morning dose. Thus, it is probably best to divide ultralente insulin into 2 doses.

The multiple-dose premeal short-acting with bedtime intermediate acting insulin regimen is popular for the following reasons:

- It offers flexibility in meal size and timing.
- It is straightforward and easy to understand and implement, because each meal and each period of the day has a well-defined insulin component providing primary insulin action.
- The introduction of insulin pens has made it more convenient.

Blood Glucose Targets. Blood glucose targets must be individualized for each patient and explicitly defined. For healthy young patients, who readily recognize hypoglycemic symptoms and spontaneously recover from hypoglycemia, such targets may approximate the levels of glycemia seen in nondiabetic individuals (Table 20.1). These targets need to be lower during pregnancy and should be raised in

Table 20.1. **REPRESENTATIVE TARGET BLOOD GLUCOSE LEVELS FOR YOUNG OTHERWISE HEALTHLY PATIENT WITH TYPE I DIABETES MELLITUS**

Time	mg/dl	mM
Preprandial	70–130	3.9–7.2
1-h postprandial	100–180	5.6–10.0
2-h postprandial	80–150	4.4–8.3
0200–0400	70–120	3.9–6.7

subjects who have difficulty perceiving hypoglycemic symptoms, who do not spontaneously recover from hypoglycemia, or in whom hypoglycemia might be particularly dangerous (e.g., patients with angina pectoris or transient ischemic attacks).

Initial Insulin Doses and Distribution. The insulin dosage required for meticulous glycemic control, in typical patients with type I diabetes within 20% of their ideal body weight, in the absence of intercurrent infections or other periods of instability, approximates $0.5–1.0 \ U \cdot kg^{-1} \cdot day^{-1}$. During the period of relative remission ("honeymoon" period) early in the course of the disease, insulin requirements generally are less. During periods of intercurrent illness, dosage requirement may increase markedly.

About 40–50% of the total daily insulin dosage is used to provide basal insulinemia. The remainder is divided among the meals either empirically, proportionate to the carbohydrate content of the meals, or by giving ~1.0–1.2 U insulin/10 g carbohydrate consumed.

Dose Alteration. Patients are provided with an action plan to alter therapy to achieve their individual defined blood glucose targets. These actions are guided by SMBG determinations and daily records.

A sample action plan for dose alteration is given in Table 20.2. The illustrative plan assumes that the preprandial and bedtime blood glucose target is 70–130 mg/dl (3.9–7.2 mM). The plan should also call for separate action in response to a pattern of glycemia occurring over several days.

Other Insulin Programs

Separately considering prandial and basal insulin needs permits flexibility in eating and activity. However, this approach requires a motivated, educated patient who carefully monitors blood glucose several (≥4) times daily. An alternative approach is to maintain day-to-day consistency both of activity and of timing and quantity of food intake. This permits the use of *1*) twice-daily administration of mixtures of short- and intermediate-acting insulin (the so-called split-mixed insulin regimen) or *2*) the morning administration of a mixture of short- and intermediate-acting insulin, with presupper regular insulin, and bedtime intermediate-acting insulin, an ap-

Table 20.2. SAMPLE PLAN FOR PREMEAL INSULIN DOSING

Once insulin dosage is stable, use the following scheme for premeal alteration of dosage of regular insulin:

- Blood glucose <50 mg/dl (<2.8 mM)
  - Reduce premeal short acting insulin by 2–3 U.
  - Delay injection until immediately before eating.
  - Include at least 10 g of rapidly available carbohydrate in the meal.
- Blood glucose 50–70 mg/dl (2.8–3.9 mM)
  - Reduce premeal short-acting insulin by 1–2 U.
  - Delay injection until immediately before eating.
- Blood glucose 70–130 mg/dl (3.9–7.2 mM)
  - Take prescribed premeal dose of short-acting insulin.
- Blood glucose 130–150 mg/dl (7.2–8.3 mM)
  - Increase premeal short-acting insulin by 1 U.
- Blood glucose 150–200 mg/dl (8.3–11.1 mM)
  - Increase premeal short-acting insulin by 2 U.
- Blood glucose 200–250 mg/dl (11.1–13.9 mM)
  - Increase premeal short-acting insulin by 3 U.
  - Consider delaying meal 15 min (to 45 min after injection).
- Blood glucose 250–300 mg/dl (13.9–16.7 mM)
  - Increase premeal short-acting insulin by 4 U.
  - Consider delaying meal 20–30 min (to 40–60 min after injection).
- Blood glucose 300–350 mg/dl (16.7–19.4 mM)
  - Increase premeal short-acting insulin by 5 U.
  - Delay meal 20–30 min (to 40–60 min after injection).
  - Check urine ketones. If moderate to large, increase fluid intake and consider extra insulin (1–2 U). Recheck blood glucose and urine ketones in 2–3 h.
- Blood glucose 350–400 mg/dl (19.4–22.2 mM)
  - Increase premeal short-acting insulin by 6 U.
  - Delay meal 20–30 min (to 40–60 min after injection).
  - Check urine ketones. If moderate to large, increase fluid intake and consider extra insulin (1–2 U). Recheck blood glucose and urine ketones in 2–3 h.
- Blood glucose >400 mg/dl (>22.2 mM)
  - Increase premeal short-acting insulin by 7 U.
  - Delay meal 30 min (to 50–60 min after injection).
  - Check urine ketones. If moderate to large, increase fluid intake and consider extra insulin (1–2 U). Recheck blood glucose and urine ketones in 2–3 h.
- Planned meal is larger than usual
  - Increase short-acting insulin by 1–2 U.
- Planned meal is smaller than usual
  - Decrease short-acting insulin by 1–2 U.
- Unusual increased activity planned after eating
  - Eat extra carbohydrate and/or decrease short-acting insulin by 1–2 U.
- Unusually decreased activity planned after eating
  - Consider increasing short-acting insulin by 1–2 U.

Plan assumes target goals in Table 20.1 and should be individualized for each patient.

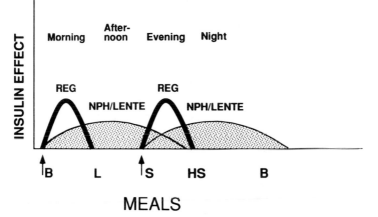

MEALS

Figure 20.4. Idealized insulin effect provided by insulin regimen consisting of 2 injections/day of short-acting (REG) and intermediate-acting (NPH or LENTE) insulin. B, breakfast; L, lunch; S, supper; HS, bedtime snack. *Arrow*, time of insulin injection, 30 min before meals.

proach used to minimize nocturnal hypoglycemia and to counteract the dawn phenomenon. These insulin programs are depicted in Figs. 20.4 and 20.5.

Generally, it is not possible to adequately control glycemia in type I diabetes with 1 or 2 injections of intermediate-acting insulin alone.

THERAPY FOR TYPE II DIABETES

Pathophysiological Defects

Patients with type II diabetes have defects in both insulin secretion and insulin action. The impairments in insulin secretion are manifest by

1. Blunted or absent first-phase insulin response to glucose, so that insulin secretion is delayed and fails to restore prandial glycemic excursions in a timely manner
2. Decreased sensitivity of insulin response to glucose, so that hyperglycemia may fail to trigger an appropriate insulin response
3. Decreased overall insulin secretory capacity, particularly in more severe type II diabetes

Chronic hyperglycemia may itself aggravate the impairment in insulin secretion. Thus, with decompensation of glycemic control in type II diabetes, there is concomitant deterioration in insulin secretory response. When hyperglycemia is corrected, there is some

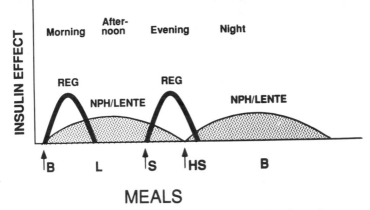

MEALS

Figure 20.5. Idealized insulin effect provided by insulin regimen consisting of morning injection of short-acting (REG) and intermediate-acting (NPH or LENTE) insulin, presupper injection of short-acting insulin, and bedtime injection of intermediate-acting insulin. B, breakfast; L, lunch; S, supper; HS, bedtime snack. *Arrow*, time of insulin injection, 30 min before meals.

reversal of the impairment in endogenous insulin response to a meal challenge. Thus, attainment of glucose control facilitates maintenance of glucose control.

Patients with type II diabetes also have impaired insulin action (insulin resistance) at target cells. This increases overall insulin requirement. Chronic hyperglycemia may aggravate the impairment in insulin action. Thus, with decompensation of glycemic control, there is concomitant diminished insulin action; when there is correction of hyperglycemia, there is some reversal of the impairment in insulin action.

Insulin Programs for Type II Diabetes

Recommended blood glucose targets for patients with type II diabetes are summarized in Table 20.3. When patients have been placed on a stable diet and activity program, they can be divided by degree of severity into four groups—mild, moderate, severe, and very

Table 20.3. BLOOD GLUCOSE TARGETS FOR TYPE II DIABETES

Normalize fasting plasma glucose: Ideally <115 mg/dl (<6.4 mM)
                                   Minimally <140 mg/dl (<7.8 mM)
Postprandial plasma glucose: Ideally <140 mg/dl (<7.8 mM)
                             Minimally <200 mg/dl (<11.1 mM)

severe—based on their level of fasting glycemia and their ability to restore postprandial glycemia to basal levels (as a measure of intactness of prandial insulin secretion).

Mild Type II Diabetes. Insulin therapy is virtually never needed for patients with mild type II diabetes, i.e., those with fasting plasma glucose <140 mg/dl (<7.8 mM).

Moderate Type II Diabetes. For patients with moderate type II diabetes, i.e., those with fasting plasma glucose 140–200 mg/dl (7.8–11.1 mM), if insulin therapy is used, basal insulin therapy alone is usually sufficient, with endogenous insulin secretion being adequate to control meal-related prandial glucose excursions. Basal insulinemia is given as 1) intermediate-acting insulin at bedtime with or without a small morning dose or 2) 1 or 2 injections/day of long-acting insulin (Figs. 20.6 and 20.7). Doses required are generally in the range of $0.3–0.4$ $U \cdot kg^{-1} \cdot day^{-1}$. The peak effect of bedtime intermediate-acting insulin coincides with the prebreakfast period, thus controlling basal (fasting) glycemia.

Severe Type II Diabetes. For patients with severe type II diabetes, i.e., those with fasting plasma glucose >200 mg/dl (>11.1 mM), around-the-clock insulinization is necessary. Thus, bedtime intermediate-acting insulin cannot be used (although twice-daily intermediate-acting insulin may be used). Most patients in this category require the addition of short-acting insulin to attain adequate glucose control. Doses required are generally in the range of $0.5–1.2$ $U \cdot kg^{-1} \cdot day^{-1}$. However, large doses, even >1.5 $U \cdot kg^{-1} \cdot day^{-1}$, may be required, at least initially, to overcome prevailing insulin resistance. High-dose therapy may be necessary only to attain control, with subsequent control maintained on lower doses, on a basal insulin program, or with oral hypoglycemic agents. Often, insulin therapy is continued at doses of $0.3–1.0$ $U \cdot kg^{-1} \cdot day^{-1}$. Premixed insulin (e.g., 30% short acting and 70% intermediate acting) may be used.

Very Severe Type II Diabetes. Patients with very severe type II diabetes are those with nonintact endogenous insulin response to meals, so that postprandial glycemia is not restored to basal levels within 5 h of meal consumption. In these individuals, fasting plasma glucose is usually quite elevated as well, i.e., >250–300 mg/dl (>13.9–16.7 mM), but may include individuals with lesser degrees of fasting hyperglycemia. There is such profound insulin deficiency that these patients initially may be difficult to distinguish from those with type I diabetes, although they generally do not manifest ketosis. Indeed, their similarity to type I diabetes indicates they are best treated like type I patients initially.

In all categories of patients with type II diabetes, pathophysiological defects improve as glycemic control is attained and maintained. This will facilitate ease of control and may permit patients initially treated with insulin to be maintained on oral hypoglycemic agents or even a diet and activity program alone. As the insulin dosage is adjusted to lower and lower amounts, a patient with type

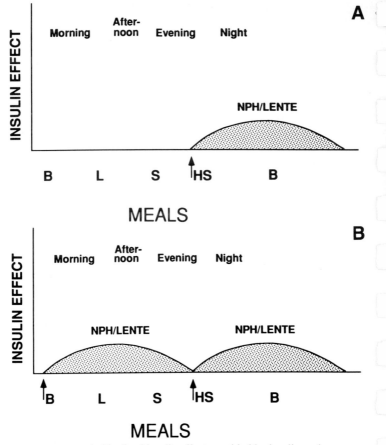

Figure 20.6. *A*: idealized insulin effect provided by insulin regimen consisting of bedtime injection of intermediate-acting insulin (NPH or LENTE). *B*: idealized insulin effect provided by insulin regimen consisting of 2 injections/day of intermediate-acting insulin. B, breakfast; L, lunch; S, supper; HS, bedtime snack. *Arrow*, time of insulin injection, 30 min before meals.

II diabetes reaching <0.3 U·kg^{-1}·day^{-1} suggests that the patient may be maintained on oral hypoglycemic agents.

Most patients with type II diabetes can be controlled with insulin if adequate doses are given and if the patient follows an appropriate diet and exercise program.

Insulin Programs for Elderly Patients

Insulin therapy is often used in the elderly as a last resort, after failure of dietary management and maximum doses of oral hypo-

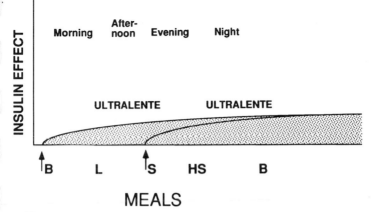

MEALS

Figure 20.7. Idealized insulin effect provided by basal long-acting insulin (ultralente). B, breakfast; L, lunch; S, supper; HS, bedtime snack. *Arrow*, time of insulin injection, 30 min before meals.

glycemic agents. The aim of therapy in the elderly is to relieve symptoms and prevent hypoglycemia and acute complications of uncontrolled diabetes, e.g., hyperosmolar states. Schedules for the injection of insulin should be kept as simple as possible, because self-administration may be difficult, and dosage errors are not uncommon. Premixed insulins may be particularly desirable because of their simplicity of use.

SUGGESTED READING

1. Hirsch IB, Farkas-Hirsch R, Skyler JS: Intensive insulin therapy for treatment of type I diabetes. *Diabetes Care* 13:1265–83, 1990
2. Schade DS, Santiago JV, Skyler JS, Rizza R: *Intensive Insulin Therapy*. Princeton, NJ, Excerpta Med., 1983
3. Skyler JS: Non-insulin-dependent diabetes mellitus: a clinical strategy. *Diabetes Care* 7 (Suppl. 1):118–29, 1984
4. Skyler JS: Insulin pharmacology. *Med Clin North Am* 72:1337–54, 1988
5. Zinman B: The physiologic replacement of insulin. *N Engl J Med* 321:363–70, 1989

21. Insulin-Pump Therapy

ROBERT S. MECKLENBURG, MD

Insulin-pump therapy, or continuous subcutaneous insulin infusion (CSII), is a highly adjustable method of injecting insulin under the skin. CSII is an alternative to multiple daily injections for people with type I (insulin-dependent) diabetes motivated to achieve excellent blood glucose control but unable to do so with 2 or 3 conventional injections daily.

The components of a subcutaneous insulin-infusion system consist of a pump and an infusion set. The pump unit contains a small syringe reservoir filled with short-acting insulin, an electromechanical assembly that advances the syringe plunger, and a microprocessor. The infusion set, coupled to the pump unit, consists of a plastic infusion tubing joined to a needle or plastic cannula inserted under the skin and secured with tape or an occlusive dressing. Insulin pumps are about the size of a stack of 15 credit cards and are carried in a pocket, on a belt, or tucked into clothing or underwear.

Insulin pumps neither measure blood glucose nor modify insulin dose to maintain euglycemia; patients adjust the amount of insulin they receive by regulating pump settings based on data from frequent self-monitoring of capillary blood glucose (SMBG).

RATIONALE

The special feature of insulin-pump therapy is the capability of providing insulin in a slow continuous basal rate, which simulates postabsorptive insulin secretion, and in boluses, which mimic normal peaks of insulin released after a meal.

Dr. Mecklenburg is Head of the Section of Endocrinology and Diabetes at the Virginia Mason Clinic, Seattle, WA.

Table 21.1. USE OF INSULIN-PUMP THERAPY

Preliminary considerations
- Test blood glucose 4×/day for best results
- Choose a treatment regimen that minimizes hypoglycemia
- Emphasize meticulous skin care to avoid infection at infusion sites
- Expect to invest more time, effort, and money than with conventional injections
- Patient must be highly motivated and reliable

Starting therapy
- Be prepared for occasional leaks and obstructions in infusion set
- Educate user of pump in basics of diabetes care
- Be able to provide technical support as health-care provider
- Review initial and ongoing costs before starting pump
- Base initial pump settings on previous doses of insulin
- Arrange backup care at home if starting pump as outpatient
- Have user practice handling pump before starting treatment
- Determine target blood glucose levels based on patient's abilities
- Arrange office visits or telephone contact after starting pump

CSII is generally more effective in improving metabolic control than 2 injections/day and is comparable in efficacy to 4 injections/day. The possible benefit of improved metabolic control in terms of preventing chronic complications of diabetes is uncertain.

Although insulin pumps more closely approximate physiological insulin secretion than do other methods of insulin administration, they share with conventional injections deficiencies in terms of mimicking normal insulin release by the pancreas. The major problem is the lack of a negative feedback component to automatically measure blood glucose and adjust insulin dosage. Another problem is unpredictable variability in absorption from subcutaneous injection sites. These features limit efficacy and safety of pump therapy when attempts are made to approach a normal metabolic state.

PRELIMINARY CONSIDERATIONS

Before initiating treatment with an insulin pump, the patient and health-care provider should be familiar with the following features of intensified insulin therapy in general and pump therapy in particular (Table 21.1).

1. Patients most likely to achieve improved glycemic control with insulin-pump therapy are those who are willing and able to monitor their capillary blood glucose concentration at least 4×/day.

2. Blood glucose target values should be selected with care to reduce the risk of hypoglycemia. Although pump therapy per se does not increase the frequency of serious hypoglycemia, attempts at achieving target blood glucose values absolutely within the normal range with intensified insulin treatment may

increase the risk of serious hypoglycemia. This is especially true for patients who do not experience symptoms of epinephrine release when hypoglycemia occurs.

3. Meticulous skin care at injection sites is important. People with a history of repeated staphylococcal skin infections or who are nasal carriers may be at higher risk.

4. Plugging of infusion sets and leaks in infusion-set connections are common. These problems can be identified with SMBG and corrected with adjustment of the infusion system, but ketoacidosis may occur if interruption of insulin delivery is not detected.

5. Insulin-pump therapy requires more effort than treatment with conventional injections. Whereas many people gain a sense of increased well-being while using a pump, those with a history of emotional problems or ongoing major stresses may be less able to meet the increased demands of intensified insulin therapy.

GETTING STARTED

A patient beginning pump therapy may require substantial support by primary-care providers, especially in the first weeks of treatment. Those prescribing insulin pumps must therefore be willing and able to devote the time and resources necessary to provide 24-h expert help to pump users. If primary-care physicians do not have these resources readily available, insulin-pump therapy is best managed by referral to a diabetes center where specialized care in intensive insulin therapy is available.

The major producer of insulin pumps in the United States is MiniMed Technologies (Sylmar, CA), whose model 504-S retails for approximately $3400. Sof-set disposable infusion sets (MiniMed) and Tegaderm occlusive dressings (3M, St. Paul, MN), usually changed every 2–3 days, cost approximately $100/mo. Insurance coverage for insulin pumps and necessary supplies is variable.

Initiating Insulin-Pump Therapy in Type I Diabetic Patients

1. The patient should be well informed and skillful in the principles and practice of conventional diabetes management.

2. Pump therapy is often initiated during a 2- to 3-day hospital stay. If pump therapy is started outside the hospital, a friend or relative should be available who could assist in the event of serious hypoglycemia. The patient should be instructed not to undertake unusual activity for several days until approximate insulin doses have been established.

3. Before using the pump, the patient should practice loading and programming the unit changing infusion sets. The best sites are usually far from bony prominences and beltlines. The

infusion set is secured with an occlusive dressing or paper tape and is generally changed every 2–3 days to avoid irritation.

4. In general, blood glucose targets are 80–140 mg/dl (4.4–7.8 mM) for the average of values taken before each meal and at bedtime. Target averages for pregnant patients are usually somewhat lower, generally not exceeding 100 mg/dl (5.5 mM). Targets for patients with a history of hypoglycemic unawareness should be higher, at least at the onset of treatment with an infusion pump.

5. The initial programming of insulin dosages is based on the total daily prepump dosages.

   - The basal rate is initially set at 50% of the total prepump dosage. Breakfast, lunch, dinner, and bedtime boluses are initially written as 16, 12, 16, and 6% of the total prepump insulin dosage. Capillary blood glucose concentrations are checked before each meal and at bedtime, and basal and bolus doses are altered by 10–20% every 1–2 days to move toward target values.

   - The basal rate is adjusted to achieve the target fasting blood glucose with multiple boluses adjusted to achieve similar values before the next meal. Peak blood glucose elevations between meals can be blunted by giving the premeal bolus 30–45 min before eating.

   - A prebreakfast increase in blood glucose may require a pre-programmed basal rate step-up in the early morning, but multiple complex changes in basal rate throughout the day are usually not necessary. In general, begin with the proportion of insulin delivered over 24 h at ~50% of the total for the basal and bolus modes to preserve flexibility in bolus doses. Advancement in basal rate and bolus doses are usually required if hyperglycemia occurs during intercurrent illness.

EXPECTED RESULTS

Benefits

Approximately 90% of patients changing from 2 conventional injections to insulin-pump therapy will achieve improvement in glycemic control (Table 21.2). Fifty percent of patients using pumps achieve at least temporary normalization of glycosylated hemoglobin concentration, and 15% are able to maintain normal yearly averages for glycosylated hemoglobin for at least 3 yr. Most appreciate the greater flexibility in terms of matching insulin administration to variations in diet and exercise.

Complications

1. Approximately 30% of patients develop infection at infusion sites, usually caused by coagulase-positive *Staphylococcus au-*

reus. Cellulitis is often responsive to dicloxicillin, 250 mg orally 4×/day for 1 wk. Abscesses should be incised and drained promptly.

2. Ketoacidosis is the second most frequent acute complication of pump therapy, occurring in 15% of patients using pumps in one large series. Capillary blood glucose determinations should be performed 4×/day. If the patient has a blood glucose level of ≥240 mg/dl (≥13.3 mM), the infusion set should be checked. Blood glucose should be rechecked in 1–2 h, and if it remains elevated, the infusion set should be changed. The infusion set should also be changed if the patient becomes ill unexpectedly and the blood glucose is ≥240 mg/dl (≥13.3 mM).

3. CSII therapy like any other intensified insulin regimen may be associated with a significantly increased incidence of hypoglycemic reactions.

Table 21.2. ADVANTAGES AND DISADVANTAGES OF INSULIN-PUMP THERAPY

Advantages
- Improved control of blood glucose
- Flexibility in matching insulin to variations in diet or exercise

Disadvantages
- Inflammation and infection at infusion sites
- Susceptibility to ketoacidosis from interrupted flow of insulin
- Increased cost compared with conventional injections

Continuous subcutaneous insulin therapy in an open-loop system and therefore requires patient input in determining/adjusting insulin dosage.

SUGGESTED READING

1. Amiel SA, Tamborlane WV, Simonson DC, Sherwin RS: Defective glucose counterregulation after strict glycemic control of insulin-dependent diabetes mellitus. *N Engl J Med* 316: 1376–83, 1987

2. Mecklenburg RS, Benson EA, Benson JW Jr, Blumenstein BA, Fredlund PN, Guinn TS, Metz RJ, Nielsen RL: Long-term metabolic control with insulin-pump therapy: report of experience with 127 patients. *N Engl J Med* 313:465–68, 1985

3. Mecklenburg RS, Benson EA, Benson JW Jr, Fredlund PN, Guinn TS, Metz RJ, Nielsen RL, Sannar CA: Acute complications associated with insulin infusion pump therapy: report of experience with 161 patients. *JAMA* 252:3265–69, 1984

4. Mecklenburg RS, Guinn TS, Sannar CA, Blumenstein BA: Malfunction of continuous subcutaneous insulin infusion systems: a one-year prospective study of 127 patients. *Diabetes Care* 9:351–55, 1986

5. Schiffrin A, Belmonte MM: Multiple daily self-glucose monitoring: its essential role in long-term glucose control in insulin-dependent patients treated with pump and multiple subcutaneous injections. *Diabetes Care* 5:479–84, 1982

22. Combination Therapy for Hyperglycemia

HAROLD E. LEBOVITZ, MD

When type II (non-insulin-dependent) diabetic patients fail to achieve their target glycemic control on diet plus sulfonylurea, metformin, or acarbose as primary therapy, the question arises as to whether they should be switched to an insulin-treatment program or a combination of oral agents. Combinations such as sulfonylurea plus metformin or sulfonylurea plus acarbose have been shown to improve glycemic control.

Another question is whether a type II diabetic patient who requires an intensive insulin-treatment program to achieve appropriate glycemic control might be controlled as well or better on a smaller dose of insulin or a more simplified insulin-treatment program if insulin therapy were combined with an oral antidiabetic agent.

RATIONALE FOR COMBINATION THERAPY

The treatment of hyperglycemia in type II diabetic patients involves correction of one or more of the following defects:

1. Increased hepatic glucose production
2. Decreased insulin secretion
3. Decreased insulin action on peripheral tissues in general and muscle in particular

Dr. Lebovitz is Professor of Medicine, Chief of Endocrinology and Metabolism/Diabetes, and Director of the Clinical Research Center at the State University of New York Health Science Center at Brooklyn, Brooklyn, NY.

Table 22.1 outlines the primary modes of action of the various antidiabetic agents. Agents with somewhat different modes of action can be combined. Contraindications and side effects are the same as for the individual pharmacological agents.

TYPES OF COMBINATION THERAPY

Table 22.2 lists the most commonly used combination therapies. Sulfonylurea plus metformin to control glycemia in type II diabetic patients who are not adequately controlled on either agent alone has been used for >30 years. Type II diabetic patients who are secondary sulfonylurea failures can be controlled as well on glyburide-metformin as on insulin. The mechanism by which hyperglycemia is reduced is different in the two regimens. Sulfonylurea-metformin therapy is not associated with a change in body weight but is associated with an increase in peripheral glucose uptake. Studies have documented that sulfonylurea-metformin therapy in type II diabetic patients with secondary sulfonylurea failure achieves a mean decrease in fasting hyperglycemia of 27% from the pre-treatment value.

Insulin-sulfonylurea therapy has led to controversial results concerning glycemic control. Concurrent therapy often leads to a decrease in insulin dosage but only in a few patients to increased glycemic control. Sequential insulin and sulfonylurea therapy seems more likely to give consistently improved glycemic control. In this treatment program, intermediate-acting insulin is given at 2200 or 2300 to suppress the increased hepatic glucose production that occurs overnight in type II diabetic patients. As a result, the morning fasting plasma glucose should be near normal. Sulfonylureas are given before breakfast and perhaps before the evening meal to control postprandial glycemia.

Sulfonylurea-acarbose treatment is relatively new and is being evaluated.

DEVELOPMENT OF COMBINATION TREATMENT STRATEGY

Sulfonylurea-Metformin

A patient who is on a maximal sulfonylurea dosage and has not achieved the target glycemic values should be kept on the sulfonylurea and started on 500 mg of metformin 1×/day. The dose of metformin should be increased to 500 mg 2× and then 3×/day at weekly intervals. The dose of metformin should not exceed 2000 mg/day. If hypoglycemia occurs, the sulfonylurea dose should be reduced and the metformin dose not increased.

Table 22.1. SITE OF ACTION OF VARIOUS ANTIDIABETIC AGENTS

Antidiabetic Agent	Carbohydrate Absorption	Insulin Secretion	Hepatic Glucose Production	Peripheral Glucose Utilization*
Sulfonylureas	0	←	→	± ←
Metformin	?	0	→	± ←
Acarbose	→	0	↓ →	0
Insulin	0	→	→	←

0, No effect; ?, unknown; ↓, decreases; ↑, increases; ±, minor effect

Table 22.2. COMMONLY USED COMBINATION THERAPIES FOR TYPE II DIABETIC PATIENTS

- Sulfonylurea-metformin
- Sulfonylurea-insulin
  - Concomitant
  - Sequential, i.e., insulin at bedtime and sulfonylureas during day
- Sulfonylurea-α-glucosidase inhibitor (acarbose)

Sulfonylurea-Insulin

Concurrent sulfonylurea-insulin therapy should only be instituted in patients who have poor glycemic control (fasting plasma glucose >200 mg/dl [>11.1 mM] and/or HbA_1 >10%) despite twice-daily insulin administration of >70 U/day. The insulin dose should be left the same, and the sulfonylurea should be started at an intermediate dose and increased weekly to the maximum dose or until appropriate glycemic control is obtained. These patients must have been failures on previous sulfonylurea therapy. As stated earlier, most patients will be able to decrease their insulin dosage by 30–50%, and a few will show improved glycemic control. For sulfonylurea-insulin therapy to be effective, the patient must have some β-cell function.

Sequential sulfonylurea-insulin therapy should be instituted in patients who are secondary sulfonylurea failures. The sulfonylurea therapy should be maintained and intermediate-acting insulin (10 U) administered at 2200 or 2300. Blood glucose should be monitored by the patient at 0300 and before breakfast. The insulin dose should be adjusted to achieve the desired fasting plasma glucose (~3–5 U every 3–4 days). The sulfonylurea dose should be maintained unless plasma glucose levels before meals become too low. The benefit of the regimen is determined by the improvement in HbA_1 or HbA_{1c}.

SUGGESTED READING

1. Bailey TS, Mezitis NHE: Combination therapy with insulin and sulfonylureas for type II diabetes. *Diabetes Care* 13:687–95, 1990
2. Groop L, Widen E, Franssila-Kallunk A, Ekstrand A, Saloranta C, Schalin C, Eriksson J: Different effects of insulin and oral antidiabetic agents on glucose and energy metabolism in type 2 (non-insulin-dependent) diabetes mellitus. *Diabetologia* 32:599–605, 1989
3. Lebovitz HE, Pasmantier R: Combination insulin-sulfonylurea therapy. *Diabetes Care* 13:667–75, 1990
4. Riddle MC: Evening insulin strategy. *Diabetes Care* 13:676–86, 1990
5. Vigneri R, Goldfine ID: Role of metformin in treatment of diabetes mellitus. *Diabetes Care* 10:118–22, 1987

23. Surgery and Anesthesia

CARLOS ARAUZ-PACHECO, MD, and PHILIP RASKIN, MD

The perioperative management of the diabetic patient is complicated by the metabolic abnormalities of the disease and by the presence of atherosclerotic disease, diabetic nephropathy, and autonomic neuropathy. There is also an increased risk of postoperative wound infection in patients with diabetes mellitus (Table 23.1).

PATHOPHYSIOLOGY

During anesthesia and surgery, there is an increase in the plasma concentrations of counterregulatory hormones. An elevation in the levels of glucagon, catecholamines, cortisol, and growth hormone is observed in nondiabetic and diabetic individuals. The increased secretion of these hormones leads to a marked increase in hepatic glucose production (due to both glycogenolysis and gluconeogenesis), a decrease in insulin-mediated glucose uptake, increased lipolysis with elevated levels of nonesterified fatty acids, and decreased insulin secretion. In nondiabetic individuals, major surgery is frequently associated with elevations in blood glucose into the range 150–200 mg/dl (8.3–11.1 mM). In diabetic individuals, insulin secretion is impaired; thus, in the presence of a major surgical stress, severe hyperglycemia with or without ketosis can occur unless adequate insulin replacement is given. The severity of the metabolic abnormality that can occur is proportional to the extent and duration of the surgical procedure and the impairment of insulin secretion. Because surgical patients are always fasting, the administration of

Dr. Arauz-Pacheco is a Clinical Research Fellow and Dr. Raskin is Professor of Internal Medicine at the University of Texas Southwestern Medical Center at Dallas, Dallas, TX.

Table 23.1. COMPLICATIONS OF DIABETES DURING SURGERY, ANESTHESIA, AND POSTOPERATIVE PERIODS

- Metabolic
  - Diabetic ketoacidosis
  - Nonketotic hyperosmolar states
  - Hypoglycemia
  - Hyperkalemia
  - Hypokalemia
- Cardiovascular
  - Hypotension (related to autonomic diabetic neuropathy)
  - Arrhythmia
  - Postoperative myocardial infarction
  - Other thrombotic phenomena
- Renal
  - Acute kidney failure
  - Volume overload
- Infections

insulin will cause hypoglycemia if an adequate and constant source of carbohydrate is not available.

The risk of postoperative myocardial infarction is higher in the diabetic population, and it is frequently asymptomatic. Diabetic nephropathy, when present, makes fluid management difficult, and electrolyte abnormalities are common. Furthermore, the nutritional status of these patients may be poor, and malnutrition can predispose to infection. Autonomic neuropathy can cause severe hypotension during the induction of anesthesia, and its presence should be evaluated before any procedure involving general and/or spinal anesthesia. The anesthesiologist must be informed about the findings of the autonomic nervous system evaluation.

EVALUATION OF DIABETIC PATIENTS BEFORE SURGERY

Metabolic Control

The degree of metabolic control should be evaluated before surgery, and attempts should be made to improve poor control on an outpatient basis before elective procedures. Chronically hyperglycemic patients are frequently dehydrated, and this condition must be corrected before surgery. Admission to the hospital to optimize metabolic control 12–16 h before elective procedures is recommended in all patients with type I (insulin-dependent) diabetes and those with type II (non-insulin-dependent) diabetes who have inadequate metabolic control. A stabilization period of 12–16 h is also recommended for semiurgent procedures if severe hyperglycemia is present. In patients with severe metabolic derangements (diabetic ketoacidosis or hyperosmolar nonketotic states) needing urgent surgical intervention, a period of 6–8 h of intensive treatment usually improves the general condition of the patient. This period also allows clarification of the diagnosis in cases of acute abdominal pain that could be the consequence of diabetic ketoacidosis rather than a surgical abdomen.

Cardiovascular Condition

Coronary artery disease and hypertensive vascular disease are common in diabetic patients. These concurrent illnesses are independent of duration of the diabetes. A thorough evaluation of the patient's cardiovascular condition, including special attention to orthostatic changes in blood pressure and changes in heart rate with respiration should be done. Abnormalities are an indication of significant diabetic cardiovascular autonomic neuropathy.

Well-controlled hypertension does not pose a major risk to surgery, but patients receiving β-blockers may develop hypoglycemia without warning symptoms and should be monitored accordingly. Type I diabetic patients receiving β-blockers are also at a greater risk for prolonged episodes of insulin-induced hypoglycemia. Diabetic patients have increased thrombotic risk, and subcutaneous 5000 U heparin every 8–12 h should be considered unless specifically contraindicated during the period of confinement to bed.

Renal Function

Measurement of blood urea nitrogen (BUN), serum creatinine, electrolytes, and proteinuria should be performed before surgery. Azotemic patients may have problems with fluid management, and monitoring of central venous or pulmonary artery wedge pressure may be necessary. Hyperkalemia with or without hyponatremia is often seen in patients with mild to moderate kidney failure, and hyperkalemia can precipitate an acute cardiac arrhythmia. This metabolic finding usually results from hyporeninemic hypoaldosteronism and diabetic autonomic neuropathy. Hypokalemia may be present, and insulin and glucose therapy may aggravate this condition.

METABOLIC MANAGEMENT AND MONITORING

Insulin and Glucose Administration During Surgery

The use of an insulin and glucose infusion is recommended in all type I diabetic patients, insulin-treated type II diabetic patients, and poorly controlled drug- or diet-treated type II diabetic patients who are undergoing general anesthesia regardless of the planned duration of the surgical procedure. Several methods of insulin administration during the perioperative period are recommended. Most of the protocols include the intravenous administration of short-acting insulin and 5–10% glucose. The subcutaneous administration of insulin is associated with unpredictable absorption and variable plasma insulin levels and is not recommended for surgical patients except for those undergoing minor procedures. In some of the protocols with intravenous insulin, the glucose and insulin are contained in the same infusion mixture. The theoretical advantage of this approach is that, if the glucose infusion is accidentally disconnected or obstructed, so is the insulin infusion, avoiding the risk of hypoglycemia. The disadvantage of this approach is that no flexibility is allowed for changes in the delivery rate of either insulin or glucose infusion.

One approach is to administer insulin and glucose in separate bags but through the same vein, i.e., to piggyback the insulin infusion onto the glucose infusion. This allows independent changes in each infusion. The insulin infusion rate is progressively increased, and the glucose infusion rate is progressively decreased according to the levels of hourly capillary blood glucose measurements. An example of such a protocol is shown in Table 23.2. With this protocol, a blood glucose level in the range of 125–200 mg/dl (6.9–11.1 mM) is easily maintained during the entire perioperative period. As with every therapeutic protocol, clinical judgment must be used. Depending on the individual patient, increases or decreases in the rate of insulin (or glucose) infusion for a given capillary blood glucose range may be necessary. Electrolyte solutions are administered as needed into the glucose infusion or with a separate infusion as needed. In patients with azotemia or other problems with fluid management or those receiving large amounts of other solu-

Table 23.2. REPRESENTATIVE PROTOCOL FOR INSULIN-GLUCOSE INFUSION FOR PERIOPERATIVE PERIODS

1. Discontinue all subcutaneous insulin after initiation of glucose-insulin infusion.
2. Measure capillary blood glucose levels at 1-h intervals.
3. Infuse 5% dextrose (D_5W) intravenously via infusion pump.
4. Make insulin solution with 0.5 U/ml short-acting insulin, i.e., 250 U regular insulin in 500 ml normal saline. Give piggyback via infusion pump into D_5W infusion.
5. Based on hourly blood glucose determination, adjust each infusion according to following schedule:

Blood Glucose (mg/dl)	Insulin Infusion ml/h	Insulin Infusion U/h	D_5W Infusion (ml/h)
<70*	1.0	0.5	150
71–100	2.0	1.0	125
101–150	3.0	1.5	100
151–200	4.0	2.0	100
201–250	6.0	3.0	100
251–300	8.0	4.0	75
>300	12.0	6.0	50

Glucose: 1 mM = 0.056 mg/dl. Modified from Rosenstock and Raskin (3).
*Give 10 ml $D_{50}W$ i.v., and repeat blood glucose measurement 15 min later.

tions, 10% dextrose ($D_{10}W$) can be substituted for the 5% dextrose (D_5W) solution. If $D_{10}W$ is not available, it can be made easily by adding 100 g $D_{50}W$ to 1000 ml D_5W.

Patients with severe fluid management problems, e.g., those with congestive heart failure or end-stage renal disease, may not tolerate the amounts of fluids administered with either a D_5W or $D_{10}W$ infusion. Thus, to provide an adequate carbohydrate supply, $D_{50}W$ must be administered through a central venous line. Table 23.3 shows a protocol for diabetic patients who are at high risk of fluid overload. Note that, for a 70-kg person, this corresponds to a glucose infusion rate of 2 mg $\cdot$ kg^{-1} $\cdot$ min^{-1}. Again, clinical judgment dictates changes in the protocol as necessary. In this circumstance, the insulin infusion rate is modified, and the glucose infusion rate is kept constant.

The blood glucose level must be monitored at hourly intervals. Bedside capillary blood glucose measurements with glucose oxidase strips and a reflectance meter done in the operating and recovery rooms are adequate for perioperative management. Hourly measurements are necessary to keep the blood glucose level between 125 and 200 mg/dl (6.9–11.1 mM).

The management of stable diabetic patients undergoing minor procedures, (e.g., endoscopic techniques or surgery done under local anesthesia) involves withholding the morning dose of insulin or oral agent if the patient is going to be fasting and measuring

Table 23.3. PROTOCOL FOR INSULIN-GLUCOSE INFUSION FOR PERIOPERATIVE PATIENTS AT RISK OF VOLUME OVERLOAD

1. Discontinue all subcutaneous insulin after initiation of glucose-insulin infusion.
2. Measure capillary blood glucose levels at 1-h intervals.
3. Infuse 50% dextrose ($D_{50}W$) intravenously into central venous line via infusion pump.
4. Make insulin solution with 0.5 U/ml short-acting insulin, i.e., 250 U regular insulin in 500 ml normal saline. Give piggyback via infusion pump into $D_{50}W$ infusion.
5. Based on hourly blood glucose determination, adjust insulin infusion according to following schedule:

| Blood Glucose | Insulin Infusion | | $D_{50}W$ Infusion |
(mg/dl)	ml/h	U/h	(ml/h)
<70*	1.0	0.5	17
71–100	2.0	1.0	17
101–150	4.0	2.0	17
151–200	6.0	3.0	17
201–250	8.0	4.0	17
251–300	10.0	5.0	17
>300	12.0	6.0	17

Glucose: 1 mM = 0.056 mg/dl.
*Give 10 ml $D_{50}W$ i.v., and repeat blood glucose measurement 15 min later.

capillary blood glucose every 2–4 h. Supplemental subcutaneous short-acting insulin can be administered following a variable insulin schedule, and the patient's usual insulin or oral agent can be resumed after surgery (Table 23.4).

Postoperative Metabolic Management

Glucose and insulin infusion should be continued until the metabolic condition of the patient is stable and the patient is able to tolerate oral feeding. The insulin and glucose infusions are stopped only after the administration of subcutaneous short-acting insulin. After major surgery, the glucose and insulin infusions should be continued until the patient is able to take solid food without difficulty. In these patients, the use of multiple subcutaneous injections of short-acting insulin before meals and intermediate-acting insulin at bedtime is recommended during the first 24–48 h after the insulin and glucose infusions are stopped and before the patient's usual insulin regimen is resumed. Table 23.5 shows an example of such an insulin-injection schedule.

The use of total parenteral nutrition (TPN) is frequently required in the postoperative period. Diabetic patients can develop serious metabolic derangements with TPN. A variable insulin-infusion schedule similar to that shown in Table 23.2 with hourly determinations of blood glucose is also recommended under these circum-

Table 23.4. DIABETES MANAGEMENT DURING MINOR SURGICAL PROCEDURES

Day of procedure (if patient NPO)
1. Withhold morning dose of insulin or oral agent.
2. Measure capillary blood glucose level before procedure and every 2–4 h.
3. Give short-acting insulin every 2–4 h as follows:

Blood Glucose (mg/dl)	Short-Acting Insulin (U)
<150	0
151–200	2
201–250	3
251–300	5
>300	6

4. Give usual afternoon insulin or oral agent dose.

Day of procedure (if breakfast allowed)
1. Give normal morning dose of insulin or oral agent.
2. Measure blood glucose levels before and after procedure.
3. Give supplemental 4 U of short-acting insulin if blood glucose >250 mg/dl.
4. Give usual afternoon insulin or oral agent dose.

Glucose: 1 mM = 0.056 mg/dl. Modified from Rosenstock and Raskin (3).

Table 23.5. POSTOPERATIVE DIABETES MANAGEMENT WHEN PATIENT TOLERATES SOLID FOOD

1. Do not discontinue intravenous insulin-glucose infusion until after 1st subcutaneous insulin.
2. Measure capillary blood glucose before meals, at 2200, and at 0300.*
3. Provide 3 meals and 3 snacks (20–30 cal · kg^{-1} · day^{-1}).
4. Administer preprandial short-acting insulin according to following variable insulin-dosage schedule:

Blood Glucose (mg/dl)	Insulin (U)			
	Breakfast	Lunch	Dinner	2200
<70	3	2	2	0
71–100	4	3	3	0
101–150	6	4	4	0
151–200	8	6	6	0
201–250	10	8	8	1
251–300	12	10	10	2
>300	14	12	12	3

5. Intermediate-acting insulin 10–20 U at 2200.

Glucose: 1 mM = 0.056 mg/dl. Modified from Rosenstock and Raskin (3).
*If hypoglycemia is present at 0300, reduce 2200 insulin dose.

stances, but additional glucose infusion is not required because it is contained in the TPN solution. Initially, the insulin should be given as a separate continuous infusion from the TPN solution. Once a stable dose of insulin is reached (usually within 24–48 h), the total amount of insulin required over 24 h can be added to the TPN bag, and the frequency of the capillary blood glucose measurements can be reduced to every 2–4 h. The doses of insulin needed during TPN are high, often >100 U/24 h.

Postoperative Cardiovascular Evaluation

Serial postoperative electrocardiograms are recommended for older diabetic patients, those with long-standing type I diabetes, and those with known heart disease. Postoperative myocardial infarction may be silent and has a high mortality. When ambulation of the patient begins, attention must be paid to the possibility of orthostatic hypotension.

Postoperative Renal Evaluation

Careful monitoring of BUN and serum creatinine levels will help to detect acute kidney failure that may occur especially after procedures with iodinated contrast material. If contrast material is to be used, the patient should be well hydrated before and after the procedure. Potassium levels may be elevated or low, and these electrolyte abnormalities must be treated aggressively.

Postoperative Infection

Wound infection is common among diabetic patients with poor metabolic control. Impaired granulocyte function due to hyperglycemia may predispose to bacterial infections. Poor circulation due to macroangiopathy or microangiopathy can also contribute to postoperative infection. Tight metabolic control during the perioperative period can decrease the risk of postoperative infection. Wound infections in diabetic individuals are usually due to mixed flora, and antibiotic coverage must include coverage for anaerobic bacteria, gram-negative enteric bacteria, and *Staphylococcus aureus*. If surgical debridement and drainage is needed, it should be performed early. Cultures should be obtained during drainage procedures and before antibiotic therapy is started. In patients with severe infections that are not responding to antibiotic therapy, *Candida* species or other fungal species should be suspected.

SUGGESTED READING

1. Alberti KGMM: Diabetes and surgery. In *Ellenberg and Rifkin's Diabetes Mellitus. Theory and Practice*. Rifkin H, Porte D, Eds. New York, Elsevier, 1990, p. 626–33
2. Burgos LG, Ebert TJ, Asiddas C, Turner LA, Pattison CZ, Wang-Cheng R, Kamysine JP: Increased intraoperative cardiovascular morbidity in diabetics with autonomic neuropathy. *Anesthesiology* 70:591–97, 1989
3. Rosenstock J, Raskin P: Surgery! Practical guidelines for diabetes management. *Clin Diabetes* 5:49–61, 1987
4. Stein PA, Tinker JH, Tarhan S: Myocardial reinfarction after anesthesia and surgery. *JAMA* 239:2566–70, 1978
5. Taitelman U, Reece E, Bessman A: Insulin in the management of the diabetic surgical patient. *JAMA* 237:658–60, 1977

24. Geriatric Patients

JEFFREY B. HALTER, MD

Diabetes mellitus is an important health problem among the elderly population. The dramatic age-related increase in the prevalence rate of diabetes mellitus is demonstrated in Fig. 24.1, indicating that >10% of people >65 yr of age have diabetes. The rapid growth of the United States aging population, which will increase from a current total of ~28 million people over age 65 yr to >50 million by the year 2020, suggests continued growth in the number of older people with diabetes mellitus. Hyperglycemia in older people is not a benign condition, because it is associated with risk for long-term diabetes complications. Thus, the management of hyperglycemia in an elderly patient with diabetes mellitus should be considered seriously.

PATHOPHYSIOLOGY AND RATIONALE FOR TREATMENT

Most older people with diabetes mellitus have type II (non-insulin-dependent) diabetes mellitus. The pathogenesis of type II diabetes in this group is similar to that in other age-groups. Many factors may contribute to the high rate of development of type II diabetes in elderly patients (Fig. 24.2). Age-related impairments of both pancreatic β-cell function and insulin action appear to be important factors in the pathophysiology of hyperglycemia in elderly people with diabetes mellitus. An age-related increase in body adiposity

Dr. Halter is Professor of Internal Medicine, Chief of the Division of Geriatric Medicine, Research Scientist and Medical Director of the Institute of Gerontology, and Director of the Geriatrics Center, University of Michigan and VA Medical Center, Ann Arbor, MI.

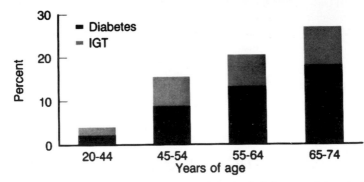

Figure 24.1. Prevalence (% of population) of diabetes and impaired glucose tolerance (IGT) in U.S. as function of age. Data are from National Health and Nutrition Examination Survey II (4). From Halter (2).

and a decrease in physical activity both contribute to the insulin resistance of aging. In addition, the prevalence of coexisting illnesses and use of various drugs may contribute to the development of hyperglycemia.

The short-term risks of poor diabetes control for elderly patients merit intervention. Marked hyperglycemia associated with glucosuria and weight loss is a catabolic state that predisposes the diabetic patient to various acute illnesses, particularly infections. The most extreme example of poor diabetes control among elderly patients

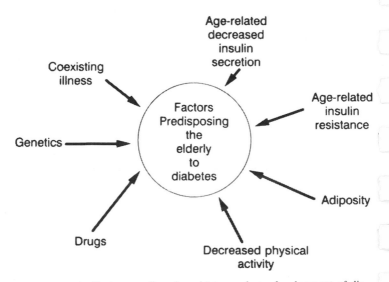

Figure 24.2. Factors predisposing older people to development of diabetes mellitus. From Halter (2).

is the syndrome of hyperosmolar coma, which is associated with a high mortality rate and requires aggressive intervention (see chapt. 22).

Elderly patients are also at risk for many long-term complications. This risk may not be simply a function of duration of diabetes, because the patient may have had asymptomatic undetected hyperglycemia for an extended period before the initial diagnosis was made. Older patients with diabetes mellitus have approximately a 2-fold increased risk for myocardial infarction, stroke, and renal insufficiency compared with patients of the same age without diabetes. The risk for amputation in an older patient with diabetes is increased almost 10-fold.

THERAPY

General Approach to Management

Severe symptomatic hyperglycemia must be treated to control excessive fatty acid mobilization and oxidation, excessive protein catabolism and muscle wasting, excessive glucose production, and urinary loss of calories in the form of glucose. Development of a rational long-term treatment plan for an elderly (>65-yr-old) diabetic patient must take into consideration 1) life expectancy, 2) presence of diabetes complications, 3) presence of coexisting medical or neuropsychiatric disorders, and 4) the patient's ability and willingness to comply with the proposed diabetes treatment program (Table 24.1). In a healthy 65-yr-old individual without associated medical problems or diabetes complications in whom a reasonable life expectancy (10–20 yr more) is anticipated, the physician should strive for the best possible glycemic control without predisposing the individual to the unnecessary risks of hypoglycemia. One approach is to strive for a fasting glucose level of 115 mg/dl (6.4 mM) and a postprandial glucose level of 180 mg/dl (10 mM). In the elderly diabetic patient with established microvascular complications (especially diabetic nephropathy and retinopathy), the likelihood of

Table 24.1. IMPORTANT FACTORS TO CONSIDER FOR DIABETES MANAGEMENT IN ELDERLY PATIENTS

- The patient's remaining life expectancy
- Patient commitment
- Availability of support services
- Economic issues
- Medical disorder
  - Psychiatric disorder
  - Cognitive disorder
  - Diabetes complications
  - Major limitation of diabetes functional status
- Complexity of medical regimen

ameliorating their progression may be less. Therefore, more conservative therapeutic targets (e.g., fasting glucose <140 mg/dl [7.8 mM] and a postprandial glucose <200–220 mg/dl [<11.1–13.3 mM]) may be more prudent. Elderly diabetic patients with serious associated medical problems, especially cardiovascular or cerebrovascular, should be treated in a manner similar to patients with underlying diabetes complications. A less aggressive approach is also advocated in patients with impaired cognitive function, neuropsychiatric disorders, or demonstrated inability to comply with the proposed therapeutic regimen.

Once a therapeutic goal for glycemic control has been established, an orderly approach to treatment, including diet, exercise, oral agents, and insulin, should be developed as described in chapters 14, 16, 17, and 20.

Diet

Dietary intervention as a primary mode of diabetes management should be considered first for an overweight elderly person because of the potential effectiveness of weight reduction and its relative safety (see chapt. 14). Even a modest amount of weight reduction in an obese elderly patient can lead to a marked improvement in the degree of hyperglycemia, presumably by reducing resistance to insulin.

Note that substantial barriers may limit the effectiveness of a weight-reducing diet in an elderly patient. Lifelong dietary habits, often based on long-standing cultural traditions, may be particularly difficult to modify. Many elderly patients have changes in taste, vision, or smell that may lead to difficulties with food preparation. Arthritis or other neurological or muscular disorders may also limit the patient's access to the most appropriate kinds of foods, and financial factors may also be important. Because of these complexities, the skills of an experienced dietitian and the help of family may be of considerable importance in instituting and maintaining an appropriate dietary regimen.

Exercise

A carefully developed exercise program can benefit elderly diabetic patients. The same principles that guide the choice of exercise program in younger diabetic patients apply to the elderly. It is important to recognize that the intensity of physical training must be commensurate with the patient's degree of physical fitness. Because of the high incidence of clinically silent coronary artery disease among the elderly, any physical training program should be based on an appropriate exercise tolerance test and carried out with careful supervision. A foot injury resulting from an exercise program could have devastating effects in an elderly patient who is at a high risk for infection and amputation. Therefore, choice of appropriate footwear is critical. As with any exercise program, the risk of hypoglycemia should be minimized (see chapt. 16).

Sulfonylureas

If the defined treatment goal is not achieved with a program of diet and exercise, it is appropriate to consider the use of a sulfonylurea drug. The dosage, mechanism of action, efficacy, and specific side effects of sulfonylurea drugs are discussed in chapter 17. Although no major differences in clinical pharmacology of these agents in older adults have been defined, a prudent approach to the use of these agents in this population is to start with a relatively small dose and increase slowly while observing the patient's response.

The most significant risk of the use of sulfonylurea drugs in elderly patients is hypoglycemia. Because of the importance of the kidneys and liver for drug elimination and the importance of the liver for glucose counterregulation, both renal and hepatic insufficiency are substantial risk factors for the development of severe hypoglycemia during sulfonylurea therapy. An age-related decline in renal function would contribute to this susceptibility.

Because many older people take multiple drugs, it is important to consider potential sulfonylurea-drug interactions (see chapt. 17). Despite the potential for hypoglycemia with use of sulfonylurea drugs, the risk appears to be small in elderly patients who have good nutritional status and who do not have major problems with renal or hepatic insufficiency. When hypoglycemia does occur, patients need to be carefully observed for a considerable period, particularly with some of the longer-acting agents. Chlorpropamide should be avoided in older people because of the concern for prolonged hypoglycemia.

Insulin

When the treatment goal for a patient has not been met by use of a weight-reduction diet, exercise, and a trial of sulfonylurea drugs, insulin therapy should be considered. Institution of insulin therapy and subsequent adjustment of the insulin regimen should be carried out as discussed in chapter 20.

Insulin does not have any major drug interactions, and there are virtually no contraindications to its use. It is important to emphasize, however, that the use of insulin requires that the patient or care provider be trained in self-monitoring of blood glucose (SMBG). Skills required for independence in insulin administration and SMBG that must be evaluated in elderly diabetic individuals are

- Sufficient cognitive function to manage a complex regimen
- Adequate vision to read labels, syringes, and glucose-monitoring equipment
- Fine motor control to draw up and use insulin

Table 24.2. **RISK FACTORS FOR HYPOGLYCEMIA IN OLDER DIABETIC PATIENTS**

- Impaired autonomic nervous system function
- Impaired counterregulatory responses
- Poor or irregular nutrition
- Cognitive disorder
- Use of alcohol or other sedating agent
- Polypharmacy
- Kidney or liver failure

Limitations in some of these areas can be overcome. Family members and home-health aides can help with administering insulin. The developing technology of SMBG can make up for limitations in vision and some of the fine motor skills.

The major risk associated with insulin administration in the elderly is the development of hypoglycemia. Treatment of this complication is discussed in chapter 20. Risk factors that may increase the likelihood of a hypoglycemic reaction in elderly patients are described in Table 24.2.

SUGGESTED READING

1. Funnell MM: Role of the diabetes educator for older adults. *Diabetes Care* 13 (Suppl. 2):60–65, 1990
2. Halter JB: *Diabetes Update: Elderly Patients With Non-Insulin-Dependent Diabetes Mellitus.* Kalamazoo, MI, Upjohn, 1990
3. Halter JB, Morrow LA: Use of sulfonylurea drugs in elderly patients. *Diabetes Care* 13 (Suppl. 2):86–92, 1990
4. Harris MI, Hadden WC, Knowler WC, Bennett PH: Prevalence of diabetes and impaired glucose tolerance and plasma glucose levels in U.S. population aged 20–74 yr. *Diabetes* 36:523–34, 1987
5. Herman WH, Teutsch SM, Geiss LS: Closing the gap: the problem of diabetes mellitus in the United States. *Diabetes Care* 8:391–406, 1985
6. Jackson RA: Mechanisms of age-related glucose intolerance. *Diabetes Care* 13 (Suppl. 2):9–19, 1990

25. Hypoglycemia in Patients With Type I Diabetes

JULIO V. SANTIAGO, MD, LUCY A. LEVANDOSKI, PA-C, and
JEANNE BUBB, MSW

Hypoglycemia is the most common complication of insulin treatment in type I (insulin-dependent) diabetes. A typical person with type I diabetes treated with two daily injections of insulin over 30 yr will experience ~1482 episodes of hypoglycemia or ~1 episode/ wk. Some will experience more, some less. In 15- to 45-yr-old type I diabetic subjects treated conventionally between 1983 and 1987, the overall incidence of severe hypoglycemia resulting in coma, seizure, or need for intravenous glucose or glucagon was ~1 episode/ 4–5 yr of diabetes. As with milder forms of hypoglycemia, considerable variation exists among patients. Fortunately, many surveys of well-trained and prudent type I diabetic patients have shown no increases in automobile accident rates compared with people without diabetes. Nevertheless, all patients treated with insulin need to be aware of the potential risks of severe hypoglycemia and need to adapt common-sense measures to avoid its occurrence.

DEFINITIONS

Biochemically, *hypoglycemia* can be defined as a venous or capillary blood glucose concentration <50 mg/dl (<3.1 mM). This definition

Dr. Santiago is Professor of Pediatrics and Director of the Diabetes Research and Training Center, Ms. Levandoski is Diabetes Research Associate and Clinical Coordinator of the DCCT, and Ms. Bubb is a Clinical Research Social Worker at the Washington University School of Medicine, St. Louis, MO. Ms. Bubb is also a Clinical Research Social Worker at St. Louis Children's Hospital.

may be precise but is not too useful because many episodes of glucose slightly below this level are undetected, particularly during sleep, and an occasional patient will develop neurological impairment at a slightly higher level. Furthermore, many patients begin to sense a low glucose value at slightly higher levels.

Clinical definitions are more useful. *Mild hypoglycemia* is defined as an episode in which the patient feels symptoms related to activation of adrenergic (tachycardia, palpitations, shakiness) or cholinergic (sweating) defense mechanisms or the effects of hypoglycemia on the nervous system (e.g., inability to concentrate, dizziness, hunger, blurred vision) but is not sufficiently impaired to interfere with normal activities. *Severe hypoglycemia* is an episode of hypoglycemia resulting in coma, seizure, or sufficient neuorological impairment so that the patient is unable to initiate self-treatment or requires the assistance of another person. *Moderate hypoglycemia* is an episode in which a person's neurological status is marked by obvious impairment of motor function, confusion, or inappropriate behavior but is still alert enough to seek self-treatment. Episodes of severe hypoglycemia will sometimes occur without warning symptoms. This is a common finding in patients with long-standing type I diabetes. Occasionally patients may have repeated episodes of hypoglycemia with coma or seizure without any warning symptoms. These patients are said to have the *hypoglycemia-unawareness syndrome*.

It is not necessary to measure blood glucose to make a presumptive diagnosis of hypoglycemia. Any episode with clinical characteristics typical of hypoglycemia that reverse soon after treatment designed to raise the blood glucose level can be presumed due to hypoglycemia.

CAUSES OF HYPOGLYCEMIA

Physiologically, most episodes of hypoglycemia can be considered due to relative or absolute hyperinsulinemia in patients with diabetes. *Absolute* insulin excess is most common before lunch and before supper, when the insulin given the previous morning is excessive, when more than usual amounts of injected insulin are absorbed at a particular time, when a meal is either delayed or has insufficient carbohydrate, or when gastric emptying is delayed. Absolute insulin excess is also common in the early morning (0100–0300), because less insulin is usually needed to normalize blood glucose levels during the predawn period than during the following hours (dawn phenomenon). *Relative* insulin excess is most commonly seen with exercise. In type I diabetes, exercise does not suppress insulin release from the pancreas thus producing a fall in blood glucose concentration. Hypoglycemia can also result from alcohol's suppression of glucose release from the liver.

Clinical Causes of Hypoglycemia

All patients should be able to list the most common causes of hypoglycemia:

1. Too much insulin
2. Delayed or inappropriate food intake
3. Exercise
4. Alcohol

With each episode of hypoglycemia, these possible causes should be noted and common-sense measures taken to reduce the chances of recurrence. However, even with perfect attention to the treatment regimen, inadvertent episodes of hypoglycemia are still common, especially among well-controlled patients maintaining their blood glucose at <180 mg/dl (<10 mM).

Sometimes, the causes of hypoglycemia are subtle. For example, at the onset of menses, a fall in progesterone level may decrease insulin requirements and contribute to a tendency to develop hypoglycemia. When patients switch to a new bottle of insulin, hypoglycemia is sometimes noted because the old insulin had lost some of its potency. Some patients with diabetes will have delayed gastric emptying, especially when a meal is difficult to digest, and this will result in hypoglycemia. Some patients report that hypoglycemia will occur after they have changed their insulin-injection site. Insulin absorption may be variable according to site of injection. Even after all of these factors have been sought, some episodes may remain unexplained. Many are due to the erratic absorption of insulin, a problem that cannot be eliminated totally even by the most careful patient and are an inherent deficiency of an imperfect mode of treatment.

HOW TO REDUCE RISK FACTORS FOR HYPOGLYCEMIA

Poor Adherence and Inadequate Training

Failure to follow a prearranged treatment plan or to make common-sense day-to-day adjustments in diet, insulin, exercise, and glucose monitoring are frequent causes of hypoglycemia. Common errors in insulin administration include

- Mistakes in measurement
- Switching the morning dose with the evening dose
- Inappropriate efforts to rapidly reduce hyperglycemia with large doses of short-acting insulin
- Taking excessive amounts of insulin at bedtime

Other factors resulting in hypoglycemia are

- Missing or delaying meals
- Reducing carbohydrate intake
- Failing to compensate for increased physical activity

Patients who are poorly trained, inattentive or careless, or have erratic life-styles can be expected to have more difficulties adhering to complex treatment plans and thus to experience more hypoglycemic reactions. For type I diabetic patients, particularly adolescents, concerns about blood glucose control may have a low priority. Simplifying a complex regimen, making it more realistic, and adjusting it to meet individual needs may be required to reduce hypoglycemia. All patients should be provided with written instructions regarding hypoglycemia, and this material should be reviewed during subsequent office visits.

Sometimes, patients feel that admitting to errors that have resulted in hypoglycemia cause family members and health professionals to "hassle" or think less of them. As a result, type I diabetic patients often fail to report even severe episodes of hypoglycemia, preferring to "take care of things" on their own and not subject themselves to being viewed as unreliable or incompetent. A straightforward nonjudgmental approach by a trusted health professional may help reduce cat-and-mouse games that some patients play with their health-care providers.

Attempts to Maintain Normoglycemia

A risk factor for hypoglycemia in type I diabetic patients is an unrealistic or inappropriate attempt to maintain normoglycemia or normal glycosylated hemoglobin values. Although near normoglycemia is a desirable goal that can sometimes be sustained for several months after initial diagnosis of type I diabetes, efforts to maintain near-normal glycosylated hemoglobin levels after the end of the honeymoon phase often lead to a different reality. A threefold increase in largely iatrogenic hypoglycemia is seen even in highly motivated, closely supervised, and unusually resourceful patients willing to take three or four daily insulin injections or use an insulin-infusion pump, follow a meal and exercise plan, and measure glucose concentrations ≥ 120 times every month of their lives. The risks are probably greater if near normoglycemia is the target goal rather than moderate glycemic control.

Normoglycemia may be an unrealistic long-term goal for many nonpregnant type I diabetic patients, and even with enormous effort, many patients cannot be expected to safely maintain blood glucose low enough to achieve normal glycosylated hemoglobin levels without serious hypoglycemic complications. Negotiation of appropriate glucose goals should be an ongoing process between the patient and the health professionals responsible for providing help and guidance.

Longer Duration of Diabetes

Longer duration of diabetes may increase the risk for severe hypoglycemia for several reasons:

1. More frequent and larger doses of insulin are necessary to maintain normoglycemia.

2. After several years, type I diabetic patients begin to lose their ability to release glucagon in response to hypoglycemia. Glucagon is the body's first defense against acute hypoglycemia due to insulin excess.

3. After ~10–15 yr of diabetes, a few patients will also begin to lose their ability to secrete epinephrine in response to hypoglycemia. This is a form of autonomic neuropathy and/or a resetting of CNS activation points for glucoregulation. Epinephrine compensates for the lack of glucagon and assumes the primary role in defense against hypoglycemia. With its loss, type I diabetic patients become virtually defenseless against even moderate degrees of hyperinsulinemia that can occur anytime. These patients are referred to as "poor glucose counterregulators" and are at increased risk for developing hypoglycemia with intensive therapy.

4. With time, type I diabetic patients who have been free of severe hypoglycemia often assume a false sense of confidence. Risk-taking behaviors, failure to note subtle changes in early warning signs of hypoglycemia, and the natural wish to "take a vacation" from diabetes management all are common. Patients may begin to feel that they can usually get away with behaviors their health professionals have branded as dangerous.

5. Increased duration of diabetes is sometimes associated with decreased warning symptoms of diabetes. This is discussed below.

Hypoglycemia Unawareness

Type I diabetic patients sometimes lapse repeatedly into coma or develop a seizure without any warning signs of hypoglycemia. These patients have lost their ability to counterregulate effectively, and they no longer recognize normal neurogenic or neuroglycopenic warning symptoms before they become so severely compromised that they can no longer seek assistance. Fortunately, this syndrome is not common.

A phenomenon in which the symptoms and signs of hypoglycemia simply change with time or become less noticeable is much more common. In some cases, subtle early warning symptoms are masked by ordinary activities such as exercise or by anxiety but may still be detectable by an experienced observer.

The reasons the symptoms of hypoglycemia change with time are complex and poorly understood. Sometimes, when patients with average blood glucose levels well above 180 mg/dl (10 mM) are treated intensively and their blood glucose is lowered substantially over several weeks, the normal counterregulatory hormonal protective mechanisms and hypoglycemia warning symptoms are blunted.

The key practical point, however, is that patients must know that changes in warning symptoms are likely to occur over time. It has been estimated that 35% of all episodes of severe hypoglycemia during waking hours occur without patients recognizing any premonitory symptoms. Fortunately, most of these patients have the ability to recognize or correctly respond to early warning symptoms of hypoglycemia on subsequent occasions.

The fact that hypoglycemia can occur without warning symptoms should be used to help motivate patients to monitor their blood glucose levels routinely, particularly when hypoglycemia is likely to occur. It is also important to teach patients that blood glucose <50 mg/dl (3.1 mM) without accompanying symptoms should be a cause of concern and should cause the patient to initiate discussions with the physician.

Nocturnal Hypoglycemia: Predawn Phenomenon

Over 50% of all episodes of severe hypoglycemia occur during the night or before breakfast. The reasons for an increased risk for hypoglycemia during the night include the following:

1. Patients when asleep are commonly unaware of the premonitory symptoms of nocturnal hypoglycemia.
2. Even modest hyperinsulinemia produces hypoglycemia in patients with poor glucose counterregulation.
3. Insulin requirements to maintain normoglycemia are 20–30% lower in the predawn period than at dawn (the predawn phenomenon).
4. Intermediate-acting insulin given before dinner to lower prebreakfast blood glucose levels often produces relative hyperinsulinemia at 0100–0300 (the waning insulin phenomenon).

Several practical measures can be used to prevent nocturnal hypoglycemia.

1. Patients predisposed to hypoglycemia should be encouraged to periodically measure blood glucose levels at 0100–0300. The frequency of early-morning blood glucose monitoring will depend on the needs of the patient. More frequent measurements may be needed if insulin doses are being adjusted to reduce prebreakfast hyperglycemia, if prebreakfast glucose levels are routinely <120 mg/dl (<6.7 mM), when patients are traveling, when keeping irregular school/work schedules, or after exercise.
2. Patients predisposed to nocturnal hypoglycemia should routinely measure their blood glucose at bedtime, before their bedtime snack. Glucose levels <120 mg/dl (<6.7 mM) at this time, particularly after increased daytime exercise, may require an increase in the size of the usual bedtime snack.

3. When attempts to reduce prebreakfast hyperglycemia cause early morning hypoglycemia, a series of corrective measures should be explored. These include increasing the bedtime snack and reducing the evening preprandial dose of intermediate-acting insulin. However, this can result in prebreakfast hyperglycemia. When this happens, the evening intermediate-acting insulin dose may be moved to bedtime, or the patient can be given a longer-acting (peakless) form of insulin (e.g., ultralente) before supper. Because of differences in formulation, human NPH or lente insulin may be more rapidly absorbed than pork insulin, making these insulins a problem for some patients with predawn hypoglycemia.

The relevance of nightmares, night sweating, nocturnal seizures, inability to arouse from sleep, unexplained morning headaches, and the need for 0100–0300 glucose monitoring on days after prolonged or severe exercise all need discussion and planning with family or roommates.

Previous Severe Hypoglycemia

Once a patient has experienced one episode of severe hypoglycemia, the risk of a subsequent episode during the next year increases severalfold. Thus, patients with repeated episodes of severe hypoglycemia should be treated with caution, even when these episodes of hypoglycemia are thought to be related to professional mismanagement.

TREATMENT

After a person has learned to correctly identify the early warning symptoms of hypoglycemia, blood glucose measurements are not necessary if the symptoms are typical for a given situation. Atypical episodes or episodes with unusual or new signs or symptoms may require verification with blood glucose measurements. When blood glucose levels are low and there are no symptoms, patients should treat themselves, especially if they are going to sleep, operate dangerous machinery, or drive a car. A common mistake is to delay or put off treatment for ≥30 min until a meal is ready or the patient has arrived at a destination. A second common mistake is to overtreat hypoglycemia because patients remain symptomatic after low blood glucose has been corrected or because they take too much carbohydrate for a mild episode.

Family members, close friends, babysitters, and someone at work or school should be taught how to recognize hypoglycemic signs and how to treat hypoglycemia. These individuals should be encouraged to firmly insist that disoriented patients take some form of carbohydrate. Family members, roommates, and school nurses should be expected to know when and how to give glucagon if a patient taking insulin suddenly loses consciousness or experiences a seizure. Glucagon-injection criteria and techniques should be reviewed regularly with those who are most likely to have reason to use it.

Mild hypoglycemic episodes and those occurring during the night, when insulin levels are only moderately elevated, may require less carbohydrate than more severe or daytime episodes caused by a skipped or late meal or strenuous exercise.

A person weighing 130 lb (60 kg) whose blood glucose level is 36 mg/dl (2.0 mM) will need ~5.0 g of glucose to raise the blood glucose concentration by 50 mg/dl (3.1 mM). With mild episodes, an additional ~5–7 g of glucose may be needed every hour, whereas with a skipped meal or severe exercise, 2–4× as much may be needed each hour.

A simple rule of thumb is that ~10–15 g of carbohydrate should be given for mild to moderate episodes of hypoglycemia. This can be in the form of

- 2 or 3 glucose tablets (5 g each)
- ⅓–½ a tube containing 30 g of glucose in gel form
- 4–6 oz of orange juice
- 4–6 oz of regular cola
- ¼–⅓ cup of raisins

These can be repeated in 15–30 min if symptoms persist and/or the measured blood glucose level falls below 60 mg/dl (3.3 mM). Twice as much may be needed if hypoglycemia is caused by a missed meal or strenuous exercise.

Severe episodes in which patients cannot or will not take food can be treated with intramuscular or subcutaneous glucagon (0.5–1.0 mg) or intravenous glucose (20–30 ml of a 50% solution). Patients given glucagon often vomit, and 50% glucose has to be administered with care to avoid painful extravasation. Blood glucose measurements at 30- to 60-min intervals and close surveillance for recurrence of hypoglycemia are indicated in treating severe episodes of hypoglycemia.

SUGGESTED READING

1. Amiel SA, Tamborlane WV, Simonson DC, Sherwin RS: Defective glucose counterregulation after strict glycemic control of insulin-dependent diabetes mellitus. *N Engl J Med* 36:1376–83, 1987
2. Casparie AF, Elving LD: Severe hypoglycemia in diabetic patients: frequency, causes, prevention. *Diabetes Care* 8:141–45, 1985
3. Cox DJ, Gonder-Frederick LA, Lee JH, Julian DM, Carter WR, Clarke WL: Effects and correlates of blood glucose awareness training among patients with IDDM. *Diabetes Care* 12:313–18, 1989
4. Cryer PE, Gerich JE: Glucose counterregulation, hypoglycemia and intensive insulin therapy in diabetes mellitus. *N Engl J Med* 313:232–41, 1985

5. DCCT Research Group: Diabetes Control and Complications Trial (DCCT): results from feasibility study. *Diabetes Care* 10:1–19, 1987

6. DCCT Research Group: The epidemiology of severe hypoglycemia in the Diabetes Control and Complications Trial. *Am J Med.* In press.

7. Hepburn DA, Eddington DQ, Patrick AW, Frier BM: Symptomatic awareness of hypoglycemia: does it change on transfer from animal to human insulin? *Diabetic Med* 6:586–90, 1989

26. Insulin Allergy and Insulin Resistance

S. EDWIN FINEBERG, MD

There is ample evidence that the insulin molecule itself induces antibodies and is the most likely cause of immunologic complications.

Other potential antigens may be obtained in pharmaceutical insulins of pancreatic and rDNA origin. Protamine antibodies have been demonstrated in ~40% of individuals treated with NPH insulins. These antibodies are rarely the cause of insulin-associated allergic phenomena but have been associated with anaphylaxis during the reversal of intraoperative heparin anticoagulation. In patients previously treated with NPH insulins, heparin anticoagulation should be allowed to spontaneously reverse, or if protamine reversal is necessary, it should be carried out with preparations for possible anaphylaxis.

Noninsulin pancreatic peptides are absent or present in vanishingly small concentrations in highly purified insulins. Insulin dimers and oxidative products form during the storage of pharmaceutical insulins, especially at high temperatures; only the former incites specific antibodies. There are few cases of zinc-related insulin allergy, despite the common demonstration of positive skin tests to zinc acetate or zinc sulfate. With regard to rDNA human insulin made via *Escherichia coli*, no individuals have been shown to have increased antibody concentrations to bacterial peptides.

In general, the order of immunogenicity is beef > pork > human insulins and repository > soluble insulins. Within species, protamine and lente insulins are equivalent with regard to immunogenicity.

Dr. Fineberg is Professor of Medicine at the Indiana University School of Medicine, Indianapolis, IN.

Local insulin-allergic phenomena are encountered in ~2–3% of patients treated with highly purified pork or human insulins, whereas systemic insulin allergy has seldom been reported with human or pork insulins. Systemic allergy has rarely been reported to be associated with pork or human insulins when individuals were begun and continued only on these insulins. Insulin-antibody–mediated insulin resistance resulting in insulin requirements of >1.5 U · kg^{-1} · day^{-1} (>10 nM · kg^{-1} · day^{-1}) in adults and >2.5 U · kg^{-1}· day^{-1} (>16.7 nM · kg^{-1} · day^{-1}) in children is an extremely rare complication of therapy and has not been associated with individuals begun and continued on human insulin or purified pork insulin therapy.

PATHOPHYSIOLOGY OF INSULIN ALLERGY

1. Insulin allergy is usually local and occurs within the first 2 wk of therapy (Table 26.1). About 90% of individuals with local allergy have spontaneous remissions within 2 mo while on the same therapy, and an additional 5% will improve within 6–12 mo.
2. Isolated wheal and flare and biphasic reactions are mediated by reaginic antibodies (IgE). The late phase of a biphasic reaction is characterized by pain and erythema.
3. Arthus reactions (inflammatory response to the deposition of antigen-antibody complexes) are uncommon and characterized by localized small-vessel injury and neutrophilic infiltrates.
4. Delayed reactions are indurated and often pruritic and painful with well-defined borders. Histologically, these lesions are associated with perivascular cuffing with mononuclear cells.
5. Systemic allergic reactions are seen most commonly in individuals with prior histories of atopy and/or intermittent insulin therapy. Anti-insulin IgG and IgE levels are not predictive of types of local reactions but are significantly elevated in individuals with systemic insulin allergy.

Table 26.1. **ALLERGIC REACTIONS TO INSULIN**

Type	Description
Local	
Isolated wheal and flare	Occurs within 30 min, resolves within 1 h
Biphasic	Wheal and flare followed by a late-phase reaction peaking in 4–6 h and persisting for 24 h
Arthus reaction	Develops over 4–6 h, peaks at 12 h
Delayed (tuberculinlike)	Develops nodule or "deep hive" over 8–12 h, peaks in 24 h
Systemic	
Urticaria to anaphylaxis	Immediate reaction

Modified from DeShazo et al. (2)

Table 26.2. THERAPY FOR PERSISTENT SEVERE LOCAL ALLERGY (PRESENT FOR 14–30 DAYS)

Rule out improper injection technique (also infection and contaminated alcohol)

↓

Switch to human insulin

↓

No improvement (2–14 doses)

↓

Skin test to select least reactive insulin, 0.02-ml intradermal injections of 1:1 dilution of U-100 human, pork, and beef NPH, lente, and regular insulins, diluted in phenol-saline; 700 μg/ml (4.3 mM) zinc sulfate, 0.1 mg/ml (0.48 mM) histamine phosphate (positive control); and phenol-saline (negative control). Observe for reactions at 20 min, 6 h, and 24 h. A positive wheal and flare is 5 mm > phenol-saline 20 min after injection, surrounded by erythema. Significant induration is >1 cm.

↓

Treat with least reactive insulin

↓

Persistent severe allergy

↓

Divide the doses and inject into multiple sites; consider delivery of regular insulin by multiple doses in continuous subcutaneous insulin infusion; may modify reaction by use of local steroids, 1 μg (2.5 mM) dexamethasone/U insulin and/or systemic antihistamines.

If reactive to zinc sulfate, consider use of zinc-free or low-zinc insulin. If reactive to NPH insulins, avoid protamine. Protamine insulins are typically low in zinc, and sodium insulin is available on a compassionate basis from Lilly. Modified from DeShazo et al. (2) and Galloway and DeShazo (4).

THERAPY FOR INSULIN ALLERGY

1. In individuals with severe persistent local allergy and individuals with systemic allergy, further therapy is indicated and is summarized in Tables 26.2–26.4.

2. Therapy of systemic allergy is based on intradermal testing to ascertain the least reactive insulin (i.e., insulin evoking the least hypersensitivity in the patient), desensitization, and, less frequently, the use of steroids and/or antihistamines.
3. With systemic or severe insulin allergy, insulin therapy must be continued to avoid future anamnestic reactions. Both human and purified pork insulins have been successfully used for desensitization. Over 94% of individuals with systemic allergy can be desensitized as described above. Steroids and/or antihistamines may rarely be required to modify insulin-allergic symptoms that persist.

Table 26.3. THERAPY FOR SYSTEMIC INSULIN ALLERGY

Is insulin necessary? ——No——→ Diet ± oral hypoglycemic agents

↓ Yes

Skin test for least reactive insulin: at 20-min intervals, 0.02 ml by intradermal injections of 0.001, 0.01, and 0.1 U (0.007, 0.07, and 0.7 nM, respectively) of human insulin diluted in sterile phenol-saline or neutral insulin-dilution fluid. If wheal and flare 5 mm > phenol-saline 20 min after injection of any dilution, test with dilutions of pork insulin then, if necessary, beef insulin. Use saline and/or insulin diluting fluid as negative-control solutions. If negative (<5 mm larger than control) test with 1 U (6.7 nM)

Positive wheal and flare reaction		Negative wheal and flare with 1 U (6.7 nM)
↓		↓
Desensitize with least reactive insulin		Treat with nonreactive insulin

Medically stable and last insulin <24 h prior	Medically unstable and/or last insulin >24 h prior
↓	↓
Administer ⅓ of last dose as same type of insulin and increase by 33 nM every 12 h until metabolic control is achieved. Then continue with long-acting insulin every 12 h (lente or NPH). If reaction occurs, reduce dose or proceed to rapid desensitization protocol (Table 26.4)	Proceed to rapid desensitization protocol (Table 26.4)

Neutral insulin-diluting fluid and empty insulin mixing vials are available from Lilly. Modified from Galloway and DeShazo (4).

Table 26.4. RAPID DESENSITIZATION PROTOCOL

Prepare serial 1:10 dilutions of least reactive insulin (after an initial 1:1 dilution of U-100 insulin, then serial 1:10 dilutions of the least reactive insulin in neutral insulin-diluting fluid of 50, 5, 0.5, 0.05 and 0.005 U/ml)

| | STEP (every 20–30 min) | | | | | | | | | | | |
| | Intradermal | | | | | | Subcutaneous | | | | | |
	1	2	3	4	5	6	7	8	9	10	11	12
Volume (ml)	0.02	0.04	0.08	0.02	0.04	0.08	0.02	0.04	0.08	0.02	0.04	0.08
U/ml	0.05	0.05	0.05	0.5	0.5	0.5	5	5	5	50	50	50
U	0.001	0.002	0.004	0.004	0.02	0.04	0.1	0.2	0.4	1	2	4

Instructions

1. Precede with skin testing as described in Table 26.3.
2. Carry out in the hospital under medical supervision. If reactions have been severe, carry out procedure in intensive-care unit.
3. Avoid concomitant use of antihistamines or steroids. Have a syringe filled with 1 ml of 1:1000 epinephrine, life-support equipment, and an allergy consultant available.
4. If patient reacts to initial dosage, begin with 0.005 U/ml.
5. If patient has more than a wheal-and-flare reaction or induration >1 cm, reduce by 2 dilution steps and then proceed again.
6. After step 12, double dose subcutaneously every 4 h until metabolic stability is established. Then long-acting insulin may be administered (lente or NPH as described in Table 26.3).

Insulin: 1 pM = 0.139 mU/ml.

Table 26.5. IDENTIFICATION AND TREATMENT OF ANTIBODY-MEDIATED INSULIN RESISTANCE

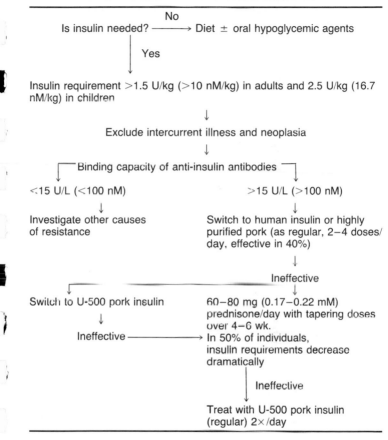

Is insulin needed? ———No———→ Diet ± oral hypoglycemic agents

↓ Yes

Insulin requirement >1.5 U/kg (>10 nM/kg) in adults and 2.5 U/kg (16.7 nM/kg) in children

↓

Exclude intercurrent illness and neoplasia

↓

Binding capacity of anti-insulin antibodies

<15 U/L (<100 nM)   >15 U/L (>100 nM)

↓   ↓

Investigate other causes of resistance   Switch to human insulin or highly purified pork (as regular, 2–4 doses/day, effective in 40%)

↓ Ineffective

Switch to U-500 pork insulin   60–80 mg (0.17–0.22 mM) prednisone/day with tapering doses over 4–6 wk.

↓

Ineffective ————→ In 50% of individuals, insulin requirements decrease dramatically

↓ Ineffective

Treat with U-500 pork insulin (regular) 2×/day

ANTIBODY-MEDIATED INSULIN RESISTANCE

1. Individuals with this complication of therapy commonly have histories of intermittent insulin therapy or atopy. Therapy with beef-containing insulins before the initiation of resistance is virtually always noted.
2. To demonstrate that antibodies are the primary cause of insulin resistance, other etiologies, including intercurrent illness, and neoplasia must be eliminated. Possible factitious resistance, e.g., resistance absent when insulin is administered by MD or RN, must also be eliminated.

3. Occasionally, insulin-antibody–mediated insulin resistance may be an early manifestation of the insulin autoimmune syndrome or the manifestation of a lymphoma. Identification and treatment of such insulin resistance is described in Table 26.5.

4. Occasionally, the use of U-500 purified pork insulin may be advantageous, in lieu of a course of steroid therapy or if such therapy fails to decrease insulin volume requirements. Because of its concentration, U-500 insulin acts as a repository insulin due to the formation of insulin hexamers.

5. In general, immunologic resistance spontaneously remits in <1 yr, but durations up to 5 yr have been reported.

6. Approximately 40–50% of patients will have substantial decreases in insulin requirements when switched to purified pork or human insulin, and of the remainder, ~50% will benefit by a tapering course of high-dose glucocorticoid (initially 40–80 mg of prednisone daily) over 2–4 wk. Occasionally, dramatic decreases in insulin-dosage requirements are seen within days after the institution of such therapy, and thus hypoglycemia must be avoided.

SUGGESTED READING

1. Davidson JK, DeBra DW: Immunologic insulin resistance. *Diabetes* 27:307–18, 1978

2. DeShazo RD, Mather P, Grant W, Carrington D, Frentz JM, Lueg M, Lauritano AA, Falholt K: Evaluation of patients with local reactions to insulin with skin tests and in vitro techniques. *Diabetes Care* 10:330–36, 1987

3. Fineberg SE, Galloway JA, Finberg NS, Goldman J: Effect of species of origin, purification levels and formulation on insulin immunogenicity. *Diabetes* 32:592–99, 1983

4. Galloway J, DeShazo R: Insulin chemistry and pharmacology; insulin allergy, resistance, and lipoclystrophy In *Ellenberg and Rifkin's Diabetes Mellitus: Theory and Practice*. 4th ed. Rifkin H, Porte D, Eds. New York, Elsevier, 1990, p. 504–508

5. Weiler JM, Freiman P, Shanath MD, Metzger WJ, Smith JM, Richerson HB, Ballas ZK, Halverson PC, Shulau DJ, Matuso S, Wilson RL: Serious adverse reactions to protamine sulfate: are alternatives needed? *J Allergy Clin Immunol* 75:297–303, 1985

27. Drugs and Hormones That Increase Blood Glucose Levels

DAVID M. KAYNE, MD, and SHERMAN M. HOLVEY, MD

The short-term and long-term complications of hyperglycemia secondary to the treatment plan are significant risks that must be weighed against the benefits of any drug therapy. Few drugs are contraindicated for use in the diabetic patient, however, most require close glucose monitoring and appropriate adjustments of the patient's hypoglycemic regimen.

HORMONES

Hormones are used for various reasons in patients with diabetes. Table 27.1 lists the hormones that cause hyperglycemia. These hormones either increase gluconeogenesis, increase glycogenolysis, or decrease the peripheral sensitivity to the action of insulin.

Glucagon

Glucagon is used therapeutically to counteract symptomatic hypoglycemia. Glucagon acts primarily by activating adenylate cyclase on hepatocytes, which leads to increased glycogenolysis and gluconeogenesis and thus increased hepatic glucose release. Once 1–2 mg of glucagon is administered, the patient's blood glucose will increase within minutes. The effect is sustained for ~30 min.

Dr. Kayne is Clinical Faculty Member and Dr. Holvey is Associate Clinical Professor at the UCLA School of Medicine. Dr. Holvey is also Director of the Diabetes Management Center, Los Angeles, CA.

Table 27.1. HORMONES THAT CAUSE HYPERGLYCEMIA

- Glucagon
- Glucocorticoids
- Growth hormone
- Epinephrine
- Estrogen and progesterone (oral contraceptives)
- Thyroid preparations

Glucocorticoids

Regardless of the dose, site, or frequency of administration (i.e., even a single intra-articular steroid injection), glucocorticoids can lead to significant and sometimes severe hyperglycemia. If a glucocorticoid must be administered to a patient with diabetes, the patient's blood glucose should be monitored even more closely, and appropriate adjustments in diabetes treatment should be made.

Growth Hormone

Growth hormone is used illicitly by adolescents and athletes to increase lean muscle mass and experimentally in the elderly to increase and sustain muscle mass. When used for physiological replacement, growth hormone causes minimal changes in blood glucose. However, when used in supraphysiological dosages, growth hormone can lead to clinically significant hyperglycemia.

Epinephrine

Catecholamines lead to hyperglycemia by increasing glucagon secretion and by directly increasing glycogenolysis and gluconeogenesis at the hepatocyte level. Catechols can also elevate blood glucose by decreasing peripheral glucose uptake. Severe elevations in blood glucose have occurred in patients after intravenous administration of epinephrine (or its analogues) for hypotension or cardiac arrest. Although the benefits far outweigh the risks of these drugs in life-threatening situations, catecholamines can cause significant hyperglycemia.

Over-the-counter epinephrinelike analogues, such as decongestants, can also significantly elevate blood glucose. Although not contraindicated for use by people with diabetes, blood glucose should be monitored and treatment adjusted if necessary.

Oral Contraceptives

The effects of oral contraceptives on glucose metabolism in nondiabetic women are unclear. Patients with increased risk factors for diabetes (e.g., obesity) may be at greater risk for developing diabetes when on oral-contraceptive therapy. These steroids cause hyperglycemia through increased insulin resistance. Oral contraceptives are not contraindicated for use in women with diabetes. Women with diabetes risk factors (i.e., a history of gestational diabetes or impaired glucose tolerance) should have their blood glucose monitored while taking oral-contraceptive agents.

Thyroid Preparations

The mechanisms for hyperglycemia are not completely clear, but insulin resistance appears to be a component. A patient who is kept chemically euthyroid on a therapeutic regimen is unlikely to develop hyperglycemia.

DRUGS

Therapy with various drugs can lead to significant hyperglycemia. Table 27.2 lists the commonly used drugs that lead to elevations in blood glucose. The drugs that are most commonly associated with a decrease in glycemic control are antihypertensive agents.

Diuretics

Diuretics, particularly thiazides, are clearly associated with elevated blood glucose, especially in patients with diabetes or those who are prone to diabetes. The mechanism appears to be related to decreased insulin secretion secondary to associated hypokalemia and

Table 27.2. DRUGS THAT CAUSE HYPERGLYCEMIA

- Thiazide diuretics
- Furosemide
- Bumetanide
- Acetazolamide
- Indapamide
- Diazoxide
- β-Blockers
- α-Agonists
- Ca^{2+}-channel blockers
- Phenytoin
- Phenobarbital sodium
- Pentamidine isethionate
- Nicotinic acid
- Cyclophosphamide
- L-Asparaginase
- Epinephrinelike drugs (decongestants and diet pills)
- Nonsteroidal anti-inflammatory agents
- Nicotine
- Caffeine
- Sugar-containing syrups
- Fish oils

the development of insulin resistance. Other diuretics, e.g., furosemide, bumetanide, acetazolamide, and indapamide, have been reported to elevate blood glucose presumably secondary to hypokalemia. To avoid the hyperglycemic effects of diuretics, closely monitor the patient's blood glucose and electrolytes, and keep potassium replenished.

Diazoxide

This is a unique nonthiazide diuretic that has both antihypertensive activity and significant hyperglycemic activity. Its hyperglycemic effect is so profound that it is the drug of choice to control hypoglycemia caused by tumors producing insulinlike substances. Diazoxide acts by decreasing insulin release from islet cells. This drug has also been known to stimulate the release of endogenous catecholamines.

β-Blockers

These drugs can lead to mild elevations in blood glucose in diabetic patients. The mechanism is secondary to increased α-adrenergic–receptor–mediated hepatic glycogenolysis and/or decreased insulin secretion. Because the hyperglycemic effect of β-blockers is mild and can usually be compensated for by adjustment in the patient's regimen, they are not contraindicated in diabetic patients. However, β-blockers are not usually recommended for diabetic patients on hypoglycemic therapy because they can prevent the awareness of a hypoglycemic reaction and may cause dyslipidemia.

Phenytoin

Phenytoin causes significant hyperglycemia in diabetic patients. In diabetic patients, phenytoin is frequently used to help treat painful neuropathy. Phenytoin elevates blood glucose by inhibiting release of insulin from islet cells and thus hyperglycemia. Phenobarbital sodium has also been reported to cause hyperglycemia in diabetic patients. However, this drug has hyperglycemic effects only in patients on sulfonylurea agents. Phenobarbital sodium increases the hepatic metabolism of sulfonylureas, thus increasing drug clearance leading to elevations in blood glucose.

Nicotinic Acid

This is the drug of choice for first-line therapy of combined hyperlipidemia (i.e., increased cholesterol and triglycerides). Dyslipidemia, particularly hypertriglyceridemia, is a common problem in diabetic patients. Reduced glucose tolerance due to nicotinic acid therapy has been reported in nondiabetic patients, and frank deterioration in diabetes control has been reported in many patients with diabetes. The mechanism for the hyperglycemia is not completely clear, but insulin resistance has been hypothesized as the cause. Because of the deleterious effects of nicotinic acid on glycemic control, fibric acid derivatives (e.g., gemfibrozil) are often the drug of choice for combined hyperlipidemia in diabetic patients. Marine fatty acids (ω-3 fatty acids) found in fish oils cause deterioration of glycemic control when used in large doses to control hypertriglyceridemia in patients with established diabetes.

Pentamidine Isethionate

Pentamidine has often been used because of its effectiveness in treating *Pneumocystis carinii* infection in patients with autoimmune deficiency syndrome. Although clinically effective, pentamidine has many serious side effects, most notably, hypoglycemia secondary to pancreatitis resulting from direct toxicity to β-cells. Paradoxically, β-cells secrete excess amounts of insulin; however, as the cells become hypofunctional, hyperglycemia and diabetes can develop.

Cyclophosphamide and L-Asparaginase

Both of these drugs cause elevations in blood glucose, but their mechanism and clinical significance remain obscure.

NONPRESCRIPTION DRUGS

Many over-the-counter drugs can also lead to clinically significant hyperglycemia. Nonsteroidal anti-inflammatory agents elevate blood glucose, but their clinical significance is minimal. Other drugs to consider are the many sugar-containing cough and cold remedies. Nicotine and caffeine in large doses have also been implicated in hyperglycemia. Smoking should be discouraged in all people with diabetes, and caffeine consumption should be moderate.

SUGGESTED READING

1. Campbell K: Medications and treatment of diabetes. *Clin Diabetes* 3:109–18, 1988
2. Garg A, Grundy S: Nicotinic acid as therapy for dyslipidemia in non-insulin-dependent diabetes mellitus. *JAMA* 264:723–26, 1990
3. Gilman AG, Goodman L, Gilman A: *Goodman and Gilman's The Pharmacological Basis of Therapeutics*. 6th ed. New York, Macmillan, 1980
4. Spellacy W: Carbohydrate metabolism during treatment with estrogen, progestogen and low-dose oral contraceptives. *Am J Obstet Gynecol* 142:732–34, 1982
5. Struthers A, Murphy M, Dollery C: Glucose tolerance during antihypertension therapy in patients with diabetes mellitus. *Hypertension* 7 (Suppl. II):II-95–101, 1985

28. Dyslipidemia

YAAKOV HENKIN, MD, and ROBERT A. KREISBERG, MD

Lipoprotein abnormalities are common in diabetes and contribute significantly to its complications. The misconception that such abnormalities are always secondary to poor glycemic control focuses most of the attention on the management of hyperglycemia. As a result, the treatment of dyslipidemia is often neglected, despite convincing evidence linking it to the development of atherosclerosis. Lipoprotein abnormalities often precede the onset of diabetes mellitus by many years and persist despite achievement of euglycemia, particularly in type II (non-insulin-dependent) diabetes. They are often aggravated by the compounding effects of age, obesity, ethanol, antihypertensive drugs, diet, and separately inherited lipid disorders. Consequently, lipoprotein disorders in type II diabetes should be considered distinct entities. Lipid abnormalities associated with type I (insulin-dependent) diabetes also predispose to atherosclerosis, but in contrast to type II diabetes, these abnormalities can often be reversed by appropriate glycemic control.

The most common serum lipoprotein abnormality in type II diabetes is elevation of very-low-density lipoprotein (VLDL) levels, which is manifested as hypertriglyceridemia with mild hypercholesterolemia. High-density lipoprotein cholesterol (HDL-C) levels are often decreased. Low-density lipoprotein cholesterol (LDL-C) levels are usually normal or even decreased in type II diabetes, although structural abnormalities in LDL have been described that may increase its atherogenicity. Other structural abnormalities include glycosylation of apoproteins and an increased unesterified cholesterol fraction in VLDL. Because LDL levels are not usually

---

Dr. Henkin is Assistant Professor of Medicine and Dr. Kreisberg is Professor of Medicine and Vice-Chairman of the Department of Medicine at the University of Alabama at Birmingham School of Medicine, Birmingham, AL.

increased by diabetes mellitus, other contributing factors should be suspected in the presence of elevated LDL-C.

TREATMENT RATIONALE

The rationale for treating diabetic dyslipidemia is based on clinical evidence that reducing the concentrations of atherogenic lipoproteins will lead to a slower rate of progression, stabilization, or even reversal of atherosclerotic lesions. In nondiabetic subjects, every 1% decrease in total serum cholesterol is associated with a 2% decrease in coronary heart disease (CHD) mortality. For every 1% increase in HDL-C, there is a corresponding 2–3% decrease in CHD mortality. Although the atherogenicity of triglycerides (or of triglyceride-rich lipoproteins) in nondiabetic patients remains controversial, there is growing evidence of a probable role for VLDL and VLDL remnants in the progression of atherosclerosis, especially in women. This trend is more pronounced in diabetic patients, in whom hypertriglyceridemia is better correlated with cardiovascular disease. For patients with severe hypertriglyceridemia, other complications may ensue, including acute pancreatitis, hepatosplenomegaly, eruptive xanthomas, and the chylomicronemia syndrome.

The development of atherosclerosis is dependant on other risk factors in addition to dyslipidemia, the most important of which include genetic traits that predispose to atherosclerosis, smoking, hypertension, and obesity. Male sex is generally considered a risk factor for this disease. Diabetic women do not have the same protection as nondiabetic women, and their age-adjusted risk for development of CHD is similar to diabetic men. Because many of the risk factors are more common in type II diabetes than in the general population, and because diabetes itself is an independent risk factor for atherosclerosis, an aggressive approach to the detection and treatment of dyslipidemia is indicated.

EVALUATION OF DYSLIPIDEMIA IN TYPE II DIABETES

This should include a comprehensive history to assess the time of onset of these abnormalities, dietary habits, use of drugs that may adversely affect lipoprotein metabolism, smoking, and response to previous lipid-lowering treatments. Clinical evidence of coexisting cardiovascular disease or other manifestations of atherosclerosis should be carefully documented. Familial dyslipidemia may be suspected by an appropriate family history and the presence of xanthomas or xanthelasmas. Other infrequent signs of dyslipidemia include lipemia retinalis and eruptive xanthomas in severe hypertriglyceridemia and tuberoeruptive and palmar xanthomas in type III hyperlipidemia. Finally, it is essential to exclude secondary causes or aggravating factors for the lipoprotein changes, because these may often respond favorably to specific measures (Table 28.1).

Table 28.1. **CAUSES OF SECONDARY DYSLIPIDEMIA**

Hypercholesterol-emia	Hypertriglyceridemia	Low High-Density Lipoprotein Cholesterol
Hypothyroidism	Obesity	Obesity
Cholestasis	Kidney failure	Smoking
Nephrotic syndrome	Nephrotic syndrome	Sedentary life-style
Porphyria	Systemic lupus	Progestins
Dysproteinemia	erythematosus	Androgens
Progestins	Glycogen storage disease	β-Blockers
Corticosteroids	Thiazides	Retinoids
Thiazides	β-Blockers	
Cyclosporine	Estrogens	
	Corticosteroids	
	Retinoids	
	Alcohol	

Guidelines issued by the National Cholesterol Education Panel (NCEP) for the detection of dyslipidemia in the general adult population recommend the use of a nonfasting serum cholesterol level for screening purposes. This approach may be misleading in type II diabetes, because the most common lipoprotein abnormalities occur in the VLDL and HDL fractions. Thus, a complete lipoprotein profile, after a 12-h fast, should be obtained in every diabetic patient. Because some diversity may occur in lipid and lipoprotein measurements due to both laboratory and patient variations, at least two sets of lipoprotein profiles should be used to establish the initial diagnosis. Chylomicrons can be detected as a yellow cream layer at the top of the serum or plasma sample, placed overnight at 4°C. Complex cases may require more sophisticated laboratory techniques, e.g., ultracentrifugation and apoprotein measurements, to further characterize the abnormality.

The NCEP guidelines advocate treatment when LDL-C levels are >160 mg/dl (>4.2 mM) in individuals without other risk factors or >130 mg/dl (>3.4 mM) in the presence of CHD or two major risk factors (male sex, family history of premature CHD, smoking, hypertension, diabetes mellitus, decreased HDL-C, obesity, or evidence of cerebrovascular or peripheral vascular disease). Most dyslipidemic type II diabetic patients have sufficient risk factors to include them in the high-risk category. In addition, measurement of LDL-C may underestimate the true number of LDL particles in diabetic patients due to structural abnormalities in the LDL particle. Thus, even lower LDL-C values may require treatment in high-risk patients, especially in the presence of elevated VLDL-C and reduced HDL-C. Although no strict guidelines exist for other lipoproteins, triglyceride levels >200 mg/dl (>2.26 mM) and HDL-C levels <35 mg/dl (<0.91 mM) probably require treatment in diabetic patients, especially those at high risk.

APPROACH TO TREATMENT

General Measures

Although improved glucose control infrequently normalizes lipoprotein abnormalities, it can be associated with marked improvement in the lipoprotein profile. Despite previous suggestion of a deleterious effect on HDL-C levels, most data show that sulfonylureas do not adversely affect lipoprotein metabolism and may often improve preexisting lipoprotein abnormalities. The use of biguanides often results in reduction of the total cholesterol, VLDL-C, and triglycerides. Insulin therapy in type II diabetes may similarly reduce the serum triglycerides and VLDL-C, with a concomitant increase in HDL-C, but normalization of lipid levels is unusual because of the continued presence of other uncorrected factors. However, normalization of serum lipids is often seen in nonobese type II diabetic patients.

Great emphasis must be placed on smoking cessation and increased level of exercise; this will not only eliminate two independent risk factors for atherosclerosis but may also be accompanied by modest increases in HDL-C. Weight loss may favorably influence lipoprotein metabolism in addition to improving glucose tolerance and blood-pressure control. Weight loss is often accompanied by lowering of serum triglycerides, VLDL-C, and LDL-C; increases in HDL-C may accompany these changes. Beneficial lipoprotein changes often appear soon after initiation of a low-calorie diet, even before achievement of a considerable weight loss (Fig. 28.1).

Specific Diets

Dietary modifications are the cornerstone of dyslipidemia management (Table 28.2). The traditional American (United States) diet contains ~450 mg/day cholesterol, with 35–40% of the calories derived from fat (14% of which is from saturated fat). Dietary cholesterol and most saturated fats suppress LDL-receptor activity, thereby reducing LDL clearance from the blood. Replacement of saturated fats with complex carbohydrates, polyunsaturated fats, and monounsaturated fats is beneficial in reducing total cholesterol and LDL-C levels. Current recommendations are: limitation of cholesterol intake to <300 mg/day, fat to <30% of total calories, saturated fats to <10% of total calories, and the remainder of fat calories equally divided between polyunsaturated and monounsaturated. This Step 1 Diet (NCEP) is identical to the diet recommended by the American Diabetes Association. If a desirable response is not achieved within 3 mo, a stricter Step 2 Diet may be used, in which saturated fat is limited to 7% of the daily calories and the daily cholesterol limited to 200 mg.

In both diets, saturated fat is largely replaced by carbohydrate, which constitutes 50–60% of the total calories. However, concern has been expressed that high-carbohydrate diets may increase the

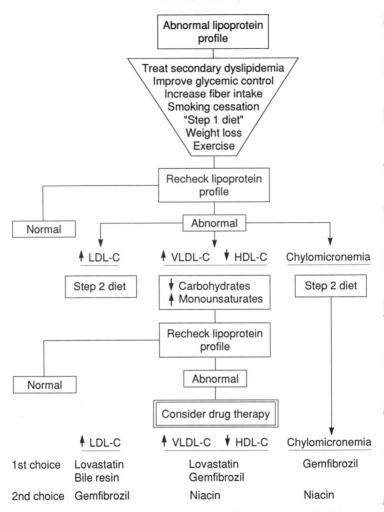

Figure 28.1. Algorithm for treatment of dyslipidemia in type II diabetes.

serum triglyceride and VLDL-C levels in susceptible individuals, especially in the presence of a low fiber intake. Thus, the NCEP offers diabetic patients an alternative diet consisting of a lower carbohydrate intake (40–45% of total calories). Excess amounts of polyunsaturated fats, while having an independent effect on lowering LDL, may also further reduce HDL-C levels. In contrast, monounsaturated fat (present in high concentrations in olive and peanut oils) has been shown to reduce LDL-C without decreasing HDL-C. Consequently, diets lower in carbohydrates and rich in monounsaturated fatty acids may result in better glycemic control, reduced triglyceride and VLDL-C levels, and higher HDL-C levels.

Table 28.2. EFFECT OF DIETARY MODIFICATION IN TYPE II DIABETES

Treatment	Lipoprotein Effects			Effect on Glucose Levels
	LDL	VLDL	HDL	
Weight reduction	↓	↓	0 ↑	↓
High-carbohydrate diet	0	0 ↑	0 ↓	0 ↓
Polyunsaturated fatty acids	↓	↓	↓	0
Monounsaturated fatty acids	↓	↓	0	0
ω-3 Fatty acids	0 ↑	↓	0	↑
Fiber	↓	↓	0	↓

LDL, low-density lipoprotein; VLDL, very-low-density lipoprotein; HDL, high-density lipoprotein. ↑, Increase; ↓, decrease; 0, unchanged.

Although the advisability and practicality of such diets are still debated, they may prove useful in type II diabetic patients with high serum triglycerides and/or low HDL-C levels.

High-fiber diets have been advocated for dyslipidemic patients. Soluble fibers can decrease LDL-C by 5–10% and reduce serum triglyceride and VLDL-C, although high quantities (15–20 g/day), which are often poorly tolerated, are required for such effects. Addition of fiber to high-carbohydrate diets may also improve glycemic control and should be recommended for diabetic patients. However, caution should be exercised in advocating high-fiber diets in the presence of autonomic gastropathy.

The ω-3 polyunsaturated fatty acids, eicosapentanoic acid (20:5), and docosahexanoic acid (22:6) are present in high concentrations in fish oil. At doses of 5–20 g/day, they have a dose-dependant triglyceride-lowering effect in hypertriglyceridemic individuals. Other potentially beneficial effects include decreased platelet adhesiveness, inhibition of eicosanoid formation, and reduction of blood pressure. Epidemiological data and some clinical trials in patients with CHD suggest that diets rich in these fatty acids can be associated with lower CHD mortality. Unfortunately, the use of high dose ω-3 fatty acids in type II diabetes has been shown to have an adverse effect on glycemic control. In addition, LDL-C and LDL apolipoprotein B (apoB) levels may paradoxically increase in hypertriglyceridemic patients treated with these agents. Therefore, until further data on their overall effects in type II diabetes accumulate, their use in high doses in these patients is not recommended.

Drug Therapy

Patients who do not respond appropriately to dietary and other nonpharmacological modifications after 3–6 mo should be initiated on drug therapy. Clinical trials in nondiabetic subjects suggest that long-term treatment of dyslipidemic subjects with nicotinic acid, bile-acid resins, or gemfibrozil can reduce the incidence of cardiovascular morbidity and mortality. Although no such studies have yet been conducted in diabetic patients, such treatments would probably be beneficial.

Hypolipidemic drugs can be categorized as those used primarily to lower LDL levels and those used primarily to lower VLDL levels, although some overlap exists (Table 28.3). Consideration should also be given to the HDL modifying effect of each drug. Bile acid sequestrants and nicotinic acid were advocated as the drugs of choice by the NCEP Adult Treatment Panel, because both have been shown to reduce cardiovascular morbidity and mortality in nondiabetic subjects and have an established record of safe clinical use. However, the efficacy and side effects of these drugs differ in diabetic patients, and modification of the NCEP guidelines in type II diabetes seems appropriate.

Nicotinic Acid. The vitamin niacin (nicotinic acid), in pharmacological doses, decreases serum triglycerides by lowering the concentrations of VLDL and intermediate-density lipoprotein (IDL). LDL-C may also decrease, although somewhat less effectively, and HDL-C usually increases. Although the exact mechanisms by which niacin affects lipoprotein metabolism remain uncertain, it is believed to decrease hepatic VLDL production by inhibition of fatty acid release from adipose tissue, reduction of hepatic triglyceride synthesis, and promotion of lipoprotein lipase activity. These versatile features theoretically make niacin the ideal drug for dyslipidemic diabetic patients.

Unfortunately, niacin has a considerable number of side effects, and its successful use requires a combination of physician skill and patient motivation. Prostaglandin-induced cutaneous flushing is the most common side effect; this can be partly ameliorated by initiating therapy with a low dose, premedication with aspirin, ingestion of the drug with food, and avoidance of concomitant hot drinks and alcoholic beverages. Gastrointestinal disturbances and abnormalities in liver function are less common, although their incidence increases with sustained-release preparations. Of greater concern in diabetes is niacin's tendency to worsen glycemic control in some patients by increasing insulin resistance. In addition, the development or aggravation of hyperuricemia may precipitate gout, a problem already more common in obese diabetic individuals. Thus, although niacin may prove useful in selected diabetic patients, its use requires caution and careful monitoring of the serum glucose and uric acid levels. Because insulin itself is believed to promote the risk of atherosclerosis, increasing the dosage to control hyperglycemia may be inadvisable, making niacin inappropriate as a first-choice drug in diabetic dyslipidemia.

Bile Acid Sequestrants. Cholestyramine and colestipol are insoluble powders (resins) that bind bile acids in the gastrointestinal tract, thus interrupting their enterohepatic circulation. Consequently, hepatic conversion of cholesterol to bile acids increases, resulting in depletion of hepatic cholesterol and stimulation of LDL receptor synthesis and expression. This results in a reduction of serum

LDL-C, making the resins useful in the treatment of isolated hyper-cholesterolemia. However, hepatocyte VLDL production usually increases, resulting in hypertriglyceridemia. Although this elevation is relatively minor in normotriglyceridemic patients, it is more prominent in patients with borderline or established hypertriglyceridemia, making the drug unsuitable for many diabetic patients.

Bile acid resins are not absorbed from the gastrointestinal tract, and systemic adverse effects are rare. However, gastrointestinal side effects are often disturbing and may be accentuated in diabetic patients with autonomic visceral neuropathy. Side effects may be reduced by initiating treatment at low doses, a high fiber intake, and administration of a stool softener during the initial phases of therapy. Bile acid resins also interfere with the absorption of drugs such as digitalis, β-blockers, thiazide diuretics, warfarin, and L-thyroxine. To prevent reduced bioavailability of these and possibly other drugs, they should not be taken 1 h before or 3 h after the resin. This may cause inconvenience for diabetic patients who require multiple drugs for concomitant diseases.

Fibric Acid Derivatives. Fibric acid derivatives constitute a class of drugs with potent triglyceride-lowering properties. Gemfibrozil and clofibrate are the only drugs of this class available for prescription use in the U.S. and Canada, whereas bezafibrate, fenofibrate, and ciprofibrate are widely used in Europe. Their major mechanism of action seems to be mediated by an increase in lipoprotein lipase activity, although decreased hepatic VLDL synthesis and enhanced LDL catabolism may also occur by unknown mechanisms. HDL-C often increases concomitant with the triglyceride reduction. Although LDL-C often decreases in normotriglyceridemic patients, it usually increases in patients with hypertriglyceridemia.

Use of gemfibrozil has been associated with reduced cardiovascular mortality, especially in patients with elevated serum triglycerides (types IIb, hypertriglyceridemia, increased LDL-C and decreased HDL-C; and type IV, hypertriglyceridemia). In type II diabetes, gemfibrozil reduces triglyceride and increases HDL-C levels, the magnitude of this HDL effect being inversely proportional to its initial concentration. However, concomitant elevations in LDL-C and LDL-apoB may attenuate these beneficial effects.

The most common side effects of gemfibrozil are gastrointestinal. Elevated liver enzymes and creatinine phosphokinase (CPK) levels are infrequent but deserve monitoring. Although gemfibrozil increases bile lithogenicity, the clinical significance of this action is uncertain. Gemfibrozil is approved by the Food and Drug Administration for treatment of patients with hypertriglyceridemia (type IV) or combined hyperlipidemia (type IIb). Because its ability to reduce LDL-C is modest, it is not a drug of choice for treatment of isolated hypercholesterolemia.

HMG-CoA Reductase Inhibitors. This new class of drugs reduces hepatic cholesterol synthesis by competitive inhibition of the rate-limiting enzyme HMG-CoA reductase. Reduction of hepatocyte cholesterol content stimulates the synthesis of LDL receptors, with

Table 28.3. DRUGS USED FOR TREATMENT OF DYSLIPIDEMIA

Drug	Daily Dose	Lipoprotein Effects (%)			Major Side Effects	Effect on Glucose Levels	Other Considerations in Diabetes
		LDL	VLDL	HDL			
Niacin	1–6 g	↓ 10–40	↓ 20–50	↑ 10–30	Flushing, itching, rash Gastrointestinal symptoms* Aggravation of duodenal ulcer Hepatotoxicity Macular edema	↑	May precipitate gout
Cholestyramine Colestipol	8–32 g 10–40 g	↓ 15–35	↑ 5–30	0↑ 5–10	Gastrointestinal symptoms*	0	May aggravate hypertriglyceridemia May interfere with drug absorption
Gemfibrozil	0.6–1.2 g	variable ↓	↓ 30–50	↑ 5–15	Gastrointestinal symptoms* Hepatoxicity	0↓	Elevates LDL-C in hypertriglyceridemic individuals

Drug	Dose					Side effects	Comments
						Myopathy Bone marrow depression	May increase bile lithogenicity
Lovastatin	10–80 mg	↓ 20–40	0↓ 10–30	0↑ 5–10	0	Gastrointestinal symptoms* Headache Hepatotoxicity Myopathy	
Probucol	500–1000 mg	↓ 8–15		↓ 15–35	0	Gastrointestinal symptoms* QT prolongation	May inhibit LDL oxidation and foam cell production Decreases "toxicity" of diabetic VLDL
Conjugated estrogens	0.625 mg	↓ 10–30	↑ variable	↑ 20–40	0↑		May aggravate hypertriglyceridemia

LDL, low density lipoprotein; VLDL, very-low-density lipoprotein; HDL, high-density lipoprotein. ↑, Increase; ↓, decrease; 0, unchanged.
*Abdominal pain, flatulence, diarrhea, constipation, etc.

consequent increased clearance of LDL and IDL from the blood. Lovastatin is currently in clinical use in the U.S., whereas other HMG-CoA reductase inhibitors (pravastatin, simvastatin) await approval. Clinical experience with lovastatin in diabetic patients has demonstrated dose-dependent reductions in serum LDL-C, LDL-apoB, VLDL-C, and triglycerides that are similar to those of non-diabetic patients; although HDL-C levels are not consistently affected, they may increase by 5–10%. The drug has no effect on glycemic control.

Lovastatin is extremely well tolerated in most patients. Its most worrisome side effect is elevation of serum CPK levels, with clinically significant myopathy occurring in ~0.5% of treated patients. The frequency of myopathy increases with concomitant use of gemfibrozil, niacin, cyclosporine, and erythromycin, and life-threatening rhabdomyolysis has been documented. Thus, patients should be warned to report any muscle weakness, soreness, or tenderness. In addition, elevations of liver function tests can occur with lovastatin use and should be monitored. Despite this, its overall efficacy and safety in type II diabetes shows great promise. In view of the problems associated with niacin and the resins, some investigators consider lovastatin to be the first-choice drug in dyslipidemic diabetic patients.

Probucol. Probucol is a highly lipophilic compound that is slowly and incompletely absorbed from the intestines. Its onset of action is slow, and several months are required to reach steady plasma levels. Being stored in adipose tissue, probucol is slowly released into the blood after therapy is discontinued, and several months are required for its effects to resolve.

Probucol has a modest LDL-C–lowering effect, due to increased LDL clearance through non–receptor-mediated pathways. Unfortunately, HDL-C levels are decreased to a greater degree, due to suppression of apoAI and apoAII synthesis. This effect is accentuated in diabetic patients who already have low HDL-C levels, making probucol treatment theoretically undesirable. On the other hand, probucol has been shown to cause regression of xanthomas in some hypercholesterolemic patients, suggesting that other mechanisms may promote its antiatherogenic effects, e.g., inhibition of LDL oxidation.

Drug Combinations. Patients with severe dyslipidemia and high cardiovascular-risk profiles, especially those with concomitant CHD, may benefit from use of combinations of hypolipidemic drugs that have different mechanisms of action. Combinations provide increased potency at lower doses and, consequently, fewer side effects. Bile acid resins are especially useful in combination with niacin, fibrates, or lovastatin; these combinations may also block the development of hypertriglyceridemia usually observed with the resins. The use of lovastatin with niacin or gemfibrozil has theoretical advantages but should be used only in carefully selected patients because of reports of increased frequency of myopathy and rhabdomyolysis with these combinations.

SPECIAL CONSIDERATIONS

Type I Diabetes

Most nonobese type I diabetic patients who are maintained at good glycemic control have normal or even better-than-normal lipoprotein profiles. This delicate balance disappears with the development of diabetic nephropathy as reflected by microalbuminuria, when abnormalities in VLDL, LDL, and HDL metabolism appear. The principles of nonpharmacological therapy in type I diabetes are similar to those in type II diabetes. Although little clinical experience exists with the pharmacological treatment of lipoprotein disorders in type I diabetes, there seems to be no reason to adopt an approach that is different from that in nondiabetic individuals.

Chylomicronemia Syndrome

Diabetic patients occasionally present with marked elevations of both VLDL and chylomicrons, resulting in severe hypertriglyceridemia. When this occurs in poorly controlled type I diabetic patients, especially in the context of ketoacidosis, the abnormalities can usually be corrected by intensive insulin therapy. In type II diabetes, these abnormalities often arise when diabetes is superimposed on a second genetic form or other secondary causes of hypertriglyceridemia (Table 28.1). Triglyceride levels >1000 mg/dl (>11.3 mM) pose a risk of acute pancreatitis. Other symptoms may include lethargy, memory loss, paresthesias, and arthralgia. Eruptive xanthomas, lipemia retinalis, hepatosplenomegaly, or lymphadenopathy may be seen on physical examination.

Prompt reduction of the serum triglycerides is mandatory in such cases. When accompanied by poor glycemic control, improvement in the latter and institution of very-low-fat diets may reduce chylomicron production. If these measures are inadequate, fibric acid derivatives are usually effective in reducing the serum triglycerides to a safe range. Niacin may be tried in cases where fibric acid derivatives are contraindicated.

Diabetic Nephropathy

In nephrosis, both hepatic overproduction of apoB-containing lipoproteins and reduced lipoprotein lipase activity are responsible for elevations in VLDL and LDL levels. In chronic kidney failure, reduced lipoprotein lipase and hepatic lipase activities are the predominant abnormalities, leading to increased VLDL and IDL and reduced HDL levels. When these abnormalities coexist with diabetes mellitus, the dyslipidemia may be accentuated.

Dietary treatment of dyslipidemia must often be modified in the presence of kidney disease because of constraints on protein intake. Furthermore, these patients may often be unresponsive to low-fat diets.

The pharmacological management of dyslipidemia in diabetic kidney disease has not been sufficiently evaluated. Fibric acid derivatives are excreted predominantly by the kidneys, and an increased risk of myopathy and rhabdomyolysis has been observed with the use of clofibrate in kidney failure. Although other fibric acid derivatives may be safer, their use in kidney failure warrants caution. Lovastatin is excreted primarily by the liver and is safe and effective in nephrotic patients. However, its use in diabetic nephropathy warrants further study.

Pregnancy

Because pregnancy alone is often associated with elevations in all of the lipoprotein fractions, it may aggravate the dyslipidemia in diabetic women. Nonpharmacological management of such lipoprotein abnormalities should remain the primary treatment in pregnant women, because the safety of hypolipidemic drugs in this situation is unknown. When severe hypertriglyceridemia cannot be controlled by such means, the use of fish oils may be tried while closely monitoring glycemic control.

SUGGESTED READING

1. Axelrod L: Omega-3 fatty acids in diabetes mellitus: a gift from the sea? *Diabetes* 38:539–43, 1989
2. Garg A, Bonanome A, Grundy SM, Zhang Z-J, Unger RH: Comparison of a high-carbohydrate diet with a high-monounsaturated-fat diet in patients with non-insulin-dependent diabetes mellitus. *N Engl J Med* 319:829–34, 1988
3. Garg A, Grundy SM: Management of dyslipidemia in NIDDM. *Diabetes Care* 13:153–69, 1990
4. Howard BV: Lipoprotein metabolism in diabetes mellitus. *J Lipid Res* 28:613–28, 1987
5. Reaven GM: Abnormal lipoprotein metabolism in non-insulin-dependent diabetes mellitus. *Am J Med* 83 (Suppl. 3A):31–38, 1987

29. Antihypertensive Therapy

JAMES R. SOWERS, MD

An estimated 2.5 million Americans have both clinical diabetes mellitus and hypertension. The prevalence of hypertension in diabetic patients increases with age. The coexisting conditions occur more frequently in men than in women before age 50 yr and more frequently in women thereafter. The prevalence of hypertension and diabetes is almost twice as great in blacks as in whites, and both conditions are more common among the socioeconomically disadvantaged. In addition to age, race, sex, and greater body mass, a longer duration of diabetes and the presence of persistent proteinuria are important determinants of hypertension.

The risk of cardiovascular disease is strikingly increased by the coexistence of hypertension and diabetes. In fact, the risk of cardiovascular death in diabetic individuals is approximately doubled in the presence of hypertension. Strokes and transient ischemic events are more frequent in these patients than normotensive diabetic individuals. Peripheral vascular disease is also increased by the coexistence of hypertension and diabetes. Both diabetes and hypertension are independent risk factors for accelerated atherosclerosis.

Hypertension in patients with diabetes is also associated with acceleration of diabetic retinopathy: a relationship exists between diastolic and systolic blood pressures and background and proliferative diabetic retinopathy. Furthermore, the progression of diabetic retinopathy is slowed with effective treatment of hypertension.

Dr. Sowers is Professor of Medicine, Physiology, and Nutrition and Director of the Division of Endocrinology and Hypertension at Wayne State University, Detroit, MI.

PATHOPHYSIOLOGY

An understanding of the pathogenesis of hypertension in the diabetic patient and of the pharmacological effects of antihypertensive drugs in these individuals will help clinicians make rational therapeutic choices. The two consistent hallmarks of hypertension in the diabetic individual are increased vascular resistance and expanded plasma volume.

Increased peripheral vascular resistance and enhanced vascular contractility responses to agonists such as angiotensin II and norepinephrine appear to be the hallmark of the diabetic hypertensive state. Exaggerated pressor responses to both agonists have also been observed in normotensive and slightly hypertensive uncomplicated diabetic patients, indicating that enhanced vascular reactivity plays a key role in the development of hypertension in patients with diabetes mellitus.

Hyperinsulinemia could theoretically increase renal tubular Na^+ reabsorption and may therefore account for increases in exchangeable sodium and volume expansion. Thus, hyperinsulinemia could be a common factor in the hypertension associated with type II (non-insulin-dependent) diabetes and that associated with obesity.

FACTORS CONTRIBUTING TO ACCELERATED ATHEROSCLEROSIS

Hyperinsulinemia may accelerate the development of atherosclerosis. It is associated with disorders of carbohydrate tolerance (e.g., essential hypertension and type II diabetes) and could accelerate atherogenesis directly and by promoting hypertension (Fig. 29.1).

The hyperinsulinemia and insulin resistance associated with essential hypertension appear to be strongly linked to body-fat distribution. Upper-body (central or android) obesity is much more strongly linked to hypertension, hyperlipidemia, diabetes, and cardiovascular risk than is lower-body (peripheral or gynecoid) obesity.

PATIENT EVALUATION

1. Diabetic patients are prone to lability in blood pressure; thus, multiple readings should be obtained over several weeks.
2. Once hypertension is satisfactorily documented, a thorough history and physical examination should be performed to assess end-organ damage and to identify secondary causes of coexistent hypertension and diabetes, e.g., primary aldosteronism, pheochromocytoma, Cushing's disease, acromegaly, and hyperthyroidism.
3. Renovascular disease is associated with the atherosclerotic process. Initial laboratory evaluation is important to assess the metabolic status of these patients before and after antihypertensive therapy (Table 29.1).

GENETIC FACTORS	ENVIRONMENTAL FACTORS
1. Cellular cation abnormalities (e.g., altered intracellular Ca^{2+} metabolism) 2. Obesity (central or android)	1. Drugs (e.g., diuretics, β-blockers) 2. Obesity (central or android) 3. Inactivity 4. Aging 5. Pregnancy/oral contraceptives 6. Stress (elevated glucocorticoids, catecholamines, and growth hormone)

↓

Insulin resistance/hyperinsulinemia

↓

Altered Ca^{2+} metabolism

↓

3. Peripheral vascular resistance	⟶	Accelerated atherosclerosis (cardiovascular disease)	⟵	7. Dyslipidemia

Figure 29.1. Insulin resistance/hyperinsulinemia as nexus between genetic/environmental factors contributing to development of hypertension, dyslipidemia, and accelerated atherosclerosis.

NONPHARMACOLOGICAL THERAPY

1. Because of the strong connections between obesity, hypertension, insulin resistance and dyslipidemia, weight reduction is generally the most important nonpharmacological approach to the treatment of many hypertensive patients with diabetes mellitus.
2. Exercise and restriction of alcohol consumption are nonpharmacological approaches to treating hypertensive diabetic patients. Exercise should be supervised by health-care professionals, because many of these patients will have underlying, perhaps asymptomatic, ischemic heart disease.
3. Because cigarette smoking is a major risk factor for ischemic heart disease, people with diabetes and hypertension should be encouraged to quit.
4. Salt restriction is generally useful in hypertensive diabetic patients because they are usually salt sensitive.

PHARMACOLOGICAL THERAPY

General Considerations

Many patients with diabetes and hypertension will require pharmacological intervention either because of noncompliance with non-

Table 29.1. **INITIAL EVALUATION**

- Complete history and physical examination
- Laboratory workup
- Complete blood count
- Serum creatinine and blood urea nitrogen
- Urinalysis
- Serum electrolytes
- Serum Mg^{2+}
- Serum uric acid
- Fasting cholesterol, high-density lipoprotein, and triglycerides
- 24-h urine sample for total protein and creatinine clearance
- ECG
- Chest X ray

pharmacological modalities or because their hypertension cannot be adequately controlled with this approach. If antihypertensive drug therapy is required, it is still important to adhere to the non-pharmacological approaches to minimize drug requirements. For example, moderate salt restriction should decrease diuretic-associated losses of potassium in the urine. Also, the utilization of patient self-monitoring of blood pressure and serum glucose will reinforce self-care. Self-monitoring increases the success in maintenance of life-style changes (e.g., weight loss) that will potentially improve the control of both hypertension and the glycemic state.

Therapeutic Goals

Appropriate blood-pressure levels in diabetic hypertensive patients have not yet been determined. However, considering the additive impact of hypertension and diabetes as cardiovascular risk factors, it appears prudent to reduce systolic and diastolic pressures to the degree recommended for nondiabetic hypertensive subjects.

Thiazide diuretics, α-adrenergic–blocking agents, angiotensin-converting enzyme (ACE) inhibitors, or Ca^{2+}-channel blockers may all be suitable for initial therapy in these patients. However, there are several factors that need to be considered (Fig. 29.2).

Adverse Effects

Adverse effects associated with antihypertensive therapy are more often observed in hypertensive diabetic patients. These patients respond with reduced baroreceptor sensitivity and a tendency to orthostatic hypotension. Accordingly, to prevent inappropriate orthostatic reduction of blood pressure with antihypertensive drug therapy, blood pressures should be monitored immediately on standing, after 1 min in the upright position, and after walking, particularly if the patient is experiencing symptoms suggestive of orthostatic hypotension. When these symptoms are present, standing blood pressure should be considered the therapeutic end point.

NONPHARMACOLOGICAL THERAPY

- Weight reduction toward ideal body weight
- Salt restriction to as close to 2 g/day as possible
- Diet adequate in fiber, K, and Ca
- Smoking cessation
- Limited daily alcohol intake to <2 oz
- Aerobic exercise

If blood pressure is controlled at <140/90 mmHg, continue on nonpharmacological program

If blood pressure is not controlled at <140/90 mmHg, add pharmacological regimen

↓

FIRST-LINE AGENTS: alone or in combination
- Ca^{2+} antagonists
- α-Blockers
- Angiotensin-converting enzyme inhibitors
- β-Blockers if postmyocardial infarction

If not controlled on combination of first-line drugs, use second-line drugs

↓

SECOND-LINE AGENTS
- Diuretics, small doses
- Central-acting agents (e.g., clonidine)
- Labetalol

Figure 29.2. Antihypertensive therapy for hypertensive diabetic patients.

Knowledge of the adverse effects of antihypertensive drugs in the hypertensive diabetic population is important to minimize the effects and optimize compliance. This is especially important with regard to combination therapy. Better blood-pressure control is often achieved by adding a second drug to small or moderate doses of the first drug rather than proceeding to maximum doses of the first drug. Smaller doses of several drugs with different pharmacological actions often produce fewer side effects than maximum doses of any one drug. In some patients, a reduction in drug dosage or elimination of the particular drug therapy may be possible after ≥6 mo of drug treatment.

Thiazide Diuretics

Thiazide diuretics are effective antihypertensive agents in diabetic patients with hypertension. However, they can induce various metabolic abnormalities, e.g., hypokalemia, hypomagnesemia, hyper-

Table 29.2. ADVANTAGES AND DISADVANTAGES OF FIRST- AND SECOND-LINE ANTIHYPERTENSIVE DRUGS

Class of Drug	Advantages	Disadvantages
Ca^{2+} antagonists	1. Maintain and may improve organ blood flow 2. Have no clinically significant effects on glucose or lipid metabolism 3. May reduce proteinuria (diltiazem and nicardipine)	1. Minimal 2. Verapamil and diltiazem should be avoided in patients with heart failure or significant blocks
Peripheral α-adrenergic blockers	1. Maintain and may improve organ blood flow 2. May improve insulin sensitivity and increase high-density lipoprotein cholesterol (prazosin and doxazosin)	1. May be associated with orthostatic hypotension, particularly in the initial period
Angiotensin-converting enzyme inhibitors	1. Maintain and may improve organ blood flow 2. May improve insulin sensitivity (captopril) 3. May reduce proteinuria	1. May cause hyperkalemia and renal-function deterioration with renal artery stenosis

β-Blockers	1. Drugs of choice for postmyocardial infarction (those without intrinsic sympathomimetic activity)	1. May further compromise peripheral blood flow 2. May worsen insulin resistance and promote dislipidemia
Diuretics	1. In low doses, may be useful as second-line drugs in difficult-to-control hypertensives; appears to be synergistic with ACE inhibitors	1. May increase insulin resistance and worsen dyslipidemia
Central-acting α-antagonists (e.g., clonidine)	1. Often effective (particularly the transdermal preparation of clonidine in the hypertensive not controlled with first-line agents) 2. Maintain or improve organ blood flow 3. No adverse effects on glucose or lipid metabolism	1. May be associated with orthostatic hypotension and CNS side effects
Labetalol	1. Maintains organ blood flow 2. No adverse effects on glucose or lipid metabolism	1. May be associated with orthostatic hypotension

uricemia, hypercalcemia, insulin resistance, and dyslipidemia. Reductions in serum K^+ and Mg^{2+} levels can alter glucose and lipid metabolism and may cause arrhythmias and increase peripheral vascular resistance. Most of the metabolic effects of thiazides are dose-related and can be negated by using low-dose therapy. However, one side effect not clearly dose related is the elevation in low-density lipoprotein cholesterol. In general, in hypertensive diabetic patients with multiple preexisting cardiovascular risk factors, therapy that adversely affects the lipid profile and carbohydrate tolerance should be avoided (Table 29.2).

β-Blockers

β-Blockers may be appropriate first-line therapy in some hypertensive diabetic patients. For example, young patients without complications and with relatively rapid pulse rates may respond well to these agents. Also, β-blockers may be useful in patients with angina who do not have heart failure. However, there are special problems associated with the use of β-blockers in the diabetic population. Because insulin secretion is mediated partly through the stimulation of $β_2$-adrenoreceptors, glycemic control can be compromised in hypertensive type II diabetic patients placed on noncardioselective agents. Even cardioselective β-blockers can potentially inhibit $β_2$-mediated insulin secretion when administered in the doses often required for treatment of hypertension. Furthermore, $β_2$-blockade during hypoglycemia may cause hypoglycemic unawareness and delay the physiological correction of hypoglycemia. Symptoms of hypoglycemia, e.g., tachycardia, tremor, and anxiety, are often diminished. Because glucagon and catecholamines mediate glycogenolysis via stimulation of $β_2$-receptors in both muscle and liver tissues, correction of hypoglycemia may be impaired (Table 29.2).

Cardioselective and nonselective β-blockers increase triglycerides and decrease high-density lipoprotein levels. Nonselective β-blockers can impair β-mediated vascular smooth muscle dilation and cause exacerbation of occult peripheral vascular disease.

Ca²⁺-Channel Blockers and ACE Inhibitors

Both Ca^{2+}-channel blockers and ACE inhibitors are often useful antihypertensive agents in patients with diabetes and hypertension, because they generally are not associated with adverse metabolic side effects. Neither class of drugs causes insulin resistance or dyslipidemia. These agents generally improve blood flow to the kidneys and other vital organs, which may be important in diabetic patients. These agents have a relatively low risk of causing sexual dysfunction—an important consideration in diabetic patients. Ca^{2+}-channel blockers are often useful in diabetic hypertensive patients who have concomitant angina. ACE inhibitors may be particularly salutary in patients with early diabetic nephropathy (proteinuria and glomerular hyperfiltration).

α-Adrenergic Blockers

Peripheral α-adrenergic–blocking agents, e.g., prazosin and dox-azosin, are also useful antihypertensive agents in hypertensive diabetic patients. These drugs do not adversely affect insulin action or lipid metabolism and do not generally cause sexual dysfunction. α-Blockers also tend to improve blood flow to vital organs. Occasionally, fluid retention occurs with use of these agents, which may necessitate concomitant administration of low-dose diuretics (Table 29.2).

SUGGESTED READING

1. Jarrett RJ: Hypertension in diabetic patients and differences between insulin-dependent diabetes mellitus and non-insulin-dependent diabetes mellitus. *Am J Kidney Dis* 13:14-16, 1989
2. Sowers JR: Relationship between hypertension and subtle and overt abnormalities of carbohydrate metabolism. *J Am Soc Nephrol* 1:539-47, 1990
3. Sowers JR, Levy J, Zemel MB: Hypertension and diabetes. *Med Clin North Am* 72:1399–414, 1988
4. Sowers JR, Zemel MB: Clinical implications of hypertension in the diabetic patient. *Am J Hypertens* 3:415-24, 1990
5. The Working Group on Hypertension in Diabetes: Statement on hypertension in diabetes mellitus: final report. *Arch Intern Med* 147:830-42, 1987

30. Skin and Subcutaneous Tissues

JEAN L. BOLOGNIA, MD, and IRWIN M. BRAVERMAN, MD

The cutaneous disorders discussed in this chapter are waxy skin and stiff joints, scleredema, diabetic dermopathy, necrobiosis lipoidica diabeticorum (NLD), disseminated granuloma annulare, eruptive xanthomas, lipodystrophy, acanthosis nigricans, diabetic bullae, necrolytic migratory erythema (NME; glucagonoma syndrome), and reactions to oral hypoglycemic drugs and insulin. Cutaneous infections, e.g., candidiasis and mucormycosis, and lower-extremity ulcerations are covered elsewhere (see chapts. 31 and 49).

PATHOPHYSIOLOGY

The underlying pathophysiology is theoretical in most of the cutaneous disorders associated with diabetes mellitus. In the skin lesions of NLD and diabetic dermopathy, there is histological evidence of microangiopathy, and this presumably plays a role in the formation of these lesions. In waxy skin associated with stiff joints, the thickened dermis may be the result of an increase in glycosylated insoluble collagen. The epidermal hyperplasia seen in lesions of acanthosis nigricans is thought to result from the action of insulin on growth factor receptors, whereas the epidermal necrosis seen in NME may be a reflection of glucagon-induced hypoaminoacidemia. Hypertriglyceridemia and eruptive xanthomas are presumably due to the effects of hypoinsulinemia on lipid metabolism in that they quickly resolve after insulin administration.

Dr. Bolognia is Assistant Professor of Dermatology and Dr. Braverman is Professor of Dermatology at the Yale University School of Medicine, New Haven, CT.

WAXY SKIN AND STIFF JOINTS

Up to 30% of young patients (aged 1–28 yr) with type I (insulin-dependent) diabetes have limited mobility of the small and large joints, and in those with diabetes for ≥4.5 yr, the severity of joint disease is correlated with microvascular complications. Involvement of the small joints of the hands can be easily demonstrated by the failure of the palmar surfaces of the interphalangeal joints to approximate (Fig. 30.1). Approximately 35% of patients with limited joint mobility have tight, thick, waxy skin over the backs of the hands that is difficult to tent. However, thickened skin has only been observed in individuals with moderate to severe joint disease. These skin findings may reverse with improved control of the diabetes; otherwise, there is no known treatment.

SCLEREDEMA

In scleredema, there is a thickening of the skin due to the deposition of mucopolysaccharides in the dermis. Areas of involvement may not be visually apparent, although they can develop a peau d'orange appearance as a result of prominent and depressed follicular openings (Fig. 30.2). The extent of involvement is best appreciated by palpation of the induration. Because scleredema is found most commonly on the upper back and posterior neck, the patient may be unaware of its presence. Less common sites of involvement include the face, upper arms, abdomen, lower back, and tongue.

Scleredema has been associated with preceding streptococcal and viral infections as well as type I and type II (non-insulin-dependent) diabetes (usually long standing, sometimes insulin resistant). In the form seen in patients with diabetes, the induration may be accompanied by erythema (Fig. 30.2), which might be misdiagnosed as treatment-resistant cellulitis.

There is no effective treatment for scleredema, although some cases, especially those in nondiabetic patients, may spontaneously resolve.

DIABETIC DERMOPATHY

Diabetic dermopathy is characterized by multiple hyperpigmented macules on the extensor surface of the distal lower extremities (Fig. 30.3). The individual lesions range in size from 0.5 to 2 cm, are oval or circular, and may have associated atrophy and scale. These skin changes have also been referred to as shin spots or pigmented pretibial patches. These skin lesions may also be seen in individuals without evidence of glucose intolerance, albeit less often. In general, the dermopathy is asymptomatic except for its appearance, and no effective treatment has been described.

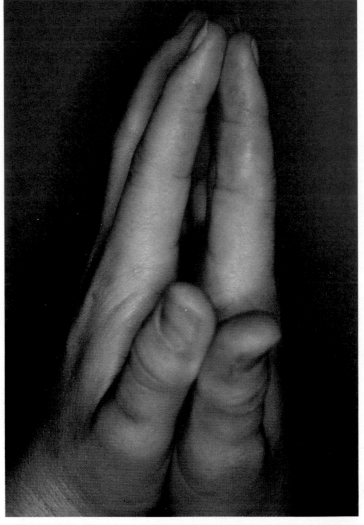

Figure 30.1. Failure of palmar surfaces of interphalangeal joints to approximate in patient with stiff joints and waxy skin.

NECROBIOSIS LIPOIDICA DIABETICORUM

NLD skin lesions are so named because of the presence of necrobiosis or degeneration of collagen in the dermis, the yellow color of most well-developed lesions due to carotene and lipid, and the association with diabetes mellitus. NLD is characterized by red to

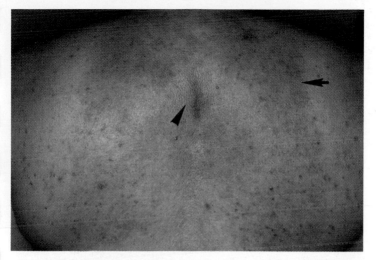

Figure 30.2. Scleredema of upper back with overlying erythema (*large arrow*) and development of peau d'orange appearance centrally (*small arrow*).

red-brown to violet plaques that enlarge and frequently become yellow centrally. In addition, there is atrophy of the epidermis, which leads to shiny transparent skin and visualization of underlying dermal and subcutaneous vessels (Fig. 30.4). The most common location of NLD is the shin, found in 90% of patients, but lesions can occur on the scalp, face, arms, and trunk. Lesions of NLD may ulcerate, especially those on the distal lower extremities.

NLD is uncommon, occurring in 0.1–0.3% of the diabetic population, usually in the third or fourth decade of life. Approximately 65% of patients who develop NLD have diabetes at the time of presentation (most for several years), and another 15% subsequently develop diabetes.

There is no well-established treatment for NLD, but some success has been reported for pentoxifylline (400 mg 3×/day), dipyridamole (50–75 mg 3–4×/day) plus low-dose aspirin (325 mg/day), and intralesional corticosteroids (triamcinolone acetonide 5 mg/ml). The latter may have mixed results in that breakdown of skin lesions after injections has been reported.

DISSEMINATED GRANULOMA ANNULARE

Granuloma annulare is characterized by annular or arciform plaques that form from the coalescence of flesh-colored, red, or red-brown papules (Fig. 30.5). The skin in the center of the lesion may be normal or erythematous in appearance. Most commonly, granuloma annulare has an acral distribution, but the lesions can be more numerous and papular and found on the trunk as well as the ex-

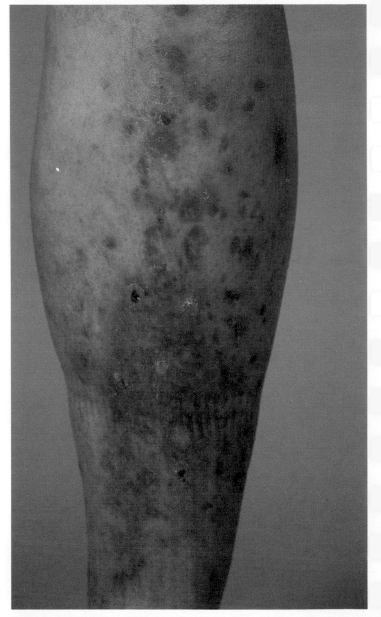

Figure 30.3. Hyperpigmented macules on shin of patient with diabetic dermopathy.

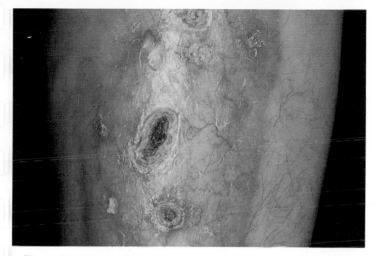

Figure 30.4. Necrobiosis lipoidica diabeticorum of anterior lower extremity with characteristic atrophy and visualization of underlying vessels.

tremities. The term *generalized* or *disseminated granuloma annulare* is used to describe these patients.

A patient with generalized granuloma annulare should be screened for glucose intolerance. The clinical diagnosis can be confirmed by performing a skin biopsy. The etiology of granuloma annulare is unknown, and the treatment is empiric and includes topical and

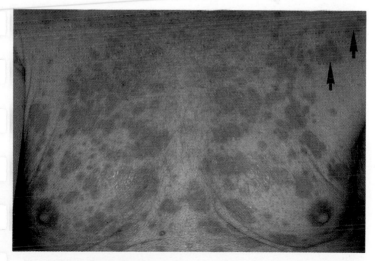

Figure 30.5. Generalized granuloma annulare. Annular shape of lesions is best seen on left shoulder (*arrows*).

intralesional corticosteroids (triamcinolone acetonide 5 mg/ml daily), niacinamide (500 mg 3×/day), and, in severe cases, dapsone (50–100 mg).

XANTHOMAS

There are several types of cutaneous xanthomas, including eruptive, tendinous, tuberous, and planar, which are reflections of hyper-cholesterolemia and/or hypertriglyceridemia. Eruptive xanthomas can appear suddenly, and the lesions are usually 4–6 mm in diameter, firm, and yellow with a red base; the elbows, knees, buttocks, and sites of trauma are the favored sites (Fig. 30.6). Biopsy findings are diagnostic and demonstrate collections of lipids within the dermis.

Administration of insulin results in a decrease in the circulating levels of triglycerides, and the xanthomas quickly resolve. If the patient is not appropriately treated, the eruptive lesions can enlarge into tuberous xanthomas. Xanthelasma (plane xanthoma of the eyelids) is the least specific marker of hyperlipidemia in that 50% of the patients have normal lipid levels. In addition, there is no clear-cut association between diabetes and xanthelasma.

LIPODYSTROPHY

Although the diseases outlined in this section are referred to as lipodystrophies, the patients have primarily lipoatrophy, and the

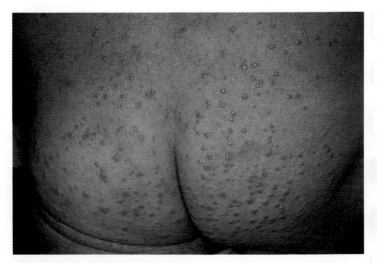

Figure 30.6. Eruptive xanthomas on buttocks of patient with poorly controlled diabetes mellitus.

lipoatrophy is divided into two major forms: total (generalized) and partial. In the generalized form, the entire body is involved, the inheritance is often autosomal recessive, and the onset is either congenital (at birth or during infancy) or acquired (during the 1st–3rd decades of life). In contrast, partial lipoatrophy usually involves the face, neck, arms, and upper trunk (above the waist); is not inherited; and has its onset from childhood to early adulthood. Occasionally, partial lipoatrophy affects only areas below the waist, and hemilipoatrophy has occurred in a few patients. In biopsy specimens of areas of subcutaneous fat loss, the fat cells are present, but the cytoplasmic fat is absent.

Both forms of lipoatrophy, total and partial, are associated with insulin-resistant diabetes mellitus. Patients with total lipoatrophy also have accelerated somatic growth and bone maturation, increased muscle mass, hypertriglyceridemia, and fatty infiltration of the liver. In addition, those with congenital total lipoatrophy have hyperpigmentation, acanthosis nigricans, and generalized hirsutism. In contrast, ~40–50% of those with partial lipoatrophy have evidence of membranoproliferative glomerulonephritis, often in association with hypocomplementemia.

ACANTHOSIS NIGRICANS

In acanthosis nigricans, velvety tan to dark-brown plaques are seen on the sides of the neck, axillae, and groin (Fig. 30.7). Additional sites of involvement include the extensor surface of the small joints

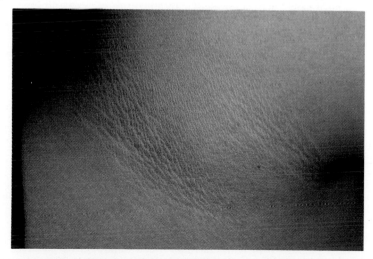

Figure 30.7. Velvety dark-brown plaques on lateral neck of patient with acanthosis nigricans.

of the hand, the elbows, and the knees. Acanthosis nigricans can be a reflection of an underlying malignancy, usually adenocarcinoma of the gastrointestinal tract, but is more commonly associated with obesity.

The clinical spectrum in obese patients can range from euglycemia with mild hyperinsulinemia and tissue resistance to insulin-requiring diabetes mellitus. Acanthosis nigricans is also a cutaneous manifestation of the insulin-resistant syndromes, types A and B as well as congenital total lipoatrophy. In obese patients, weight loss and improvement of tissue resistance to insulin has improved their acanthosis nigricans. Otherwise, treatment is limited to topical agents such as retinoic acid (0.05–0.1%) and urea (10–25%), which can improve the cosmetic appearance.

BULLOSIS DIABETICORUM

The spontaneous formation of bullae in a primarily acral location (forearms, fingers, feet, and toes) is an uncommon manifestation of diabetes mellitus. The lesions arise from normal noninflamed skin and range in size from a few millimeters to several centimeters (Fig. 30.8). The blisters are usually tense and contain clear viscous fluid that is sterile. There is no history of antecedent trauma, and the lesions may recur. Two major forms exist and are distinguished by the site of blister formation: *1*) the blister is intraepidermal and heals without scarring, or *2*) it is subepidermal and may heal with atrophy and mild scarring. Both types are found predominantly in middle-aged to elderly patients with long-standing diabetes. Other than local care, there is no specific treatment to recommend.

NECROLYTIC MIGRATORY ERYTHEMA

Patients with NME have bright erythematous patches that are most frequently seen in the girdle area (lower abdomen, groin, buttocks, and thighs), perioral region, and extremities (Fig. 30.9). The cutaneous finding that distinguishes NME from other migratory eruptions is the presence of superficial bullae at the active borders. Because the bullae rapidly break, only denuded areas and crusts may be observed clinically. These areas then heal with superficial desquamation as the erythema advances.

Histologically, swollen and necrotic keratinocytes are seen in the superficial layers of the epidermis, findings similar to those seen in acrodermatitis enteropathica. In addition to the cutaneous eruption, the patients frequently have glossitis, anemia, weight loss, and diarrhea, as well as diabetes mellitus.

Most patients with NME have an α-cell tumor of the pancreas and markedly elevated serum glucagon levels; removal of the tumor can result in prompt resolution of the cutaneous eruption. Other-

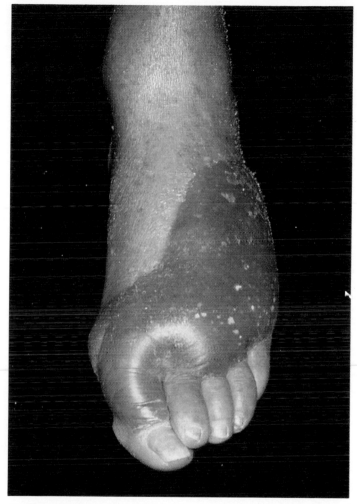

Figure 30.8. Tense large bulla on dorsum of foot characteristic of bullosis diabeticorum. From Braverman (1).

wise, the lesions are treatment resistant, although they do wax and wane spontaneously.

DRUG REACTIONS TO ORAL HYPOGLYCEMIC AGENTS AND INSULIN

Administration of oral hypoglycemic agents can lead to commonly recognized drug reactions such as pruritus, urticaria, erythema mul-

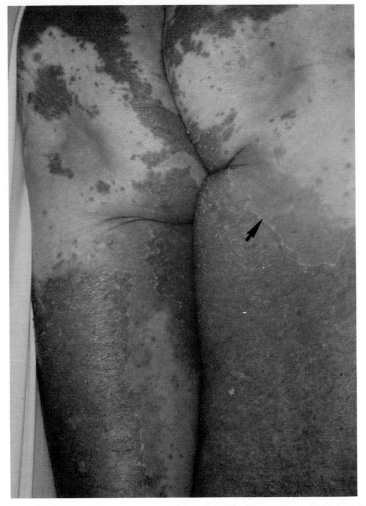

Figure 30.9. Angular erythematous patches on buttocks and thighs of patient with glucagonoma of pancreas; note peripheral desquamation (*arrow*). From Braverman (1).

tiforme, and morbilliform eruptions. Phototoxic (dose-related exaggerated sunburn) and photoallergic (idiosyncratic eczematous dermatitis in a photodistribution) eruptions are additional potential cutaneous side effects and are related to the sulfur moiety found in these compounds. A unique reaction is the chlorpropamide alcohol flush, which is similar to the disulfiram alcohol flush.

The cutaneous reactions to insulin can be divided into localized, generalized, and lipoatrophy/lipohypertrophy. The localized reactions include erythema, induration, and, occasionally, ulceration at the insulin-injection site. They are secondary to either an idiosyncratic reaction or dermal rather than the subcutaneous injections. Allergic local reactions vary from the immediate formation of an urticarial lesion at the injection site to the appearance of a pruritic papule or nodule 24–48 h after the injection. The latter lesions represent a delayed hypersensitivity reaction and, as such, heal slowly over a week or more and often leave residual hyperpigmentation. They frequently cease to form after several weeks or months. The primary treatment of persistent localized reactions is a switch to purer forms of insulin; if this is unsuccessful, the possibility of a zinc allergy should be considered.

Generalized reactions are uncommon and are characterized by pruritus, erythema, and urticaria/angioedema. If the patient has to receive insulin, a referral to specialists in diabetes and immunology should be made.

Lipoatrophy at injection sites is seen with older less-purified forms of insulin and is rare with purified pork or biosynthetic human insulin. Improvement in the areas of subcutaneous fat loss has been reported after injection of purified insulin into the edge of the lipoatrophy. Lipohypertrophy, i.e., an increase in the amount of subcutaneous fat, can also be seen at the site of insulin injection. Treatment consists of rotation of injection sites and the use of purified insulin.

SUGGESTED READING

1. Braverman IM: *Skin Signs of Systemic Disease*. 2nd ed. Philadelphia, PA, Saunders, 1981
2. Huntley AC: The cutaneous manifestations of diabetes mellitus. *J Am Acad Dermatol* 7:427–55, 1982
3. Jelenick JE: *The Skin in Diabetes*. Philadelphia, PA, Lea & Febiger, 1986
4. Rosenbloom AL, Silverstein JH, Lezotte DC, Richardson K, McCallum M: Limited joint mobility in childhood diabetes mellitus indicates increased risk for microvascular disease. *N Engl J Med* 305:191–94, 1981

31. Infections

JOHN R. GRAYBILL, MD

Host immune defenses are altered in the diabetic patient through several mechanisms. Hyperglycemia and acidosis alter the functions of phagocytic cells and result in changing their movement toward the site of an infection and impairing their microbicidal activity. Subtle alterations in cell-mediated immunity predispose the patient toward tuberculosis, coccidioidomycosis, and cryptococcosis. The diabetic host's metabolic state also favors the specific nutritional requirements of some microbes. High glucose concentrations in blood and body fluids promote the overgrowth of certain fungal pathogens, particularly *Candida* species and Zygomycetes. Zygomycetes also grow more rapidly in a state of acidosis. Finally, mechanical factors largely contribute to the increased susceptibility of the diabetic patient to infections (Table 31.1).

SUPERFICIAL TISSUE INFECTIONS

Minor trauma to tissues affected by vascular insufficiency often initiates superficial tissue infection. In addition, peripheral sensory neuropathy facilitates the occurrence of an insensibility to minor injuries and delays their care. Infection may take the form of a cellulitis, soft tissue necrosis, draining sinus, or osteomyelitis. Although the feet are most commonly involved in these infections, a similar process can occur in skin beneath pressure points (bedsores). In both situations, tissue undermining can be extensive.

These infections are caused by both aerobic and anaerobic organisms, e.g., *Escherichia coli*, *Proteus*, various other Enterobac-

Dr. Graybill is Professor of Medicine and Clinical Chief of Infectious Diseases at the Audie L. Murphy Veterans Hospital, San Antonio, TX.

Table 31.1. **MECHANICAL FACTORS CONTRIBUTING TO INFECTIONS IN DIABETIC PATIENTS**

Physiological Change	Disease Process	Result
Ischemic changes	Chronic diabetic vascular disease	Mixed bacterial foot infections
Depressed cough reflex	Cerebrovascular insults	Pneumonia
Impaired bladder emptying	Autonomic neuropathy	Urinary tract infections
Fecal incontinence	Autonomic neuropathy	Cutaneous maceration
Impaired mobility	Various	Decubitus ulcers

teriaceae, various *Streptococci*, *Staphylococcus*, *Streptococci* A and B, *Peptostreptococcus*, and *Bacteroides fragilis*.

Several organisms produce gas, resulting in the development of crepitation in the patient with "diabetic foot." This must be distinguished from the much less common and more acutely devastating clostridial gas gangrene and necrotizing fasciculitus.

The infectious process is insidious, and the serious threat it poses must be recognized. Antimicrobial treatment should be directed at the pathogens identified by cultures. However, empiric therapy for the most likely organisms should be initiated promptly and used until the results of cultures are available. "Swarming" of *Proteus* may obscure other pathogens on culture plates also including *Staphylococci*, *Streptococci*, anaerobic *Streptococci*, and *Bacteroides*, and common enteric gram-negative organisms. Useful antibiotics are listed in Table 31.2. Unless the patient is clearly septic, the use of aminoglycosides is not recommended because of their nephrotoxicity and the likelihood that patients with diabetes may have underlying kidney disease.

GANGRENE

Diabetic patients are susceptible to more severe infections such as streptococcal gangrene. This is marked by a rapid progression from cellulitis to the development of vesicles and bullae over a hemorrhagic base. The overlying cutaneous tissues rapidly necrose, and the process may spread quickly within a few days. Group A *Streptococci* may be recovered from the lesions and the blood. Antibiotics alone are insufficient, and wide excision or guillotine amputations may be necessary. Mortality is >10% and has not changed much in the antibiotic era. When use of antibiotics is indicated, $18-21 \times 10^6$ U penicillin/day i.v. should be given. In penicillin-allergic patients, 1 g vancomycin/12 h i.v. should be given. Much lower doses of either drug should be given in patients with kidney failure; ane-

Table 31.2. ANTIMICROBIAL THERAPY OF INFECTIONS IN DIABETIC PATIENTS

Agent	Dose	Comment
Superficial infections		
Cefoxitin	1 g/8 h i.m.*	
Ceftriaxone	1 g/12 h i.m. or i.v.	
Cephalosporins	Various	Gram-positive, gram-negative, and anaerobic activity
Amoxicillin + metronidazole	500 mg/8 h orally	
Penicillin + clindamycin	500 mg orally 4×/day 600 mg orally 2×/day	
Malignant otitis externa		
Ticarcillin*	3 g/4 h i.v.	
Gentamicin*	6–8 mg · kg^{-1} · day^{-1} in 2–3 doses	
Amikacin*	500 mg/12 h i.v. (15–20 mg · kg^{-1} · day^{-1} in 2 doses)	
Imipenem	500 mg/8 h i.v.	
Ciprofloxacin	750 mg orally 2×/day	Resistance may occur
Urinary tract infections		
Trimethoprim-sulfa*	1 double strength orally 2×/day	Common first choice
Ciprofloxacin	500 mg orally 2×/day	Excellent for gram-negative organisms
Norfloxacin	400 mg orally 2×/day	Excellent for gram-negative organisms
Ampicillin	500–1000 mg orally/6 h	For *Streptococci*
Amoxicillin	500 mg orally 3×/day	For *Streptococci*
Amoxicillin with clavulanate (Augmentin [Beecham])	500 mg orally/8 h	Increases spectrum among gram-negative Enterobacteriaceae
Fungal infections *Candida*		
Flucytosine*	50–75 mg · kg^{-1} · day^{-1} for 2 wk	
Fluconazole*	100 mg/day orally for 2–4 wk	No data on urinary tract infections; excreted by urinary route
Amphotericin B*	50 mg/L for bladder irrigations	Efficacy uncertain
Amphotericin B* with flucytosine*	20–30 mg/day i.v.	For severe or refractory infections

Table 31.2. (*continued*)

Agent	Dose	Comment
Zygomycetes		
Amphotericin B*	$1-1.5$ mg $\cdot$ kg^{-1} $\cdot$ day^{-1} i.v. or 50 mg/L of 5% glucose to irrigate debrided areas	High doses cause kidney failure
Pulmonary infections		
For tuberculosis		
INH, rifampin, and PZA for 2 mo followed by INH and rifampin for 4 mo	300 mg/day/INH orally 600 mg/day rifampin orally $15-20$ mg $\cdot$ kg^{-1} $\cdot$ day^{-1} PZA orally	
For coccidioidomycosis		
Amphotericin B*	$2-3$ g total dose given at 50 mg i.v. $3\times$/wk	Nephrotoxicity, anemia, fever, chills
Ketoconazole	400 mg/day orally for $9-12$ mo	Nausea, vomiting, advent suppression dose related
Itraconazole	400 mg/day orally for $\geq 9-12$ mo	

PZA, pyrazinamide.
*Must reduce dosage with impaired renal function.

phric patients should be given a maximum of $6-8 \times 10^6$ U penicillin/day or 1 g vancomycin/$7-10$ days.

Antimicrobial therapy alone is commonly insufficient for serious infections in diabetic patients. Local debridement is frequently helpful. Tenuous vascular supply and poor tissue healing often necessitate amputation more proximal than the obviously infected tissue. Because of the danger of gangrene and possible necessity of amputation, diabetic patients with foot infections should be promptly hospitalized for treatment.

A related but more slowly advancing process is synergistic gangrene. This often begins at surgical suture sites and involves microaerophilic or anaerobic *Streptococci* and *Staphylococcus aureus*. Occasionally, enteric gram-negative bacilli such as *Proteus* may also be present. The process is a gradually enlarging area of necrosis with fistulous tracts tunneling under the skin to emerge elsewhere.

MALIGNANT OTITIS EXTERNA

Malignant otitis externa is an infection caused by *Pseudomonas aeruginosa* that occurs virtually exclusively in diabetic patients. It is a chronic erosive process that initially involves the soft tissue and cartilage around the external auditory canal. There is pain and drainage of purulent material and progressive destruction as the process works into the temporal and petrous bones and mastoids. The infection progresses regardless of tissue planes and ultimately reaches cranial nerves and/or the meninges or sigmoid sinus. Paralysis of nerves V, VII, and VIII may occur. Death may result from epidural abscess or rupture into the meningeal space. Treatment is with local debridement of necrotic tissue and prolonged therapy with antipseudomonal antibiotics. Because osteomyelitis is usually present, the course of therapy should be at least 4–6 wk. Useful agents are listed in Table 31.2.

URINARY TRACT INFECTIONS

Urinary tract infections (UTIs) frequently occur in patients with diabetes. *E. coli* and *Streptococci* are the most common bacteria involved, and *Candida* and *Torulopsis glabrata* are common fungal pathogens in part because of the high urine glucose concentration. Women are at higher risk for UTIs than men because of the short urethra. The neurogenic bladder associated with diabetic neuropathy provides a reservoir for infection and poses a dilemma for management because catheterization is often necessary for drainage, which poses the risk of ascending catheter infection. Intermittent catheter drainage has been recommended as a compromise but is not always possible.

UTIs are the most common nosocomial infections and are especially likely to occur in the catheterized patient. Although bacteriuria can be delayed for up to a month via closed drainage systems, even short-term catheterization results in 10–30% of patients developing symptomatic UTIs.

Asymptomatic bacteriuria in the catheterized patient is best treated by removal of the catheter if possible. Antibiotics are not given. If catheters are left in place, they should be changed periodically to avoid buildup of concretions, which are a nidus for persistent bacterial colonization. Antimicrobials should be used only if the catheterized patient is symptomatic. Useful agents are listed in Table 31.2.

For the patient with fever and back pain, pyelonephritis is the likely diagnosis, especially if urinary bacteria are antibody coated. Hospitalization and parenteral antimicrobial therapy are necessary in the diabetic patient with suspected pyelonephritis. Aminoglycosides should be avoided because they aggravate renal insufficiency. However, they may be necessary in the patient with hypotension or with a history of repeated UTIs treated previously with other agents. If they must be used, aminoglycosides should only be given until in vitro antimicrobial susceptibilities are available and possible alternatives are identified.

FUNGAL INFECTIONS

Candida and *Torulopsis glabrata* Infection

The most common fungal infections seen in diabetic patients are UTIs with *Candida* and *T. glabrata*, a related organism. *Candida* urinary tract colonization is common, and it is especially difficult to distinguish infection from colonization. Neither antibody coating, counts of >10⁵/ml, or mycelial versus yeast form are useful in distinguishing upper- from lower-tract infection or colonization. *Candida* are probably present in significant numbers if >10⁴/ml, but this is uncertain. A major problem is the difficulty of obtaining uncontaminated specimens from obese diabetic women. A catheterized urine specimen is preferable in this situation. If *Candida* are repeatedly isolated from the urine of a catheterized patient, the best treatment is to remove the catheter. If this cannot be done, the catheter should be replaced and consideration given to a short course of antifungal therapy. Because of nephrotoxicity, amphotericin B should be avoided. See Table 31.2 for appropriate agents for the treatment of *Candida* UTIs. *T. glabrata* tend to be more refractory to treatment.

Zygomycetes Infection

Much less common but much more devastating is infection by the Zygomycetes. The syndrome most often seen in diabetic patients is rhinocerebral mucormycosis. This is an invasive process caused by the mycelia of the genera *Mucor, Absidia, Rhizopus*, and *Cunninghamella*. The conidia of the organisms are unable to regenerate if ingested by normal macrophages, and the organisms are essentially nonpathogenic in the normal host. The growth of *Rhizopus* is inhibited by normal human serum. However, these fungi can grow remarkably rapidly in the presence of high concentrations of glucose and in an acid environment. Both conditions prevail in the patient with ketoacidosis. In such patients, these organisms are able to germinate at the site of infections, probably the nares and the sinuses, and to begin the phenomenally rapid necrotizing process that characterizes rhinocerebral zygomycosis. Within a few days, the process may extend from a small eschar on the nasal septum to involve the paranasal sinuses and orbit. The infection proceeds without regard for tissue planes and rapidly erodes into the nerves and blood vessels. It can track into the brain within a few days, and if the infective process is not stopped before this happens, the result is lethal.

Diagnosis is by prompt aggressive surgical biopsy, including tissues deep to the area of necrosis. Zygomycetes are different from other fungi in that they stain better with hematoxylin and eosin than with methenamine silver. Identification of irregular pleomorphic nonseptate branching hyphae is pathognomonic. Zygomycetes must be differentiated from *Aspergillus*, which are the most similar in appearance and also can cause sinusitis. The hyphae of *Aspergillus* are more regular and bamboo shaped, with hyphae that have septa and branch at 45° angles. They do not stain well with hematoxylin and eosin. Treatment of zygomycosis infection includes

- Correction of ketoacidosis
- Vigorous and repeated surgical debridement
- Antifungal therapy with amphotericin B

Azole antifungal drugs are not effective against Zygomycetes. A new preparation, amphotericin B in lipid complex, may be useful in the future.

PULMONARY INFECTIONS

These may include chronic bacterial pneumonia and cavitary pulmonary disease from *Mycobacterium tuberculosis* and the fungus *Coccidioides immitis*. Management is by short-course chemotherapy for tuberculosis. Coccidioidomycosis may be treated with amphotericin B or ketoconozole (Table 31.2). Itraconazole is not yet licensed in the United States but is the drug of choice based on efficacy and reduced toxicity. Fluconazole is not approved for coccidioidomycosis but is effective in 50% of patients when given at 200–400 mg/day for >6 mo.

32. Visual Loss

LLOYD M. AIELLO, MD, and
JERRY D. CAVALLERANO, OD, PhD

To achieve the goal of reducing the risk of visual loss, patients at risk must be identified and directed to appropriate ophthalmologists for laser photocoagulation.

CLINICAL CONSIDERATIONS

All patients with diabetes should be advised that they are at risk for visual loss; they should also be advised that appropriate and timely treatment can substantially reduce the risk of visual loss. As a routine part of the health history, all diabetic patients should be asked if they notice any visual symptomatology (Table 32.1), i.e.,

- Any loss of visual acuity (either at distance or near)
- Diplopia
- Fluctuation of vision
- Floating spots or flashing lights in field of view
- Any metamorphopsia or apparent warping of straight lines

There are numerous etiologies for reduced vision—some benign and some requiring immediate treatment. In general, patients who report floating spots in their view, flashing lights, or the sensation of a curtain or veil crossing their vision should be referred for immediate ophthalmological attention, because they may be reporting the symptoms of a vitreous hemorrhage, retinal detachment, or retinal hole. Patients reporting metamorphopsia may have sig-

Dr. Aiello is Director and Dr. Cavallerano is a Staff Optometrist at the Beetham Eye Institute of the Joslin Diabetes Center, Boston, MA.

Table 32.1. **VISUAL SYMPTOMS IN DIABETIC PATIENTS REQUIRING FURTHER EVALUATION AND TREATMENT**

Symptom	Possible Etiology	Management Strategy
Blurred vision	Poorly controlled diabetes mellitus	Control diabetes; no new glasses prescription for 4–6 wk
	Cataract	Referral for comprehensive eye exam
	Macular edema	
Double vision	Diabetic mononeuropathy	Neuroophthalmological and neurological evaluation; neurological referral frequently
	Other etiology	
Floaters	Vitreous hemorrhage	Urgent referral for complete ocular evaluation
	Retinal detachment	
	Retinal hole	
Ocular pain	Corneal abrasion	Emergency referral for complete ocular evaluation
	Neovascular or angle-closure glaucoma	
	Iritis	

nificant macular edema or traction in the macular area and should be referred for ophthalmological evaluation, preferably within 1 wk.

Fluctuating vision is probably the result of poor blood glucose control. Elevated blood glucose levels may lead to a myopic shift, enabling presbyopic individuals to read without their glasses, whereas their distance vision becomes blurred; for some who never wore glasses, distance vision may become blurred, and for those with hyperopia, glasses may no longer be needed for clear distance vision. Blurred vision can also be a symptom of macular edema, cataract, or other ocular conditions. In general, if the vision clears with a pinhole, the condition is most likely refractive, and referral is not urgent.

Patients complaining of pain in or above the eye should be evaluated for possible neovascular or angle-closure glaucoma, especially if there is a loss of corneal reflex, irregularity in shape and response of the pupil, or acute redness of the eye. Also, a painful or red eye may reflect a corneal abrasion or corneal erosion. In most cases, patients with anterior-segment complaints should be examined with a slit-lamp biomicroscope to rule out any form of glaucoma, a foreign body, a corneal abrasion, or iritis. Tonometry to measure intraocular pressure is also advisable. Emergency referral to an ophthalmologist is critical.

Patients with new-onset double vision require neuroophthalmic and often neurological evaluation. Any patient who shows neovascularization of the optic nerve head or elsewhere in the retina or hard exudates or microaneurysms in the macula area should be referred for complete ophthalmological evaluation. If proliferative retinopathy is present, immediate referral is warranted (Table 32.2).

Table 32.2. OCULAR SIGNS REQUIRING REFERRAL
FOR MANAGEMENT

Sign	Management
Retinal neovascularization	Immediate referral for comprehensive ocular examination and possible laser surgery
Vitreous hemorrhage	Immediate referral for comprehensive ocular examination and possible laser and/or vitrectomy surgery
Hard exudates or microaneurysms in macular area	Timely (1–2 wk) referral for comprehensive ocular examination and possible laser surgery for clinically significant macular edema
Cataract	Referral for comprehensive ocular examination depending on patient history, symptoms, and examination

Because diabetic eye disease cannot be prevented, strategies must address proper management of proliferative retinopathy and diabetic macular edema. All patients should be informed of the potential ocular complications of diabetes and should be advised to have a comprehensive annual eye examination with pupil dilation, with appropriate referral for management and treatment as indicated.

33. Ocular Complications

LLOYD M. AIELLO, MD, and
JERRY D. CAVALLERANO, OD, PhD

Type I (insulin-dependent) diabetic patients experience more frequent and severe ocular complications. In fact, after 5 yr, 23% of type I diabetic patients have retinopathy. After 10 yr, this incidence increases to almost 60%, and after 15 yr, 80% have retinopathy. Proliferative diabetic retinopathy (PDR)—the most threatening form of the disease—is present in 25% of type I diabetic patients after 15 yr and often remains asymptomatic beyond the optimal stage for treatment.

An estimated 700,000 Americans have PDR, and 500,000 have diabetic macular edema (DME). The annual projected incidence of new cases of PDR and DME is 65,000 and 75,000, respectively. About 8000 new cases of blindness a year in the United States are caused by complications from diabetes.

Diabetic retinopathy is often asymptomatic in its most treatable stages. Unfortunately, only 45% of the diabetic population receives adequate ophthalmic care. Early detection and treatment of diabetic retinopathy are critical. Laser surgery can ameliorate the devastating effects of diabetic retinal disease, particularly when laser surgery is initiated in a timely fashion. Timely laser photocoagulation treatments can reduce the risk of severe visual loss from high-risk (new-vessel) PDR by ≥60%, thus lowering the overall risk of such loss to <10%. Timely laser surgery of DME can reduce the risk of moderate visual loss by 50%. Vitrectomy can restore useful vision to some people who have lost vision due to diabetes. Emphasis must therefore be placed on early detection of retinal disorders, with appropriate referral for management and treatment.

Dr. Aiello is Director and Dr. Cavallerano is a Staff Optometrist at the Beetham Eye Institute of the Joslin Diabetes Center, Boston, MA.

DIABETIC RETINOPATHY

Pathophysiology

Elevated blood glucose levels result in structural, physiological, and hormonal changes that affect the retinal capillaries, causing the capillaries to become functionally less competent. Six clinical pathological processes are recognized in diabetic retinopathy. Clinically, these processes are manifested as either PDR or nonproliferative diabetic retinopathy (NPDR) (Table 33.1):

- Loss of pericytes of retinal capillaries
- Outpouchings of the capillary walls to form microaneurysms
- Closure of retinal capillaries and arterioles
- Increased vascular permeability of retinal capillaries
- Proliferation of new vessels and fibrous tissue
- Contraction of vitreous and fibrous proliferation with subsequent retinal detachment due to traction.

Diabetic retinopathy also may alter the structure of the macula, significantly altering function, in the following ways:

- DME, i.e., a collection of intraretinal fluid in the macular area with or without lipid exudates and with or without cystoid changes
- Nonperfusion of parafoveal capillaries with or without intraretinal fluid
- Traction in the macula by fibrous tissue proliferation causing dragging of the retinal tissue, surface wrinkling, or detachment of the macula
- Intraretinal or preretinal hemorrhage in the macula
- Lamellar or full-thickness hole formation
- Combinations of the above

DME can be associated with any stage of diabetic retinopathy. Proper evaluation dictates stereoscopic examination of the macula with slit-lamp biomicroscope and/or fundus photography. Loss of vision from diabetes usually results from nonresolving vitreous hemorrhage, PDR leading to fibrous tissue formation and subsequent traction retinal detachment, or DME.

Clinical Care

Proper management of diabetic retinopathy has been influenced by results of three major clinical trials. These studies helped establish the minimum standard of eye care for diabetic patients to reduce the threat of visual loss from diabetes.

The Diabetic Retinopathy Study (DRS) definitively established the beneficial effects of scatter (panretinal) laser photocoagulation. The Early Treatment Diabetic Retinopathy Study (ETDRS) demonstrated the benefit of focal laser treatment for DME and provided insight into the most appropriate timing for retinal laser surgery. The study also demonstrated that the use of aspirin is unlikely to

Table 33.1. CLINICAL MANIFESTATIONS OF RETINOPATHY

Diabetic macular edema (DME) occurring at any level of diabetic retinopathy
  Nonproliferative diabetic retinopathy (NPDR)
  • Mild—one or more of the following:
    −Few scattered retinal microaneurysms and hemorrhages
    −Hard exudate
  • Moderate—one or more of the following:
    −More extensive retinal hemorrhages and/or microaneurysms
    −Mild intraretinal microvascular abnormalities (IRMA)
    −Early venous beading
  • Severe to very severe—one or more of the following:
    −Severe hemorrhages and/or microaneurysms in all 4 quadrants
    −More extensive IRMA or venous beading in at least 2 quadrants
  Proliferative diabetic retinopathy (PDR)
  • Early
    −Minimal new vessels on disk (NVD) <1/4 disk area without preretinal or vitreous hemorrhage
                              or
    −New vessels elsewhere on retina (NVE) without preretinal or vitreous hemorrhage
  • High risk
    −NVD >1/4 disk area with or without preretinal or vitreous hemorrhage
                              or
    −NVE with preretinal or vitreous hemorrhage

have any effect on the progression of diabetic retinopathy. Finally, the Diabetic Retinopathy Vitrectomy Study (DRVS) established guidelines on the timing of surgical intervention after visual loss from vitreous hemorrhage.

In the DRS, scatter photocoagulation treatment was demonstrated to be so effective that the DRS research group modified their study protocol early in the study to allow treatment for all eyes with sight-threatening retinopathy. Furthermore, investigators determined that specific retinal lesions pose a significant threat for severe visual loss (visual acuity reduced to the 5/200 level). These lesions comprise high-risk PDR, which mandates immediate referral to a retinal specialist for scatter photocoagulation (Table 33.2).

Despite results of DRS, photocoagulation does not completely eliminate the risk of visual loss. To determine modalities to further

Table 33.2. HIGH-RISK CHARACTERISTICS

• Neovascularization at or within 1 disk diameter of optic nerve head ≥¼ disk area
• Neovascularization >1 disk diameter from optic nerve head accompanied by fresh hemorrhage
• Neovascularization at disk <¼ disk area in extent accompanied by fresh hemorrhage

reduce this risk, ETDRS was designed to test the effects of a daily dose of 650 mg aspirin, laser surgery for DME, and the most appropriate timing and modality of scatter laser treatment for proliferative retinopathy. ETDRS determined that

1. Focal laser surgery is effective to treat DME.
2. Scatter laser photocoagulation reduces the risk of severe visual loss, whether applied early or at the development of high-risk PDR.
3. Aspirin treatment does not alter the progression of diabetic retinopathy.

Diagnosis

Retinopathy rarely occurs before 5 yr duration of type I diabetes. After 10 yr, however, at least some degree of retinopathy is present in 60% of the diabetic population, and the figure approaches 100% by 15–17 yr. PDR is unusual before 10 yr but is present in 26% of type I diabetic patients after 15 yr. After 20 yr, PDR is present in ~56% of the type I diabetic population.

In type II (non-insulin-dependent) diabetes, diabetic retinopathy is present in ~20% of cases at diagnosis, and this figure increases to 60–85% after 15 yr. PDR is present in 3–4% of patients in <1 yr, and after 15 yr, it is present in 5–20% of the type II diabetic population. Thus, patients with type II diabetes are more likely to have diabetic retinopathy at diagnosis and are more likely to develop diabetic retinopathy sooner after diagnosis than those with type I diabetes.

NPDR

Mild. Mild NPDR, characterized by several microaneurysms with or without occasional blotch hemorrhages, is relatively benign and virtually ubiquitous after 15–17 yr of diabetes. Microaneurysms may resolve with time or show little or no change over months. Older microaneurysms may have a yellowish white appearance, imitating the appearance of hard exudates. Dot hemorrhages and microaneurysms can be considered clinically as one type of lesion. They are actually indistinguishable from one another by ophthalmoscopic examination without fluorescein angiography, but such invasive testing is not warranted at this stage of retinopathy unless macular edema threatening central vision is present. Rare flecks of hard exudates, representing small white or yellowish white deposits generally with sharp borders, may be present in the intermediate layers of the retina. Hard exudates are lipid deposits leaked from microaneurysms or compromised capillary beds, and may be present at any stage of NPDR and PDR.

The microaneurysms represent outpouchings of blood vessel walls, possibly secondary to weakness of the capillary wall from loss of pericytes or from increased intraluminal pressure. These lesions are essentially intravascular or perivascular in nature. Patients with mild NPDR can safely be followed every 9–12 mo unless macular edema is present (Table 33.1).

Moderate. Moderate NPDR is characterized by more significant retinal lesions. These lesions represent not only changes in vascular and perivascular tissue but also changes within the retina associated with the effects of relative retinal hypoxia and circulatory changes. More abundant retinal hemorrhages and microaneurysms are present (Fig. 33.1). Early venous caliber abnormalities may also be present, reflected clinically as tortuous vasculature with varying lumen size. Venous caliber abnormalities may be caused by either greater adhesiveness of blood platelets resulting in more sluggish blood flow or actual blood vessel wall weakening secondary to the diabetic condition.

Another vascular change with moderate NPDR is intraretinal microvascular abnormalities (IRMAs) (Fig. 33.2). IRMAs represent either an abnormality of preexisting retinal vessels or a type of intraretinal neovascularization. Cotton-wool spots may also be present at this stage, which represent necrosis in the nerve fiber layer of the retina caused by hypoxia after microinfarct in retinal capillaries. Cotton-wool spots are the ophthalmoscopic manifestation of infarcts of capillaries within the nerve fiber layer, and it is not unusual to see IRMAs distal to cotton-wool spots. Cotton-wool spots tend to disappear as NPDR becomes more severe.

Patients with moderate NPDR have more significant retinal disease. These patients are at greater risk for progression to vision-threatening retinopathy and should be followed every 4–6 mo.

Severe. Severe NPDR is characterized by an abundance of preproliferative lesions that include venous beading (Fig. 33.3), IRMAs (Fig. 33.2), and extensive hemorrhages and microaneurysms (Fig. 33.1). The progression to very severe NPDR represents more widespread retinal ischemia, but frank new-vessel growth on the retina is not present. Consultation with an ophthalmologist experienced in the management of diabetic eye disease for possible early laser surgery is urgent, particularly if extenuating circumstances exist, e.g., pregnancy or cataract, or if the patient seems to be noncompliant or careless about follow-up examination. Rates of progression to high-risk PDR approach 45–50% in 2 yr and 75% in 5 yr if untreated.

PDR

PDR represents a severe form of retinopathy. It is characterized by the growth of new vessels on the optic disk or within 1 disk diameter of the optic disk (NVD), the growth of new vessels elsewhere on the retina (NVE), or preretinal fibrous tissue proliferation. These vessels grow over the retinal surface and on the posterior surface of the vitreous. They are fragile and rupture easily, causing preretinal and vitreous hemorrhage. The vessels can rupture sponta-

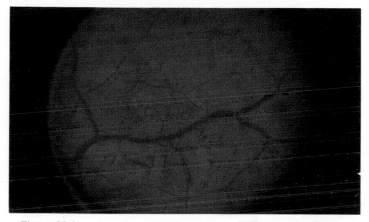

Figure 33.1. Extent of hemorrhages or microaneurysms in all 4 quadrants constitutes severe nonproliferative diabetic retinopathy. Standard photograph 2A.

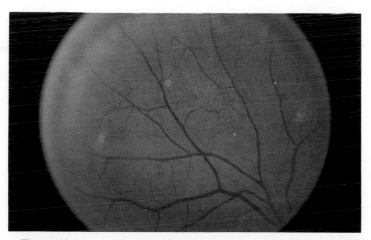

Figure 33.2. This extent of intraretinal microvascular abnormalities in ≥2 quadrants constitutes severe nonproliferative diabetic retinopathy. Standard photograph 8A.

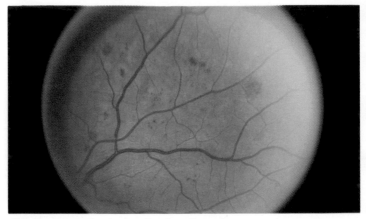

Figure 33.3. Venous beading in ≥2 quadrants constitutes severe non-proliferative diabetic retinopathy. Standard photograph 6B.

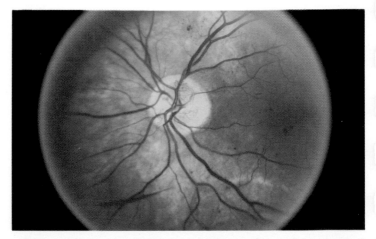

Figure 33.4. New vessels on disk ≥¼ disk area with or without preretinal or vitreous hemorrhage constitutes high-risk diabetic retinopathy. Standard photograph 10A.

neously, even while a person is asleep, or with vigorous exercise, straining, coughing, and sneezing.

High-risk PDR puts a person at significant risk of visual loss (Table 33.2). DRS revealed a 25–40% risk of severe visual loss over a 2-yr period if high-risk PDR is present. Scatter laser treatment can reduce this risk by ~60%. High-risk PDR is characterized by any one of the following lesions:

1. NVD > standard photo 10A of the modified Airlee House classification of diabetic retinopathy (i.e., NVD that covers ¼ to ⅓ of the disk area) (Fig. 33.4)
2. NVD < standard photo 10A if preretinal or vitreous hemorrhage is present
3. NVE if preretinal or vitreous hemorrhage is present

Patients with high-risk PDR are candidates for immediate emergency scatter laser photocoagulation. These patients should be referred immediately for laser treatment to a retinologist or ophthalmologist skilled in the treatment of diabetic retinopathy. These patients should not wait more than a few days for laser surgery.

ETDRS demonstrated that scatter laser treatment applied when a person approaches or reaches high-risk PDR can reduce the 5-yr risk of severe visual loss to <10%. In full scatter treatment, at least 1200–2000 lesions are applied to the posterior pole. Two or more sessions are normally required to complete the treatment. The treating ophthalmologist applies the 500-μm laser burns ~500 μm apart. Major retinal vessels and scarred areas are avoided.

The response to full scatter photocoagulation varies depending on the retinal and medical status of the patient. There may be *1*) regression of active neovascularization, *2*) persistent neovascularization without further progression, *3*) continued growth of the neovascularization, or *4*) recurrent vitreous hemorrhage. Careful follow-up evaluation by the treating ophthalmologist with additional scatter or local laser photocoagulation may be indicated, especially if continued new-vessel growth or recurrent vitreous hemorrhage occurs.

Fibrous tissue proliferation leads to traction, which may cause a retinal detachment that may not be visible if a view of the posterior pole is obscured by vitreous hemorrhage. Ultrasound examination may be necessary. Nonresolving vitreous hemorrhage and traction retinal detachments, particularly those threatening detachment of the macula, may be indications for vitrectomy surgery.

PDR usually extends through an active phase, followed by remission. In the remission phase, fibrous tissue will form, usually along abnormal vessels, but also between the retina and posterior vitreous surface. A goal of scatter laser surgery is to shorten the active phase of retinopathy, leading to remission before major vitreous hemorrhage or fibrous tissue proliferation. Patients who undergo scatter laser surgery for PDR may have activation of retinopathy in the future and require further laser treatments.

Laser photocoagulation is not without potential complications. DRS documented a minor decrease in visual acuity levels and peripheral visual fields, particularly in eyes treated with the xenon-arc photocoagulator. These risks need to be weighed against the potential benefits of laser surgery. Most scatter photocoagulation is performed with an argon laser.

Many factors affect the progression of retinopathy, including duration of diabetes and retinopathy status in type I diabetic patients, pregnancy, the use of diuretics, and glycosylated hemoglobin levels. In type II diabetic patients, the age of the patient, severity of retinopathy, diuretic usage, lower intraocular pressure, smoking, and lower diastolic blood pressure may be risk factors.

DME

DME can be present at any stage of retinopathy. It is a leading cause of moderate visual loss from diabetes (i.e., a doubling of the visual angle down to a level of ~20/200). DME is a collection of fluid or thickening in the macula, hard exudates within the macula area, nonperfusion of the retina inside the temporal vessel arcades, or any combination of these lesions. Patients with or suspected to have DME should be referred to an ophthalmologist for evaluation for clinically significant DME and treatable lesions of DME. Clinically significant DME is characterized by any of the following retinal lesions:

- Retinal thickening at or within 500 μm from the center of the macula
- Hard exudates at or within 500 μm from the center of the macula if accompanied by thickening of the adjacent retina
- A zone or zones of thickening $\geq$1 disk area in size, any portion of which is <1 disk diameter from the center of the macula

Patients with clinically significant DME should be referred to an experienced retinologist or ophthalmologist. The urgency for treatment of DME is not as acute as for high-risk PDR, but consultation and referral should occur within 1 mo.

DME can only be evaluated properly through dilated pupils and with stereoscopic examination of the macula. Stereo fundus photography is an important adjunct examination for patients who have or are suspected to have DME.

Patients with clinically significant DME are candidates for focal laser photocoagulation. The goal of treatment is to maintain acuity at approximately the same level as before treatment by preventing or limiting further leakage in the retina and allowing the leakage already present to resorb. With fluorescein angiography when possible, the ophthalmologist will determine whether treatable lesions are present and apply focal or grid laser surgery. Focal treatment should be applied to focal leaks contributing to DME. Grid treatment should be applied to areas of diffuse leakage or areas of nonperfusion in the macula area.

ETDRS demonstrated that, in eyes with edema involving the center of the macula, the risk of moderate visual loss was 50–60% less for eyes treated with focal laser compared with eyes assigned to deferral of treatment. Focal photocoagulation reduced the risk of moderate visual loss, increased the chance of visual improvement, decreased retinal thickening, and was not associated with any major adverse effects.

NONRETINAL OCULAR COMPLICATIONS

The ocular manifestations of diabetes that receive most attention are those related to diabetic retinopathy and maculopathy, because these changes are usually responsible for the most devastating visual threat from diabetes. Diabetic eye disease, however, represents an end-organ response to a generalized medical condition. Consequently, all structures of the eye are susceptible to the deleterious effects of diabetes. Following are some of the ocular problems in addition to retinopathy that are associated with diabetes:

- Mononeuropathies of cranial nerves III, IV, or VI
- Higher incidence of glaucoma
- Earlier and more rapidly progressing cataracts
- Susceptibility to corneal abrasions and recurrent corneal erosions
- Early presbyopia
- Blurred or fluctuating vision

Lenticular Opacities

Cataracts occur at a younger age and progress more rapidly in the presence of diabetes. Cataracts are $1.6 \times$ more common in people with diabetes. This increased risk of cataract development occurs in both type I and type II diabetic populations.

Reversible lenticular opacities related to diabetes mellitus can occur in different layers of the lens and are most frequently related to poor glycemic control. The so-called true diabetic cataracts are usually bilateral and are characterized by dense bands of white subcapsular spots that look like snowflakes or fine needle-shaped opacities. Because diabetic cataracts are related to prolonged periods of hyperglycemia and untreated diabetes, they are rarely seen.

Management of diabetic cataracts involves the same treatment strategies as those for age-related cataracts. For visual impairment not requiring surgery, optimum refraction is mandatory. Glare-control lenses and the use of sunglasses may relieve cataract-induced visual symptoms. Fortunately, cataract extraction with and without lens implantation is 90–95% successful in restoring useful vision, but the surgery has potential complications unique to diabetes. Intraocular lens implants provide the most natural postsurgical refractive correction, although the younger age of some diabetic patients may preclude the use of lens implantation. Careful patient education and consultation with the cataract surgeon is indicated.

A further consideration for the diabetic patient requiring cataract surgery involves the status of diabetic retinopathy. Diabetes is associated with an increased incidence of postoperative rubeosis iridis and neovascular glaucoma after intracapsular cataract extractions, regardless of the degree of retinopathy before surgery. If active PDR is present before intracapsular cataract surgery, the risk of subsequently developing rubeosis iridis, neovascular glaucoma, and vitreous hemorrhage is greater.

To provide appropriate preoperative care, physicians must determine diabetic retinopathy status before cataract extraction. Scatter laser photocoagulation is indicated for patients with high-risk PDR. With cataracts developing in the presence of severe NPDR or PDR without high-risk PDR, early laser treatment may be indicated. Laser treatment may be required a few days after surgery if active PDR is present.

Extracapsular cataract extraction with posterior chamber intraocular lens may reduce the potential problems of intracapsular cataract extraction. However, any ocular surgery presents a risk for the progression of diabetic retinopathy. The outcome of this procedure is affected by the retinal status and the presence or absence of DME.

Glaucoma

Open-angle glaucoma is 1.4× more common in the diabetic population. The prevalence of glaucoma increases with age and duration of diabetes, but medical therapy for open-angle glaucoma is generally effective. Argon-laser trabeculoplasty may normalize intraocular pressures in some patients if medical therapy proves ineffective. Treatment of open-angle glaucoma for the diabetic patient is essentially the same as for the nondiabetic patient.

Neovascular glaucoma is more severe and sometimes occurs in eyes with severe diabetic retinopathy or retinal detachments or occasionally after cataract surgery. It results from a proliferation of new vessels on the surface of the iris. These vessels are usually first observed at the pupillary border. If rubeosis progresses, a fine network of vessels may grow over the iris tissue and into the filtration angle of the eye. This growth results in peripheral anterior synechiae, and closure of the angle by this fibrovascular network results in neovascular glaucoma. In some cases, intraocular pressure may be elevated before angle involvement because of protein and cellular leakage from the proliferative vessels. Occasionally, iris neovascularization may be present in the filtration angle while not at the pupillary border.

Neovascular glaucoma is difficult to manage and requires aggressive treatment. Treatment modalities for rubeosis iridis and neovascular glaucoma include

- Scatter photocoagulation

- Goniophotocoagulation
- Topical antiglaucoma drugs
- Systemic antiglaucoma drugs
- Filtration surgery
- A combination of these therapies

Early recognition and prompt retinal photocoagulation may prevent full development of this devastating condition.

EXAMINATION CRITERIA AND FREQUENCY

Patients with diabetes mellitus should be examined *1*) at least within 5 yr of diagnosis for those with type I diabetes and at least yearly thereafter and *2*) on diagnosis for those with type II diabetes and at least yearly thereafter.

Pregnancy, nephropathy, hypertension, hypercholesterolemia, and other medical conditions may dictate more frequent examination. The presence of DME and diabetic retinopathy greater than very mild NPDR indicate a need for more frequent examination. Tables 33.3 and 33.4 outline the examination and guidelines for the care of diabetic patients.

VISUAL AND PSYCHOSOCIAL REHABILITATION

Patients with significant retinal disease or those who have lost vision from retinopathy should be encouraged to continue with regular eye care. Vitrectomy surgery can restore usable vision for some individuals who have lost sight from vitreous hemorrhages or fibrous tissue proliferation with traction retinal detachment. Proper refraction, low-vision evaluation and optical aids, and other techniques and devices are available to enable a person to use even severely limited vision. Referral to low-vision specialists may be appropriate. Support groups for the visually impaired and organizations providing vocational rehabilitation exist in most areas. All practitioners

Table 33.3. **EYE EXAMINATION SCHEDULE**

Age of Diabetes Onset (yr)	Recommended Time for First Examination	Routine Minimum Follow-Up*
0–30	5 yr after onset†	Yearly
≥31	At time of diagnosis	Yearly
During pregnancy	During 1st trimester	At physician's discretion

Adapted from the American Diabetes Association clinical recommendations
*Abnormal findings dictate more frequent follow-up examinations (Table 33.4).
†<5 yr if in immediate postpubescent stage.

Table 33.4. MANAGEMENT RECOMMENDATIONS

Diabetic Status of Retina	Follow-Up (monthly)	Color Fundus Photography	Fluorescein Angiography	Laser
1. Normal or minimal NPDR	12	No	No	No
2. Mild to moderate NPDR without DME	6–12	Rarely	No	No
3. Mild to moderate NPDR with clinically insignificant DME	4–6	Occasionally	Occasionally	No
4. Mild to moderate NPDR with CSME	3–4	Yes	Yes, if CSME	Yes
5. Severe to very severe NPDR	3–4	Yes	Yes, if CSME	Consider
6. Non–high-risk NPDR	2–3	Occasionally	Yes, if CSME	Consider
7. High-risk PDR	3–4	Yes	No	Yes
8. High-risk PDR not amenable to photocoagulation	1–6	If possible	No	Occasionally in connection with vitrectomy

NPDR, nonproliferative diabetic retinopathy; DME, diabetic macular edema; CSME, clinically significant macular edema; PDR, proliferative diabetic retinopathy. Adapted from American Academy of Ophthalmology preferred practice patterns for diabetic retinopathy.

should be familiar with appropriate referral sources for their patients with visual impairment.

Unlike many other eye conditions, diabetic retinopathy is not solely an eye problem but an end-organ response to a devastating systemic condition affecting the other organs, e.g., the heart and kidney. Multiple psychological and social issues may be present. Health-care providers must be alert to these issues and assist in their appropriate management.

In its earliest stages, diabetic retinopathy causes no symptoms. Visual acuity may be excellent and, on evaluation and diagnosis, a patient may deny the presence of retinopathy. At this stage, the physician should initiate a careful program of education and follow-up. If the retinal disease progresses, visual acuity may be compromised by DME or episodes of vitreous hemorrhage. Difficulty in the work or home environment may result. Although denial may continue, anger may result. Fear of blindness and other complications of diabetes, including death, may also develop.

If the visual acuity drops to 20/200 or worse, a patient may remain in a stage of uncertainty until the retinopathy is in quiescence either secondary to laser treatment or vitreoretinal surgery. Once the retinopathy is in remission and the vision stable, the patient is in a position to accept his/her situation and to make the appropriate psychological and social adjustments. At this time, visual and vocational rehabilitation are usually more successful.

Communication among all members of a patient's health care team is of paramount importance in dealing with the physical and psychological stresses of visual loss from diabetes.

SUGGESTED READING

1. Aiello LM, Rand LI, Sebestyen SG, Weiss JN, Bradbury MJ, Wafai MZ, Briones JC: The eyes and diabetes. In *Joslin's Diabetes Mellitus*. 12th ed. Marble A, Eds. Philadelphia, PA, Lea & Febiger, 1985, p. 600–34
2. The Diabetic Retinopathy Study Research Group: Photocoagulation treatment of proliferative diabetic retinopathy: the second report of diabetic retinopathy study findings. *Ophthalmology* 85:82–106, 1978
3. The Diabetic Retinopathy Study Research Group: Photocoagulation treatment of proliferative diabetic retinopathy: clinical application of Diabetic Retinopathy Study findings: DRS report no. 8. *Ophthalmology* 88:583–600, 1981
4. Diabetic Retinopathy Vitrectomy Study Research Group: Early vitrectomy for severe proliferative diabetic retinopathy in eyes with useful vision: results of randomized trial: Diabetic Retinopathy Vitrectomy Study report no. 3. *Ophthalmology* 95:1307–20, 1988
5. Diabetic Retinopathy Vitrectomy Study Research Group: Early vitrectomy for severe proliferative diabetic retinopathy in eyes with useful vision: clinical application of results of a randomized trial: Diabetic Retinopathy Vitrectomy Study report no. 4. *Ophthalmology* 95:1321–34, 1988

6. Early Treatment Diabetic Retinopathy Study Group: Early Treatment Diabetic Retinopathy Study report no. 1: photocoagulation for diabetic macular edema. *Arch Ophthalmol* 103:1796–806, 1985

7. Early Treatment Diabetic Retinopathy Study Group: Treatment techniques and clinical guidelines for photocoagulation of diabetic macular edema: Early Treatment Diabetic Retinopathy Study report no. 2. *Ophthalmology* 94:761–74, 1987

8. Klein BEK, Davis MD, Segal P, Long JA, Harris WA, Hawg GA, Magili YL, Syrjala S: Diabetic retinopathy: assessment of severity and progression. *Ophthalmology* 91:10–17, 1984

9. Klein R, Klein BEK, Moss SE, Davis MD, DeMets DL: The Wisconsin Epidemiologic Study of Diabetic Retinopathy. II. Prevalence and risk of diabetic retinopathy when age at diagnosis is less than 30 years. *Arch Ophthalmol* 102:520–26, 1984

10. Klein R, Klein BEK, Moss SE, Davis MD, DeMets DL: The Wisconsin Epidemiologic Study of Diabetic Retinopathy. III. Prevalence and risk of diabetic retinopathy when age at diagnosis is 30 or more years. *Arch Ophthalmol* 102:527–32, 1984

11. Klein R, Moss SE, Klein BEK, Davis MD, DeMets DL: The Wisconsin Epidemiologic Study of Diabetic Retinopathy. XI. The incidence of macular edema. *Ophthalmology* 96:1501–10, 1989

34. Drug-Induced Renal Dysfunction

WILLIAM M. BENNETT, MD

A knowledge of common drug-induced renal syndromes and their recognition and prevention are essential for the primary-care physician caring for diabetic patients.

SUSCEPTIBILITY TO KIDNEY INJURY

Two factors make the kidneys a frequent target organ for drug toxicity. First, they receive a high fraction (20–25%) of the cardiac output relative to their weight, so that drugs transit the kidneys in large amounts. Second, the renal countercurrent concentrating mechanism for water also concentrates drugs and chemicals within the filtered tubular fluid. Thus, local concentrations of these substances in contact with renal epithelium may exceed that in peripheral blood.

In diabetes, there is often subclinical preexisting renal dysfunction even when blood urea nitrogen (BUN) and serum creatinine are within the normal range. These tests are insensitive to pathological processes, e.g., diabetes-related macrovascular or microvascular disease, until substantial kidney damage is present. This is particularly true in the hypertensive diabetic patient.

Several factors affect prescribing for the diabetic patient:

1. If proteinuria without other explanation is present, diabetic nephropathy can be assumed.

Dr. Bennett is Professor of Medicine and Pharmacology and Co-Head of the Division of Nephrology and Hypertension at the Oregon Health Sciences University, Portland, OR.

2. Diabetic retinopathy is almost invariably associated with some degree of nephropathy.

3. In a patient with a history of upper urinary tract infections, bladder dysfunction, or stones, the clinician should be alert for renal papillary necrosis and underlying interstitial renal disease.

For these patients, a measured or estimated creatinine clearance is essential to avoid overdosage. The estimated clearance relates the serum creatinine to the patient's body habitus and age by the formula

$$\text{estimated creatinine clearance} = \frac{(140 - \text{patient age})(\text{body wt in kg})}{72(\text{serum creatinine in mg/dl})}$$

This formula is accurate except in patients with massive edema, ascites, or pregnancy; the final value should be multiplied by 0.85 for women. Note also that not all renal dysfunction in diabetes is due to the underlying diabetic renal disease; i.e., diabetic patients are as susceptible as nondiabetic individuals to glomerulonephritis or interstitial nephritis. A careful urinary sediment examination to exclude hematuria, cellular casts, and pyuria helps to exclude other processes in these patients.

NEPHROTOXINS

Radiographic Contrast Media

Diabetic patients are at increased risk of renal dysfunction when diagnostic procedures, e.g., intravenous pyelography, angiography, or computed tomography, are performed with iodinated dyes. Contrast agents, including nonionics, are promptly excreted by the kidney and produce acute increases in BUN and creatinine. The known risk factors for contrast nephropathy have in common relative kidney underperfusion, which may be aggravated by the reduction of vasodilatory renal prostaglandins (Table 34.1).

Some patients with contrast-associated renal failure also have permanent impairment of renal function, with some requiring di-

Table 34.1. **CLINICAL RISK FACTORS FOR CONTRAST NEPHROPATHY**

- Large amount of contrast material
- Several studies performed
- Abnormal baseline serum creatinine
- Preexisting renal disease
- Diabetes mellitus
- Abnormal liver function
- Proteinuria
- Hypertension
- Vascular disease

alysis. Virtually all of these patients will have preexisting renal disease. Contrast-associated nephropathy is rarely the only etiologic factor in acute renal insufficiency, but the patients at greatest risk are clearly those with diabetic nephropathy, chronic renal failure, or congestive heart failure.

Clinical Presentation. Contrast-associated nephropathy usually begins within 24 h after performance of a contrast study and can be defined as a change in serum creatinine of ≥50% from baseline or an absolute increase of 1 mg/dl (88.4 μM). Serum creatinine peaks within 3–5 days of the study, and oliguria is observed in only 30% of patients. Formed elements in urinary sediment, although frequent, are insensitive markers of injury and of little diagnostic value. Although the fractional excretion of sodium is frequently low, it has little prognostic value because most patients recover from contrast nephropathy without clinical consequences. The most practical way to evaluate a patient in the absence of oliguria is to monitor serum creatinine daily in high-risk patients, especially if two or more risk factors are present (Table 34.1).

Prevention and Management. To select an imaging study, always use the least invasive procedure that will provide adequate diagnostic information. The following recommendations can be used for patients whose serum creatinine is ≥2 mg/dl (≥176.8 μM) at baseline:

1. One hour before the study, begin a 20-ml/h infusion of 500 ml 20% mannitol with 200 mg furosemide added.
2. Continue this infusion uninterrupted for 6 h after completion of the study.
3. Half-normal saline in 5% dextrose and water (D_5W) with 30 meq/L potassium is used to replace urine output on a milliliter-for-milliliter basis.

Although this regimen has not been validated by controlled studies, it appears to be safe. In addition, many clinicians recommend the use of nonionic low-osmolar contrast agents in diabetic patients with renal insufficiency to further reduce the risk of significant renal ischemia. Evidence on the value of this approach is not available to justify the considerable cost of the newer agents.

Nonsteroidal Anti-Inflammatory Drugs (NSAIDs)

The adverse effects of NSAIDs on the kidney are usually confined to the clinical settings of relative renal ischemia that frequently coexists with diabetes. In diverse conditions such as congestive heart failure, cirrhosis, nephrosis, or diuretic use, there are increases in angiotensin II, catecholamines, and vasopressin. Both angiotensin II and vasopressin stimulate production of vasodilatory prostaglandins (PGE_2 and prostacyclin), which balance the vasoconstrictor actions of these agonists. Administration of NSAIDs causes selective inhibition of prostaglandin synthesis; an unmodulated vasoconstrictor response to angiotensin II, vasopressin, and catecholamines; and a reduction in renal blood flow and glomerular filtration rate. In addition to patients who have edema-forming states, others notably at risk include those with atherosclerotic cardiovascular disease.

Clinical Features. Clinical renal syndromes associated with NSAID use include the spectrum of drug-induced renal failure: hemodynamically mediated acute renal dysfunction, allergic interstitial nephritis with nephrotic syndrome, hyperkalemia due to hyporeninemic hypoaldosteronism, and sodium retention with diuretic resistance. The most common clinical presentation of NSAID-induced dysfunction is hemodynamically mediated acute renal dysfunction in patients with the aforementioned preexisting conditions of relative renal ischemia.

Hyperkalemia. NSAIDs frequently reduce the antihypertensive efficacy of diuretic agents, whereas the combination of NSAIDs with triamterene or other diuretics is additive and may produce a particularly severe form of acute renal failure. Diabetic patients with renal dysfunction are at particular risk of hyperkalemia with NSAIDS (Table 34.2). Elderly patients are at particularly high risk for problems with these agents, possibly because the frequency of their use is 3× that of patients under age 60 yr.

Acute interstitial nephritis. A more common clinical presentation is that of acute interstitial nephritis with nephrotic-range proteinuria. There seems to be no clinical situation that predisposes to this reaction. Onset may be weeks or months after starting NSAID therapy and is marked by proteinuria of ≥3 g/24 h. It is usually reversible on discontinuation of the NSAID. However, in the occasional patient who fails to respond promptly with a return of normal creatinine, a short course of high-dose steroids, i.e., 60 mg prednisone given over 3 days with rapid tapering over the next week, can speed recovery of the filtration rate.

Renal papillary necrosis and chronic tubulointerstitial disease. These conditions are associated with analgesic use and abuse in amounts

Table 34.2. **DRUG INTERACTIONS IN DIABETIC PATIENTS THAT PREDISPOSE TO SERIOUS HYPERKALEMIA**

Drug	Mechanism
β-Blockers	Inhibit renin-angiotensin system; block β-agonist movement of K^+ into cells
Amiloride	Blocks renal K^+ secretion
Triamterene	Blocks renal K^+ secretion
Spironolactone	Blocks renal K^+ secretion by blocking aldosterone action
Angiotensin-converting enzyme inhibitors	Inhibit conversion of angiotensin I to angiotensin II
Nonsteroidal anti-inflammatory drugs (NSAIDs)	Inhibit prostaglandin-mediated renin responses

>2 kg cumulatively. This can add to the papillary ischemia that occurs in some diabetic patients with bladder dysfunction and urinary tract infections. There is loss of renal concentrating capacity and the presence of electrolyte-wasting syndromes, e.g., renal sodium wasting and hyperkalemic renal tubular acidosis. Analgesic-associated nephropathy should be suspected in middle-aged diabetic women with complaints of recurrent headaches or back pain. Although many will deny intake, some confess to taking aspirin, acetaminophen, or combination analgesics in amounts >4–6 tablets/day. As with NSAIDs, the treatment of choice is withdrawal of the agents. For chronic analgesic abuse, the entity will not be reversible, but many patients will plateau at their current level of function. Avoidance of these drugs in high-risk patients and the careful monitoring of serum creatinine are of benefit.

Antibiotics and Anti-Infective Agents

Most antibiotics in clinical use have a low nephrotoxic potential except for the rare idiosyncratic acute interstitial nephritis produced by penicillin, sulfonamide, and cephalosporin derivatives. Others, e.g., amphotericin B and the aminoglycosides are significantly nephrotoxic.

Aminoglycoside Antibiotics. Aminoglycosides are valuable therapeutic agents for the treatment of serious gram-negative infections However, 10–15% of all therapeutic courses are complicated by reversible renal dysfunction, even when peak and trough serum levels are kept within the desired therapeutic range. In addition, ototoxicity, both cochlear and vestibular, is frequent, particularly in elderly patients with preexisting renal dysfunction. Various risk factors that predispose to the development of aminoglycoside nephrotoxicity have been identified (Table 34.3).

Nonoliguric renal insufficiency is the most common manifestation of aminoglycoside nephrotoxicity. Less common are various isolated tubular syndromes, e.g., nephrogenic diabetes insipidus, Fanconi syndrome, and renal potassium or magnesium wasting. Fortunately, severe oliguric renal failure requiring dialysis is rare from aminoglycosides alone. A drug-induced concentrating defect characterized by polyuria and secondary thirst stimulation precedes the detectable

Table 34.3. **RISK FACTORS FOR AMINOGLYCOSIDE NEPHROTOXICITY**

- High dose and long duration of treatment
- Recent courses of aminoglycoside therapy
- Age >60 yr
- Concomitant nephrotoxins
- Volume depletion
- K^+ depletion
- Mg^{2+} depletion
- Preexisting renal dysfunction
- Liver disease

rise in BUN and serum creatinine that will occur in as many as 30% of hospitalized patients given >5–7 days of aminoglycoside treatment. Granular casts and mild proteinuria occur frequently but are not of diagnostic assistance. The renal histological picture associated with aminoglycoside nephrotoxicity is one of patchy proximal tubular necrosis. In addition, in patients who satisfy the clinical criteria for aminoglycoside nephrotoxicity, cellular autophagocytosis has been observed with electron microscopy.

Aminoglycosides are often necessary for management of the diabetic patient. Loading doses should be sufficient to achieve high peak levels to maximize bacterial killing. Because the elimination half-life of aminoglycosides, normally 2 h, is markedly prolonged as renal function falls, maintenance-dose intervals should be carefully extended in patients with existing renal dysfunction when aminoglycosides are required. Extending the interval between doses is safer than reducing the size of individual doses in patients with renal insufficiency. Correctable risk factors should be minimized, and in high-risk patients, the less nephrotoxic congeners should be considered. Among the clinically available aminoglycosides, the spectrum of nephrotoxicity is gentamicin > tobramycin > amikacin > netilmicin. Monitoring of peak serum levels will ensure efficacy, whereas elevation of the trough level, showing drug accumulation, will often precede a rise in the less-sensitive serum creatinine measurements.

Amphotericin B. Amphotericin B is a polyene antibiotic with activity against a broad spectrum of fungi. However, renal function becomes impaired in ≥80% of patients given amphotericin B. This nephrotoxicity is dose-related and probably inevitable in cumulative doses >5 g in adults. Patients at high risk include elderly patients, particularly those with depleted extracellular volume.

The usual clinical presentation of amphotericin B nephrotoxicity is characterized by defects in renal tubular function. Occasionally, this condition will progress to nonoliguric renal failure. Modest proteinuria associated with a relatively normal urinary sediment is the initial finding. Frank azotemia is preceded by hypokalemia, renal tubular acidosis, and impaired urinary concentrating capacity. In addition, the presence of a magnesium-wasting syndrome is a prominent feature of amphotericin nephrotoxicity. Repetitive courses of amphotericin B may cause permanent impairment of renal function.

Although there is no universally accepted way to prescribe amphotericin B, the following schedule is commonly used:

1. Give a test dose of 1 mg in 200 ml of D_5W over 2–4 h.
2. Observe the patient for acute adverse effects, e.g., headache, chills, fever, nausea, vomiting, and generalized muscle pain.
3. If no problems are recognized, an additional 5 mg amphotericin B in 500 ml of D_5W can be given over 4–6 h. Increase the dose by 5 mg/day with the same 500-ml infusion over 4–6 h until a daily dose of 0.4–0.75 mg/kg is reached.

4. For critically ill patients, a dosage schedule of 0.25 mg/kg on day 1, increasing to 0.5 mg/kg on day 2, and finally achieving $0.75 \text{ mg} \cdot \text{kg}^{-1} \cdot \text{day}^{-1}$ by day 3 can be used provided there is no adverse reaction to the test dose.
5. Frequent monitoring of serum creatinine is recommended. If toxicity occurs, the amphotericin dosage can be reduced to the previous level, it can be interrupted for 2 days, or a double dose can be given on alternate days. A doubling of the baseline serum creatinine is indicative of serious nephrotoxicity.

Sodium supplementation in the form of intravenous saline can be used as a safe and effective means of reducing the risk of amphotericin nephrotoxicity to ~10%. Sodium (150 meq/day) can be administered as follows: 500 ml normal saline 30 min before amphotericin B administration and a second 500 ml given during the 30 min after completion of the amphotericin infusion. The goal is to achieve a urinary sodium excretion of 250–300 mmol/day.

Angiotensin-Converting Enzyme (ACE) Inhibitors

With emerging evidence that treatment of systemic hypertension and concomitant lowering of intraglomerular pressure has a beneficial effect on the course of renal disease in diabetes, ACE inhibitors have been advocated as the antihypertensive therapeutic class of choice. Although these compounds are generally well tolerated, acute renal dysfunction can occur in the presence of atherosclerotic vascular disease involving the main renal arteries or in any other situation where renal hemodynamics are maintained by angiotensin-mediated constriction of postglomerular vessels.

Other examples of this clinical physiology include severe congestive heart failure, diuretic-induced extracellular volume depletion, or stenosis of an artery to a solitary kidney. A chemistry panel should be checked on all patients within 5–7 days of drug initiation, particularly those over age 50 yr and those with any predisposing condition. If renal dysfunction occurs, dosage reduction or reduction of any concomitantly administered diuretic dosage usually improves renal hemodynamics.

SUGGESTED READING

1. Bennett WM: Guide to drug dosage in renal failure. *Clin Pharmacokinet* 15:326–54, 1988
2. Bennett WM: Mechanisms of aminoglycoside nephrotoxicity. *Clin Exp Pharmacol Physiol* 16:1–6, 1989
3. Bennett WM, Porter GA: Nephrotoxicity of common drugs used by urologists. *Urol Clin North Am* 17:145–56, 1990
4. Berkseth RO, Kjellstrand CM: Radiologic contrast-induced nephropathy. *Med Clin North Am* 68:351–70, 1984
5. Cooper K, Bennett WM: Nephrotoxicity of common drugs used in clinical practice. *Arch Intern Med* 147:1213–18, 1987

35. Nephropathy

RALPH A. DeFRONZO, MD

Diabetic nephropathy develops in ~40% of patients with type I (insulin-dependent) diabetes mellitus with diabetes for ≥20 yr. Clinically significant renal disease is less common in type II (non-insulin-dependent) diabetes, occurring in 5–10% of patients. However, in certain populations with an increased prevalence of type II diabetes, e.g., American Indians, Hispanics, and blacks, the prevalence of renal disease is much greater.

Diabetic nephropathy is the most common cause of end-stage renal failure (ESRF) in the United States and is responsible for ~30% of all new patients entering ESRF programs. Although dialysis and transplantation prevent death from uremia (see chapt. 36), 5-yr survival approaches 20%, which is much worse than in nondiabetic patients. Therefore, it is important to recognize the earliest stages of diabetic nephropathy and to institute appropriate therapy. Once proteinuria has become established, relentless progression to ESRF is inevitable. A program for monitoring renal function is proposed in Table 35.1.

PATHOGENESIS

A rational approach to the therapy of diabetic renal disease depends on understanding its pathogenesis (Table 35.2). Most diabetic patients who develop renal insufficiency demonstrate poor glycemic control. Genetic factors also are important; diabetic nephropathy tends to aggregate in families. Hemodynamic abnormalities, exac-

Dr. DeFronzo is Chief of the Diabetes Division at the University of Texas Health Science Center, San Antonio, TX.

Table 35.1. MONITORING RENAL FUNCTION IN POSTPUBERTAL PATIENTS

Test	Initial Evaluation	Follow-Up
Urinary microalbumin (timed collection)	After initial glycemic control (within 3 mo of diagnosis)	Type I diabetes: yearly after 5 yr
		Type II diabetes: yearly
Creatinine clearance		Every 2 yr until <100 ml·min^{-1}·1.73 m^{-2}, then yearly*
24-h urinary protein		Type I diabetes: yearly after 5 yr
		Type II diabetes: yearly
Serum creatinine		Yearly*

*More frequent evaluation is indicated in patients with a creatinine clearance <70–80 ml/min or serum creatinine >1.5–1.6 mg/dl (>133–141 μM).

erbated by excessive protein intake and systemic hypertension, have been postulated to contribute to the demise of renal function. Metabolic disturbances also have been implicated in the pathogenesis of diabetic nephropathy.

NATURAL HISTORY OF DIABETIC NEPHROPATHY

Type I Diabetes

At diagnosis of type I diabetes, there are no renal histological abnormalities, but renal blood flow (RBF) and glomerular filtration rate (GFR) are elevated (Fig. 35.1). Within 3 yr, histological changes (increased mesangial matrix material and glomerular basement membrane thickening) of diabetic nephropathy become evident.

Table 35.2. CAUSES OF DIABETIC RENAL DISEASE

- Poor glycemic control (fasting plasma glucose levels >180–200 mg/dl [>10–11.1 mM])
- Genetic factors
- Hemodynamic abnormalities (increased renal blood flow, glomerular filtration rate, and intraglomerular pressure)
- Excessive protein intake
- Systemic hypertension
- Metabolic disturbances (abnormal polyol metabolism and formation of advanced glycosylation end products)
- Release of growth factors
- Abnormalities in carbohydrate/lipid/protein metabolism
- Structural abnormalities (glomerular hypertrophy, mesangial expansion, glomerular basement membrane thickening)

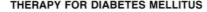

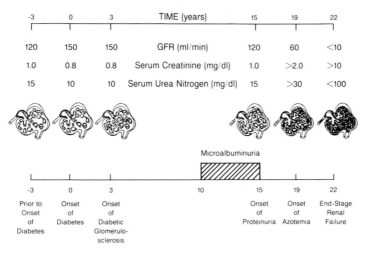

Figure 35.1. Natural history of diabetic nephropathy in insulin-dependent diabetes mellitus. GFR, glomerular filtration rate.

Over the subsequent 10–15 yr, there is progressive histological damage, but renal hyperfiltration persists, and laboratory data do not suggest renal involvement. Approximately 15 yr later, albuminuria (>250–300 mg/day) is detected, and the elevated RBF and GFR return to normal. This ominous sign heralds the onset of progressive renal insufficiency. At this stage, no intervention has been shown to prevent the eventual progression to ESRF. Within 4 yr after onset of proteinuria, ~50% of individuals experience a halving of GFR, and within ~3 yr, these patients progress to ESRF. At or just before onset of albuminuria, most patients develop hypertension, and the increase in blood pressure markedly accelerates the progression of renal disease. Effective treatment of hypertension is the only intervention that will slow, although not prevent, progression to ESRF. Once albuminuria develops, tight glycemic control cannot prevent progression to renal insufficiency.

A "preclinical" stage of diabetic nephropathy, characterized by microalbuminuria, has been recognized. Microalbuminuria, or the 25-250 mg/day range of albumin excretion, is abnormal, cannot be detected by routine means, and is the first laboratory evidence of diabetic renal disease. Fortunately, screening urine tests for microalbuminuria exist. Tight glycemic control with insulin during the microalbuminuric stage may prevent the development of diabetic nephropathy.

Type II Diabetes

The natural history of diabetic nephropathy in type II diabetes is less well characterized. Albuminuria, or microalbuminuria, is common at diagnosis, but most white patients with type II diabetes do not progress to ESRF. Rather, albuminuria may be a greater predictor of death from stroke and myocardial infarction; ~80% of these individuals die from cardiovascular complications within 10 yr.

EVALUATION OF LOSS OF RENAL FUNCTION

Every diabetic patient with proteinuria or elevated serum creatinine levels should have a thorough evaluation to exclude other causes of renal failure.

The patient history and physical examination should focus on drugs taken (nonsteroidal anti-inflammatory drugs and analgesics), toxin exposure, administration of radiographic contrast media, hereditary diseases, history of renal disease, allergic manifestations, skin rash, arthritis, fever, and involvement of other organ systems. Intravascular volume and cardiac status should be assessed to ensure adequate renal perfusion. Symptoms indicative of urinary tract obstruction (especially in men) or neurogenic bladder should be elicited. History of oliguria suggests another cause of the renal failure.

Diabetic nephropathy does not occur in the absence of retinopathy. If examination of the dilated pupil by an eye specialist fails to document evidence of diabetic retinopathy, another cause of the renal failure is likely. Proteinuria is the hallmark of diabetic nephropathy, and in its absence, the diagnosis cannot be made.

Laboratory assessment should include urinalysis, which is usually benign, although occasionally erythrocytes may be seen. Numerous erythrocytes or erythrocyte casts indicate glomerulonephritis. Leukocytes and bacteria imply urinary tract infection, and renal tubular epithelial cells suggest one of the tubulointerstitial causes of renal disease. Heavy proteinuria is consistent with diabetic renal disease or glomerulonephritis. The absence of proteinuria virtually excludes diabetic nephropathy.

Serum urea nitrogen and creatinine concentrations help exclude prerenal and postrenal causes of renal failure. In intrinsic renal disease, they increase in parallel in a ratio of 10–15:1. A disproportionate increase in serum urea nitrogen is observed with intravascular volume depletion, congestive heart failure, and urinary tract obstruction. Hyperkalemia and hyperchloremic metabolic acidosis, in the absence of a significant increase in the serum creatinine concentration (<3–4 mg/dl [<265–354 μM]), suggest interstitial nephritis or hypoaldosteronism. The latter is common in diabetic nephropathy. Serum Ca^{2+} and uric acid concentrations should be measured to exclude hypercalcemic and uric acid nephropathy, respectively.

Peripheral eosinophilia suggests an allergic interstitial nephritis. In patients with suspected glomerulonephritis, total serum complement and C3, anti-nuclear antibody, antistreptolysin O titer, antiglomerular basement membrane antibody titer, and cryoglobulins should be obtained. A very high erythrocyte sedimentation rate suggests vasculitis.

Renal ultrasound is a simple noninvasive method to exclude urinary tract obstruction and quantify kidney size. Small kidneys imply chronic advanced renal disease. Patients with early diabetic nephropathy have normal or increased kidney size. Radionuclide imaging with radiolabeled technetium allows assessment of renal blood flow. If, after a thorough evaluation, the course of the renal failure remains undefined, a renal biopsy should be considered.

TREATMENT

Antihypertensive Therapy: Therapeutic Goals

Hypertension is the most important factor known to accelerate the progression of renal failure. In type I diabetes, onset of hypertension characteristically occurs at onset of microalbuminuria. In type II diabetes, hypertension can occur at any time and parallels the patient's age and obesity index. Increased total body Na^+ content and enhanced responsiveness to angiotensin II and norepinephrine play important roles in the development of hypertension. Recent studies implicate insulin resistance and hyperinsulinemia in the pathogenesis of hypertension.

Treatment of hypertension at the microalbuminuric stage may completely arrest the progression of renal disease in some patients, whereas treatment at the stage of clinical proteinuria (>250 mg/day) can only slow the rate of deterioration. The most prudent goal is to lower the patient's blood pressure to the level present before the onset of proteinuria and/or renal insufficiency. If the patient's normal blood pressure is not known, the recommended goal should be 120–130/80–85 mmHg. Special caution is advised in elderly patients who may have underlying cerebrovascular and cardiovascular disease.

The goal of therapy is to normalize blood pressure. Weight loss and regular physical activity should be stressed, and a low NaCl intake (4–5 g/day or 68–85 meq/day) should be prescribed. Blood pressure should be assessed weekly, and the antihypertensive drug dosage should be doubled until maximum dosage is attained. If the blood pressure remains elevated, a second antihypertensive drug should be added. Patients should monitor their blood pressure daily in the home and communicate the results to the physician on a weekly basis.

All hypertensive diabetic patients with albuminuria, renal insufficiency, or evidence of hypertensive organ system damage (i.e., retinopathy, congestive heart failure, or nephropathy) should be referred to a nephrologist or a diabetes specialist with expertise in treating diabetic nephropathy. Accelerated or malignant hypertension is cause for immediate referral and hospitalization for parenteral antihypertensive treatment.

Nonpharmacological Intervention

Weight loss and exercise effectively lower blood pressure, particularly in obese type II diabetic patients. They have the added advantages of causing enhanced insulin sensitivity, lower plasma insulin levels, increased high-density lipoprotein (HDL) cholesterol levels, and reduced low-density lipoprotein (LDL) cholesterol and triglyceride concentrations (see chaps. 14 and 16).

If blood pressure is not reduced to normotensive levels, pharmacological therapy is indicated. The ideal antihypertensive agent should slow or halt the progression of renal disease and be metabolically neutral, i.e., not aggravate insulin resistance, hyperinsulinemia, and dyslipidemia.

Angiotensin-Converting Enzyme (ACE) Inhibitors

This class of drugs represents a very effective and rational approach to therapy. ACE inhibitors decrease peripheral vascular resistance by inhibiting angiotensin II production, decrease intraglomerular pressure, retard glomerular hypertrophy, reduce proteinuria and microalbuminuria, slow the rate of decline in GFR, improve insulin sensitivity, and promote a more favorable serum lipid profile.

ACE inhibitors may cause hyperkalemia, especially in patients with underlying hypoaldosteronism. In some patients (i.e., those with renal artery stenosis, severe congestive heart failure, and advanced renal insufficiency), ACE inhibition may cause a precipitous decline in GFR. Deterioration in renal function and hyperkalemia usually occur shortly after starting the drug. Therefore, patients should have their serum K^+ and creatinine concentrations checked ~1 wk after initiation of therapy. Currently available ACE inhibitors and specific doses are listed in Table 35.3.

Ca²⁺-Channel Antagonists

In hypertensive diabetic patients, intracellular Ca^{2+} concentration is increased (related to decreased activity of Ca^{2+}-ATPase), and this enhances the pressor responsiveness to vasoactive hormones, e.g., angiotensin II and norepinephrine. This pathophysiological derangement provides the rationale for use of Ca^{2+}-channel antagonists, which are very effective in reducing blood pressure in hypertensive diabetic patients. Certain Ca^{2+}-channel blockers may also decrease proteinuria and improve renal function in diabetic patients with established renal disease. This class of drugs does not adversely affect the plasma lipid profile or impair glucose tolerance, although nifedipine may aggravate insulin resistance. Peripheral edema may occur during therapy.

Specific doses of currently available Ca^{2+}-channel blockers are listed in Table 35.3. Ca^{2+}-channel antagonists, along with ACE inhibitors, are the drugs of choice in the treatment of hypertensive diabetic patients with proteinuria or renal insufficiency.

Table 35.3. RECOMMENDED ANTIHYPERTENSIVE AGENTS FOR HYPERTENSIVE DIABETIC PATIENTS

Drug	Usual Dose Range (mg)	Significant Side Effects	Other Considerations
Angiotensin-converting enzyme inhibitors			
Captopril	25–50 2 ×/day	Rash	Can improve insulin sensitivity, glucose tolerance, and plasma lipid levels. If total daily dose of enalapril and benazepril is >20 mg, split into 2 daily doses.
Enalapril	5–40/day	Neutropenia	
Benazepril	20–80/day	Proteinuria	
		Hyperkalemia	
		Fall in GFR	
Ca²⁺-channel antagonists			
Verapamil	40–120 3 ×/day	Increases serum digoxin level	Long-lasting formulations of these drugs are or will soon be available. No significant adverse effects on glucose or lipid metabolism are known.
		Negative inotropic effect	
		May cause A-V block	
Diltiazem	30–90 3 ×/day	Constipation	
		May cause A-V block	
Nicardipine	20–40 3 ×/day	Peripheral edema	
Nifedipine	10–30 3 ×/day	Peripheral edema	
Diuretics			
Hydrochlorthiazide	12.5–50/day	Hyponatremia	Thiazides are not effective when GFR decreases to <40–50 ml/min. Higher doses of furosemide may be required when nephrotic syndrome and/or renal insufficiency are present.
Chlorthiazide	500–2000/day	Hypokalemia	
Chlorthalidone	12.5–50/day	Glucose intolerance	
Metolazone	2.5–10/day	Increased low-density lipoprotein cholesterol and triglycerides	
Furosemide	20–80/day up to 40–160 2 ×/day		

Ethacrynic acid	25–100/day up to 50–200 2×/day	Decreased high-density lipoprotein cholesterol
Bumetanide	0.5–2/day up to 1–4 2×/day	Insulin resistance
β₁-Selective antagonists		
Metoprolol	50–100 2×/day	May cause A-V block	At higher doses, β₁-selectivity is lost; bronchospasm may be precipitated, hypoglycemia may occur, symptoms of hypoglycemia are masked. Severe hypertension may occur during hypoglycemic episodes.
Atenolol	50–100/day	May exacerbate congestive heart failure	
Central adrenergic antagonists		
Clonidine	0.1–0.6 2×/day	Drowsiness	Rebound hypertension may occur if these drugs are abruptly stopped.
Guanabenz	4–16 2×/day	Dry mouth	
Methyldopa	250–500 2–3×/day		
Peripheral α₁-antagonists		
Prazosin	1–5 2–3×/day	Orthostatic hypotension	These can improve insulin sensitivity and plasma lipid profile.
Terazosin	1–5/day at bedtime	First-dose phenomenon of syncope	
Doxazosin	1–8/day at bedtime		
Vasodilators		
Apresoline	10–50/3–4×/day	Headache	
		Reflex tachycardia	
Minoxidil	5–30 2×/day	Excess hair growth	Minoxidil is very effective in patients with refractory hypertension and renal insufficiency

A-V, arteriovenous; GFR, glomerular filtration rate.

Diuretics

Diabetic hypertensive patients, especially those with proteinuria and renal insufficiency, have an increase in total-body Na^+ content. This enhances the vascular responsiveness to angiotensin II and norepinephrine. Based on the central role of Na^+ retention in diabetic hypertension, diuretic therapy presents a rational therapeutic option. However, diuretics cause deterioration in glucose tolerance, worsened insulin resistance, increased LDL cholesterol and triglyceride levels, and decreased HDL cholesterol. Because of these adverse metabolic side effects and because other antihypertensive agents are equally effective, their primary use should be reserved for patients with evidence of Na^+ overload and/or renal insufficiency. Blood glucose and lipid levels should be monitored closely after the start of diuretic therapy. Concomitant use of ACE inhibitors may offset the deleterious effect of diuretics on glucose tolerance and serum lipids. Diuretics also have the undesirable side effect of hypokalemia, which increases peripheral vascular resistance and causes arrhythmias. Frequent determination of serum electrolytes and appropriate KCl supplementation can effectively correct this side effect.

The choice of diuretic agents and their recommended dose ranges are shown in Table 35.3. With serum creatinine >1.8–2.0 mg/dl (>159–177 μM), thiazides become ineffective, and loop diuretics (furosemide and ethacrynic acid) are required to promote diuresis. K^+-sparing diuretics (spironolactone, triamterene, amiloride) are not advocated for the diabetic patient who may have underlying hypoaldosteronism.

β-Adrenergic Blockers

β-Adrenergic blockers can effectively reduce blood pressure and slow the progression of diabetic nephropathy. However, they predispose to hypoglycemia, impair recovery from hypoglycemia, exacerbate hypoglycemic unawareness, inhibit insulin secretion, cause hyperkalemia, exacerbate insulin resistance, worsen glucose tolerance, and induce adverse changes in the plasma lipid profile. Consequently, β-adrenergic antagonists are not good first-line or even second-line drugs for diabetic hypertension. β-Blockers may be warranted in combination with other agents in the diabetic hypertensive patient with progressive renal insufficiency and severe hypertension that is unresponsive to multiple-drug therapy. The hypertensive diabetic patient with angina may also require β-blocking agents, but the plasma glucose and lipid profiles should be monitored closely after the institution of such therapy.

When β-adrenergic antagonists must be used, selective $β_1$-blockers are recommended because they have less prominent metabolic side effects. Recommended doses of atenolol and metoprolol are shown in Table 35.3. At higher doses, both of these agents start to lose their β-selectivity.

Vasodilators

If an adequate response to combined therapy with ACE inhibitors, Ca^{2+}-channel blockers, and diuretics is not achieved, a peripheral vasodilator can be added. In diabetic patients with renal failure and severe refractory hypertension, minoxidil is particularly effective. The major side effect of minoxidil is hair growth.

Adrenergic Antagonists

Several central adrenergic antagonists (methyldopa, clonidine, and guanabenz) and peripheral α_1-antagonists (prazosin, terazosin, and doxazosin) are available for the treatment of hypertension in the diabetic patient (Table 35.3). With the onset of renal sufficiency, these agents tend to become less effective.

OTHER INTERVENTIONS

Glycemic Control

In type I diabetes, patients in the highest quartile for hyperglycemia have a four- to fivefold increased risk of developing proteinuria and renal insufficiency compared with those in the lowest quartile. In type II diabetes, hyperglycemia is also an important predictor of clinical proteinuria. In type I patients with albuminuria or renal insufficiency, tight glycemic control has not been shown to alter the progression to ESRF. However, it has been shown that, in type I patients with microalbuminuria, tight glycemic control with insulin (glycosylated hemoglobin [GHb] <7.5%) can prevent the development of clinical proteinuria. Therefore, strict glycemic control, if implemented early, may prevent the progression to ESRF. Thus, type I patients with a normal urinary albumin excretion rate, and especially those with microalbuminuria, should be aggressively treated with insulin to maintain a near-normal glycemic profile and to achieve a GHb level <7.0–7.5% (Table 35.4). This intensive therapy requires a highly motivated patient, multiple insulin injections, and self-monitoring of blood glucose. At least 6–12 mo are needed to see a reduction in microalbuminuria.

Diabetic patients with clinically overt nephropathy (urinary albumin excretion >250–300 mg/day or serum creatinine >1.8–2.0 mg/dl [>159–177 µM]) should strive for moderate glycemic control (GHb <8.5%; Table 35.4). There is little evidence that intensive insulin therapy slows the progression of renal disease at this stage, and the risk of hypoglycemia is increased because of decreased insulin clearance, impaired glucose counterregulation, and hypoglycemic unawareness related to autonomic neuropathy.

Dietary Protein

A low-protein diet slows the decline of GFR in patients with all types of chronic renal disease, including diabetic nephropathy. In

Table 35.4. **GUIDELINES FOR GLYCEMIC CONTROL**

	Glycosylated Hemoglobin (%)	Fasting Plasma Glucose (mg/dl)	2-h Postprandial Glucose (mg/dl)
Patients at risk for nephropathy: albuminuria not elevated or microalbuminuria (25–250 mg/day)	<7.0–7.5	80–110 (4.4–6.1)	<160–180 (<8.9–10)
Patients with nephropathy: dipstick + proteinuria, albuminuria >250–300 mg/day, or serum creatinine >1.8–2.0 mg/dl (>159–177 μM)	<8.5	100–140 (5.6–7.8)	<200 (<11.1)

Values in parentheses are in mM.

microalbuminuric diabetic patients with normal renal function, a low-protein diet causes a reduction in urinary albumin excretion without any change in GFR. Thus, moderate protein restriction $(0.6–0.8 \text{ g} \cdot \text{kg}^{-1} \cdot \text{day}^{-1})$ is advocated in diabetic patients with overt renal disease and microalbuminuria (Table 35.5). Replacement of animal protein with vegetable protein is advocated because this also slows GFR decline in patients with diabetic nephropathy. Patients with normal renal function and microalbuminuria should avoid a high protein intake and substitute vegetable protein for animal protein. In diabetic patients who are poorly nourished, low-protein diets should be avoided even when renal insufficiency is present. In patients with overt diabetic nephropathy, a decline in urine albumin excretion and stabilization or increase in GFR should be observed within 2–3 mo if the diet is strictly followed.

Urinary Tract Infection

Infection of the urinary tract is common in diabetic patients, especially women, and unusual gram-negative organisms and *Candida* often appear. In adults, urine should be studied at every office visit, and if leukocytes are noted, a culture should be obtained. Prompt and appropriate antibiotic therapy should be instituted based on known sensitivities. Hyperglycemia interferes with phagocytosis by leukocyte function and may make eradication of the infection difficult. Therefore, tightened glycemic control is indicated.

Papillary Necrosis

Impaired blood flow to the medullary tissues can lead to anoxic damage and eventually necrosis of the papilla. If the papilla sloughs, it can obstruct the renal pelvis, and the patient will present with flank pain and a clinical picture similar to that observed with a renal

Table 35.5. RECOMMENDATIONS FOR DIETARY PROTEIN INTAKE

	Protein Intake ($g \cdot kg^{-1} \cdot day^{-1}$)	Other Considerations
Patients at risk for nephropathy: no albuminuria and no microalbuminuria (25–250 mg/day)	1.0 to <1.2 (avoid high intakes)	It has not been determined whether protein restriction is beneficial. Substitute animal protein with vegetable protein.
Patients with nephropathy: serum creatinine >1.8–2.0 mg/dl (>159–177 μM); dipstick + proteinuria or albuminuria (>250–300 mg/day), microalbuminuria (25–250 mg/day)	0.6–0.8 (moderately severe restriction)	Diet should remain isocaloric. Substitute animal protein with vegetable protein. Protein restriction is not recommended for patients who are nutritionally compromised.

calculus. Hematuria will be present. The diagnosis can be established with a renal ultrasound or an intravenous pyelogram, if necessary. If the patient is afebrile and does not appear toxic, symptomatic treatment with analgesics and hydration is usually sufficient for the papilla to be passed. However, if the obstruction persists and there is accompanying infection, antibiotic therapy and surgical intervention may be necessary.

Hyperkalemia

Hyperkalemia is common in diabetic patients with nephropathy and results from disturbances in both extrarenal and renal K^+ metabolism. Insulin, aldosterone, and epinephrine all enhance K^+ uptake by extrarenal tissues, and these hormones are often deficient in diabetic patients. In addition, hypertonicity (hyperglycemia) causes a shift of K^+ from the intracellular to extracellular environment. Concomitant metabolic acidosis, secondary to either aldosterone deficiency or chronic renal failure, exacerbates the hyperkalemia as H^+ moves into cells to be buffered in exchange for K^+. Diabetic patients with nephropathy often have the syndrome of hypoaldosteronism, which impairs renal K^+ excretion. Aldosterone deficiency is magnified if concomitant renal failure exists and tubular mass is reduced sufficiently to impair K^+ secretion.

Treatment of hyperkalemia involves redistribution of K^+ into cells and augmentation of urinary K^+ excretion. The insulin regimen should be optimized to restore normoglycemia, which will redistribute K^+ back into cells and may improve the defect in aldosterone secretion. Metabolic acidosis should be corrected with sodium bicarbonate, 1.8–4.8 g/day (24–64 meq/day). The maintenance dose can be adjusted empirically depending on the change in plasma bicarbonate concentration. In patients with hypoaldosteronism, renal tubular K^+ secretion becomes critically dependent on Na^+ and fluid delivery to the distal nephron segments. Therefore, adequate intake of salt and water should be administered to maintain renal perfusion and GFR. Dietary K^+ intake should be reduced to <60 meq/day. In most patients, these measures will be sufficient to restore normokalemia. If significant hyperkalemia (≥6.0 meq/L) persists and if there are electrocardiographic or neuromuscular signs, 0.1–0.2 mg/day of fludrocortisone should be considered. In hyperkalemic patients with hypoaldosteronism, higher doses of fludrocortisone may be required. If Na^+ retention and congestive heart failure become a problem, fludrocortisone should be discontinued and more severe dietary K^+ restriction instituted. In some patients, it may be necessary to continue the fludrocortisone and start diuretic therapy to prevent Na^+ retention. Drugs that predispose to hypoaldosteronism (nonsteroidal anti-inflammatory agents, ACE inhibitors, β-adrenergic blockers, or heparin) or inhibit renal tubular K^+ secretion (spironolactone, triamterene, or amiloride) should be avoided in the hyperkalemic diabetic patient.

SUGGESTED READING

1. Buhler FR, Julius S, Reaven GM: A new dimension in hypertension: role of insulin resistance. *J Cardiovasc Pharmacol* 15 (Suppl. 5): S1–3, 1990
2. Castellino P, Shohat J, DeFronzo RA: Hyperfiltration and diabetic nephropathy: is it the beginning or is it the end? *Semin Nephrol* 10:228–53, 1990
3. DeFronzo RA, Ferrannini E: Insulin resistance: a multifaceted syndrome responsible for NIDDM, obestity, hypertension, dyslipidemia, and atherosclerotic cardiovascular disease. *Diabetes Care* 14:173–94, 1991
4. Ferrannini E, Buzzigoli G, Bonadonna RC, Giorico MA, Oleggini M, Graziadei L, Pedrinelli R, Brandi L, Bevilacqua S: Insulin resistance in essential hypertension. *N Engl J Med* 317:350–57, 1987
5. Mogensen CE: Prediction of clinical diabetic nephropathy in IDDM patients. *Diabetes* 39:761–67, 1990
6. Mogensen CE: Prevention and treatment of renal disease in insulin-dependent diabetes mellitus. *Semin Nephrol* 10:260–73, 1990
7. Stein PP, Black HR: Drug treatment of hypertension in patients with diabetes mellitus. *Diabetes Care* 14:425–48, 1991
8. Tuttle KR, Stein JH, DeFronzo RA: The natural history of diabetic nephropathy. *Semin Nephrol* 10:184–93, 1990
9. Tuttle KR, DeFronzo RA, Stein J: Diabetic nephropathy: a rational approach to therapy based upon pathophysiology. *Semin Nephrol* 11:220–35, 1991

36. Chronic Renal Failure

ELI A. FRIEDMAN, MD

Diabetic nephropathy may progress to renal failure in both type I (insulin-dependent) and type II (non-insulin-dependent) diabetes. After years of hyperglycemia typically accompanied by hypertension, diabetic nephropathy may reduce renal function to the extent that life is no longer possible without replacement therapy, i.e., dialysis or kidney transplant. Chronic renal failure (CRF) in a diabetic person may develop suddenly. In the absence of a history of kidney disease, a vascular catastrophe (atheroembolic disease) or treatment with a nephrotoxic antibiotic may result in CRF. The usual course of diabetic nephropathy, however, entails months to years of a nephrotic syndrome (proteinuria >3.5 g/day and anasarca) followed by azotemia, which signals the onset of CRF. End-stage renal disease (ESRD) is the usual termination of CRF. Severe CRF induces a multiplicity of symptoms, physical signs, and abnormal laboratory values that, in the aggregate, constitute the uremic syndrome. Untreated uremia results in orange-yellow skin discoloration, wasting of muscle and fat, and a blunted, dull, affect stressed by a reversed diurnal sleep pattern. Anemia, acidosis, and azotemia are the cardinal laboratory findings in CRF. Agonal CRF may present with fibrinous pericarditis and pericardial tamponade, bowel ulceration (colitis, gastritis), and neurological syndromes (grand mal seizures, cortical blindness, motor nerve paralysis). When treated by hemodialysis, peritoneal dialysis, or kidney transplantation, life extension for years is attainable for most diabetic individuals who develop CRF.

Dr. Friedman is Professor of Medicine and Chief of the Division of Renal Diseases at the State University of New York Health Science Center, Brooklyn, NY.

THERAPY

Management strategies of diabetic nephropathy have three main objectives:

1. Detect and eliminate potentially reversible factors that can decrease renal functional reserve.
2. Minimize the rate of glomerular filtration rate (GFR) by modulating blood pressure, metabolic control, and dietary protein intake.
3. Prepare the patient and his/her family for kidney-replacement therapy while preserving work, school, or home activities when uremia supervenes. These decisions include
   • Whether to have an intrafamilial kidney transplant
   • Selection of dialysis technique (peritoneal or hemodialysis)
   • Election of locale for hemodialysis (home or facility)
   • Advising the patient of the timing and circumstances (creatinine level) when uremia therapy should be started

When constructing this "life plan," there is opportunity to fortify the patient for the components of kidney-replacement therapy by explaining the body's reliance on renal function and the nature of dialysis and kidney transplantation. Key components of therapy are given in Table 36.1.

Preserving Renal Functional Reserve

Caution in the use of nephrotoxic drugs will avoid superimposed iatrogenic injury. Drugs that should not be administered to patients with azotemia include nitrofurantoin, spironolactone, amiloride, triamterene, and phenformin. Abruptly deteriorating renal function

---

Table 36.1. THERAPY FOR AZOTEMIC DIABETIC PATIENT

1. Discontinue nephrotoxic drugs.
2. Detect and treat urinary infection.
3. Correct electrolyte imbalance.
4. Expand plasma volume if contracted.
5. Control hypertension to blood pressure of $\leq 130/80$ mmHg.
6. Restrict dietary protein to 40–60 g/day.
7. Correct hyperlipidemia by diet or pharmacological means.
8. Control hyperphosphatemia by diet and phosphate binders.
9. Reduce hyperuricemia if >12 mg/dl or at lower values if symptomatic gout.
10. Add oral bicarbonate 1.2–4.8 g/day for severe acidosis.
11. Administer synthetic vitamin D.
12. For symptomatic anemia, when hematocrit is $<30\%$, after excluding blood loss and other extrarenal causes, administer recombinant erythropoietin 50–150 U/kg s.c. $3\times$/wk.
13. Avoid volume depletion, contrast media, nephrotoxic drugs, and bladder catheterization.

may be the consequence of interstitial nephritis caused by captopril, cimetidine, methicillin sodium, allopurinol, phenylhydantoin, and furosemide. The angiotensin-converting enzyme (ACE) inhibitors enalapril, lisinopril, and captopril may reversibly worsen azotemia and precipitate hyperkalemia in up to 20% of diabetic individuals. Dosage reductions of cyclophosphamide, cimetidine, clofibrate, digoxin, and many antibiotics (particularly aminoglycosides) are required for azotemic patients.

Because of the risk of urinary infection, bladder catheterization in an azotemic diabetic patient should be restricted to instances when the information to be gained is unobtainable by other means.

There is serious risk of worsening renal insufficiency when radiographic contrast medium is administered to diabetic patients with serum creatinine levels >2.5 mg/dl (>227.3 μM). When radiographic contrast medium must be given, prior hydration and mannitol infusion (25 g in 2 L 0.45% saline solution) may protect against renal injury (see chapt. 34).

Minimizing Rate of GFR Loss

The rate of renal functional decline in diabetic nephropathy is slowed by normalization of hypertension and dietary protein restriction (see chapt. 35). Preservation of bone integrity is the objective of treatment with intestinal phosphate binders. Hypertension due to diabetic nephropathy is often associated with intravascular volume expansion and anasarca resulting from nephrotic-range proteinuria. Reduction of the excess fluid burden is a vital component of blood pressure control. Diuresis can usually be affected by graded doses of furosemide (40–120 mg 2 ×/day). Metolazone (5–20 mg/day or 2 ×/day) induces diuresis even when the creatinine clearance has fallen to <10 ml/min. Close observation of the patient, with recording of daily weight, is mandatory when prescribing a potent diuretic regimen. Once reduction in edema is accomplished, doses of metolazone and furosemide should be decreased to avoid dehydration and vascular collapse.

For hypertension resistant to diuretics, ACE inhibitors and Ca^{2+}-channel blockers or a trial-and-error regimen of vasodilators and β-blockers may be attempted. Minoxidil in doses of 5–50 mg/day almost always reduces blood pressure to <140/90 mmHg, but careful observation for tachycardia and fluid retention is required. Single daily doses of long-acting drugs such as nifedipine (Ca^{2+}-channel blocker) and lisinopril (ACE inhibitor) improve patient compliance over that attained in multidose regimens.

Dietary protein may retard the course of glomerulosclerosis. Trials in small groups of patients with progressive renal disorders, including diabetic nephropathy, show that a diet containing 40–60 g/day protein (with or without addition of essential amino acids or their precursor α-keto derivatives) slows renal functional loss. The prudent physician may opt to prescribe a diet containing ≥100 g/day dietary protein while suggesting modest protein restriction (40–60 g/day).

Maintenance of Metabolic Environment

Perturbed lipid metabolism is characteristic of diabetic patients with nephropathy, especially when accompanied by a nephrotic syndrome. Hypertriglyceridemia and low levels of high-density lipoprotein (HDL) are typical of azotemic patients with diabetic nephropathy; the risk of coronary artery disease expressed as the ratio of total cholesterol to HDL cholesterol is elevated. Partial correction of these lipid abnormalities may be affected with a low-lipid diet, nicotinic acid, gemfibrozil, lovastatin, or probucol.

As GFR falls below 20 ml/min, hyperphosphatemia may cause reciprocal hypocalcemia and hyperparathyroidism. Hyperphosphatemia can be controlled by limiting phosphate intake to 500–800 mg/day; dairy products are high in phosphate content. Premeal ingestion of intestinal phosphate-binding drugs, e.g., aluminum hydroxide and aluminum carbonate or magnesium hydroxide (1–2 g 3×/day), and calcium supplementation (calcium carbonate 1–3 g 3×/day) will lower the serum phosphate concentration to ≤5 mM. Unfortunately, while reducing serum phosphate concentration to normal, treatment with phosphate binders may be complicated by hypermagnesemia, hypercalcemia, aluminum-induced vitamin D–resistant bone disease, and neurological disorders. Aluminum toxicity is also associated with a syndrome of dementia and anemia.

Hypocalcemia in the absence of marked hyperphosphatemia can also be treated by administration of 1,25-dihydroxyvitamin D_3. Treatment with this vitamin before symptomatic bone disease appears prevents renal bone disease and reverses secondary hyperparathyroidism.

In advanced diabetic nephropathy, attention to the amount of dietary Na and K is important as the GFR falls below 15 ml/min. A small subset of patients—those with a component of interstitial renal disease—will lose large quantities of Na, similar to "saltwasting" individuals with Addison's disease. By contrast, most azotemic diabetic individuals have predominantly glomerular disease causing retention of salt and water. Defining a correct dietary salt prescription for the individual patient requires a process of trial and error termed *salt balancing*. Daily weights are the keystone to the regimen, which begins with a 40-g protein 2-g salt diet. The salt waster's weight will decrease, necessitating supplementation with sodium bicarbonate tablets (600 mg) given up to 4×/day. With continued weight loss, the amount of sodium bicarbonate is increased by 1.2-g/day increments, until a stable weight results. At the other extreme, the nephrotic salt retainer may evince pulmonary congestion and peripheral edema with the initial 2-g salt prescription, in which case furosemide (40–80 mg 3×/day) is added.

Dietary K restriction is rarely required before the daily urine output falls below 1 L or the patient is under treatment with drugs that impair K^+ excretion, e.g., an ACE inhibitor. Hyperkalemia <6 meq/L can usually be managed by reducing dietary citrus fruits, bananas, and potatoes. More severe K^+ retention requires administration of a cation-exchange resin, e.g., sodium polystyrene sulfonate. Discontinuance of ACE inhibitors and other K^+-retaining drugs is a key step in management of hyperkalemia.

Anemia in diabetic individuals with reduced renal function is mainly the consequence of diminished renal secretion of erythropoietin. In patients with ESRD who are sustained by hemodialysis or peritoneal dialysis, correction of anemia can be accomplished by thrice-weekly injections of recombinant erythropoietin. The exact indications for erythropoietin administration have not been defined in predialysis patients, although profound anemia (hematocrit <28%), coronary artery disease, and inordinate fatigue will benefit from an increased erythrocyte mass.

Comprehensive management of declining renal function involves reduction of hyperphosphatemia with phosphate binders, administration of synthetic 1,25-dihydroxyvitamin D_3, and raising the hematocrit with recombinant erythropoietin. Measurements of patient weight, hematocrit, blood urea nitrogen, serum creatinine, serum phosphorus, and serum Ca^{2+} should be performed at each visit. Insulin and other small peptide hormones are partially degraded by the kidney. On reduction of GFR to ≤25 ml/min, insulin catabolism within the kidney lessens to the extent that progressively intensive hypoglycemic episodes may interfere with metabolic control. When the serum creatinine level increases to >5 mg/dl (>455 μM), the need for kidney-replacement therapy is urgent.

HEMODIALYSIS

Maintenance hemodialysis is the kidney-replacement regimen used in >80% of diabetic people who develop ESRD in the United States. To perform maintenance hemodialysis requires vascular access to the circulation. Creation of the standard access—an internal arteriovenous fistula in the wrist—is usually more difficult in a diabetic than in a nondiabetic person because of systemic atherosclerosis. For many diabetic patients with peripheral vascular calcification and/or atherosclerosis, establishment of an access for hemodialysis necessitates use of synthetic (Dacron) prosthetic vascular grafts. In both sexes and in all age-groups, survival of diabetic individuals treated by maintenance hemodialysis is distinctly inferior to that of nondiabetic patients. The main concerns of establishing maintenance hemodialysis for diabetic patients are listed in Table 36.2.

PERITONEAL DIALYSIS

Peritoneal dialysis has been effectively used to sustain life in ~20% of diabetic individuals who develop ESRD. Continuous ambulatory

Table 36.2. CONCERNS ON MAINTENANCE HEMODIALYSIS IN DIABETIC NEPHROPATHY

Establishment of vascular access
- Internal arteriovenous fistula
- Bovine carotid arteriovenous heterograft
- Teflon arteriovenous graft

Metabolic regulation
- Frequent fingerstick glucose measurements (type I diabetes)
- Fractional insulin doses or insulin pump (type I diabetes)
- Reeducate about diet and exercise
- Normalize weight

Propensity to hypotension
- Minimize intradialytic weight gain
- Bicarbonate dialysate
- Gradual ultrafiltration

Preservation of vision
- Collaboration with ophthalmologist
- Low heparin dosage
- Two or more pillows for head elevation during active retinopathy

Preservation of lower extremities
- Wearing heel "booties"
- Collaboration with podiatrist

Obstipation complicating use of phosphate binders
- Prescribe detergent with antacid gel for phosphate sorption
- Metoclopramide

Depression
- Membership in patient self-help organizations
- Full explanation of therapy

peritoneal dialysis (CAPD), a self-treatment, has grown rapidly in application because of its advantages (compared with home hemodialysis) of rapid training, reduced cardiovascular stress, and avoidance of heparin (Table 36.3); home hemodialysis requires 3–16 wk of training. As a facilitating procedure, an intraperitoneal catheter is sewn in place ≥1 day before CAPD is begun. Motivated diabetic patients, including those who are blind, are able to learn to perform CAPD at home within 10–15 days. In practice, patients exchange 2–3 L of commercially prepared sterile dialysate 3–5×/day. Insulin, antibiotics, and other drugs can be added by the patient to each dialysate exchange.

Simplification of peritoneal dialysate exchanges has been brought about by use of a mechanical cycler in the therapeutic variation called continuous cyclic peritoneal dialysis (CCPD). Both CAPD and CCPD subject the diabetic patient to the constant risk of peritonitis and a gradual decrease in peritoneal surface area. Peritonitis has an incidence rate of about once every 10 mo of peritoneal dialysis.

KIDNEY TRANSPLANTATION

Kidney transplantation is the preferred therapeutic option for selected patients with ESRD due to diabetic nephropathy. Both pa-

Table 36.3. CONTINUOUS AMBULATORY PERITONEAL DIALYSIS FOR DIABETIC PATIENTS

Advantages
- Rapid establishment as home therapy
- Partner not essential
- Few profound hypotensive episodes
- Insulin regimen simplified by addition to dialysate
- Enthusiastic patient acceptance of freedom from machine
- Minimal stress on cardiovascular system; no extracorporeal circulation

Disadvantages
- Intra-abdominal catheter related
  - Pain, bleeding, dialysate leak
  - Obstruction of catheter
  - Perforation of abdominal viscus during catheter insertion
- Mechanical
  - Abdominal hernia
  - Hydrothorax, ascites
- Peritoneal
  - Peritonitis
  - Peritoneal thickening (sclerosis) and loss of dialyzing surface
- Neuropsychiatric
  - Depression over daily necessity for multiple exchanges
  - Boredom with regimen and altered self-image
- Time commitment

tient survival and degree of rehabilitation in diabetic transplant recipients is sharply superior to results attained by dialytic therapy. With cyclosporin as the main immunosuppressive drug for kidney transplantation, patient survival at 1 and 2 yr is equivalent in diabetic and nondiabetic recipients, whereas kidney-graft survival is ~10% lower in diabetic than in nondiabetic recipients at 2 yr.

Kidney-replacement therapy is more difficult to obtain, and the course is stressful in diabetic patients because of the impact of extrarenal disease. Variables in selecting therapy are presented in Table 36.4. Preparation for a kidney transplant in a diabetic subject, for example, requires careful cardiac evaluation to detect and treat coronary artery disease, the major cause of death in the azotemic diabetic patient. An exercise stress test with thallium imaging will suffice, if normal, as a prelude to a transplant. Cardiac catheterization and corrective coronary artery angioplasty or bypass grafting will preempt unanticipated death from heart disease during the posttransplant period.

Consultations with an ophthalmologist and a podiatrist familiar with abnormalities of the diabetic eye and foot, respectively, are also desirable during transplant evaluation.

REFERRAL TO SPECIALIST

First referral to a nephrologist is advisable when urinary protein excretion is constant at amounts to >500 mg/day. Initial renal eval-

Table 36.4. COMPARISON OF OPTIONS IN KIDNEY-REPLACEMENT THERAPY

	Kidney Transplant	CAPD/CCPD	Maintenance Hemodialysis
Advantages	Cure of uremia during graft function	Rapid initiation; avoids major surgery; simplifies insulin administration	Avoids major surgery; broad experience
	Freedom from treatment facility	Minimal burden to cardiovascular system	Can be performed at home after suitable training
	Superior rehabilitation	Can be learned in days to weeks; easy travel	Highly efficient extraction of solutes and water
	Once- or twice-daily oral drugs in most instances	Daily treatment minimizes fluid shifts	Thrice-weekly treatment increases free time
Disadvantages	Risk of surgery; toxicity of immunosuppressive regimen	Peritonitis; bowel puncture during catheter insertion; abdominal hernia, fluid leakage	Exsanguination from dislodged needles; air embolism; infected or thrombosed vascular access
	Sepsis from immunosuppression	Protein and nutrient loss	Risk of trace-element (aluminum) toxicity (water contamination)
	Hypertension and worsened metabolic control (steroids)	Gradual reduction of peritoneal surface area	Exhaustion of vascular access sites
	Recurrent glomerulosclerosis in allograft	Boredom, devalued self-image; fatigue, failure to thrive	Repetitive hypotensive episodes; fatigue, failure to thrive; restricted travel

CAPD, continuous ambulatory peritoneal dialysis; CCPD, continuous cyclic peritoneal dialysis.

uation will be directed toward quantifying renal reserve and excluding causes of nephropathy other than diabetes. Subsequent nephrology consultations at yearly intervals will inventory renal function, proteinuria, and regulation of blood pressure. The use of synthetic vitamin D and erythropoietin to manage hyperphosphatemia (hypocalcemia) and anemia should be guided by a kidney specialist. Once azotemia is noted, the frequency of contact with a nephrologist should increase. When it is anticipated that dialytic therapy or a kidney transplant will be needed within 6 mo (serum creatinine ≥ 5 mg/dl), the main responsibility for management should shift to the collaborating nephrologist.

SUGGESTED READING

1. Adamson JW, Eschbach JW: Treatment of the anemia of chronic renal failure with recombinant human erythropoietin. *Annu Rev Med* 41: 349–61, 1990
2. Klahr S: Effects of protein intake on the progression of renal disease. *Annu Rev Nutr* 9:87–96, 1989
3. Lockwood AH: Neurologic complications of renal disease. *Neurol Clin* 7:617–24, 1989
4. Malluche H, Faugere M-C: Renal bone disease 1990: an unmet challenge for the nephrologist. *Kidney Int* 38:193–97, 1990
5. U.S. Renal Data System: *USRDS 1990 Annual Data Report*. The National Institutes of Health, National Institute of Diabetes and Digestive and Kidney Diseases, Bethesda, MD, August 1990

37. Painful or Insensitive Lower Extremity

MICHAEL A. PFEIFER, MD

Complaints of pain and/or muscular weakness in lower extremities are common expressions of neuropathy in diabetic patients. Onset of peripheral neuropathy is insidious, and the disease is progressive; therefore, early detection is important to prevent further nerve damage.

PATHOPHYSIOLOGY

The etiology of diabetic neuropathy is not completely understood. Figure 37.1 illustrates the self-sustaining mechanism that accounts for some of the metabolic alterations. Hyperglycemia interferes with cell metabolism in two ways: *1*) It stimulates the polyol pathway, an alternative pathway for glucose metabolism, causing intercellular accumulation of sorbitol; and *2*) it competitively inhibits *myo*-inositol uptake. Both result in decreased nerve *myo*-inositol, an important membrane component. Na^+-K^+-ATPase activity is decreased when membrane *myo*-inositol is decreased. This further aggrevates Na^+-dependent *myo*-inositol uptake. In addition, there is increased glycosylation of neural proteins. The cumulative effect is impaired nerve conduction and axonal transport. Ischemia caused by vascular disease may further decrease nerve function.

Dr. Pfeifer is Director of the Diabetes Center of Excellence,Humana Hospital Lexington, and of the Diabetes Research and Analysis Association, Inc., Lexington, KY.

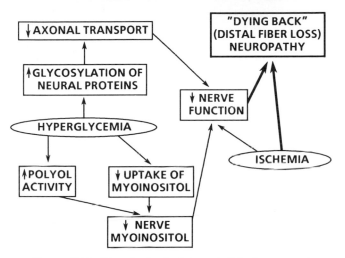

Figure 37.1. Hypothesis of etiology of diabetic neuropathy.

RISK FACTORS AND SYMPTOMS

Several risk factors have been identified, including

- Stature (height)
- Male sex
- Age
- Hypertension
- Duration of diabetes
- Glucose control
- Cholesterol level
- Smoking

Because peripheral neuropathy may not be painful, all diabetic patients should be evaluated yearly. Exams should include

- Pinprick
- Proprioception
- Reflexes
- Two-point discrimination
- Light touch

Vibratory and thermal testing can further identify and document sensory deficits. Nerve conduction velocities confirm motor abnormalities. Ankle-brachial index by Doppler testing assesses the degree of vascular disease. Several other conditions that mimic or contribute to the symptoms of diabetic neuropathy include

- Pernicious anemia
- Vitamin B_6 intoxication

- Alcohol
- Uremia
- Chemical toxins
- Nerve entrapmnent and compression (carpal or tarsal tunnel syndrome)

These conditions should be ruled out before making a diagnosis of diabetic neuropathy.

PREVENTION AND TREATMENT

Currently, prevention and education are the first line of treatment. The metabolic alterations can be prevented or reversed, if no structural changes have occurred, by good glycemic control.

Patients should be warned that concurrent insult to the nerves by alcohol and chemical toxins may aggrevate the development and/or hasten the progression of diabetic neuropathy. The patient should be educated about methods for and the importance of preventing foot injury (see chapt. 47).

Treatment is available to relieve painful neuropathy. Often, improving glycemic control provides relief. Figure 37.2 is an algorithm for assessing the etiology of pain and its treatment. Therapy is

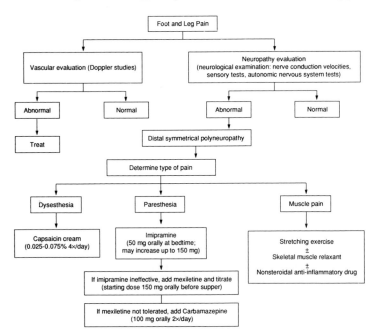

Figure 37.2. Algorithm for diagnosis and treatment of foot and leg pain. Based on pain model developed by D. Ross, MD (unpublished).

directed toward the type of peripheral nerve pain (e.g., dysesthesia, paresthesia, muscle) according to the Ross pain model. Thus, it is important that an individual familiar with diabetic painful neuropathy treatment initiate therapy. A careful neurological exam and detailed patient report will establish the type of pain present. Dysesthesia is commonly described as pain caused by contact with objects that normally do not cause pain, e.g., clothing or bedding. Paresthesias are described by the patient as pins and needles and/or burning sensations. Typical patient complaints of muscle pain are a bandlike feeling; dull, achy night cramps; and/or shooting pains.

Capsaicin cream, 0.075% 4×/day, applied to affected areas has been effective in relieving dysesthesia. Paresthesias are treated with imipramine (50–150 mg orally at bedtime) and/or mexiletine. Mexiletine is contraindicated for patients with conduction abnormalities, so an ECG should be done before treatment. Dosage should be increased over a 3-day period, with rhythm strip done before each increase. Initial dosage is 150 mg orally before supper, increased to 10 mg/kg orally 4×/day before breakfast, lunch, supper, and evening snack. If the combination of imipramine and mexiletine fail, then mexiletine may be replaced with carbamazepine (100 mg orally 2×/day for 1 day, increased to 200 mg 2×/day). The muscle pain requires physical therapy and many also need skeletal muscle relaxants and/or nonsteroidal anti-inflammatory drugs. The physical therapist can instruct the patient in stretching exercises that help relieve pain.

SUGGESTED READING

1. Corbin DOC, Young RJ, Morrison DC, Hoskins P, McDicken WN, Housley E, Clarke BF: Blood flow in the foot, polyneuropathy and foot ulceration in diabetes mellitus. *Diabetologia* 30:468–73, 1987
2. Greene DA, Lattimer SA, Sima AAF: Pathogenesis and prevention of diabetic neuropathy. *Diabetes Metab Rev* 4:201–21, 1988
3. Pfeifer MA, Schumer MP, Jung S, Pohl SL: Diabetic autonomic neuropathy and painful somatic neuropathy. *Curr Ther Endocrinol Metab.* In press
4. Sosenko JM, Gadia MT, Fournier AM, O'Connell MT, Aguiar MC, Skyler JS: Body stature as a risk factor for diabetic sensory neuropathy. *Am J Med* 80:1031–34, 1986

38. Mono-/Amyoradiculopathy

DOUGLAS A. GREENE, MD

Focal and multifocal diabetic peripheral neuropathies are neurological deficits confined to the distribution of single or multiple peripheral nerves (Table 38.1). They are called diabetic mononeuropathy and diabetic mononeuropathy multiplex, respectively. A focal neurological deficit in nerve distribution at the brachial or lumbosacral plexus is known as diabetic plexopathy or, when at the nerve root, diabetic radiculopathy. Diabetic mononeuropathy or mononeuropathy multiplex can involve cranial and peripheral nerves, which is known as diabetic cranial neuropathy.

These syndromes are uncommon, of sudden onset, and generally but not always self-limited and tend to occur in older diabetic patients. The third cranial nerve is frequently involved. Patients often present with diabetic ophthalmoplegia, i.e., unilateral pain, diplopia, and ptosis with pupillary sparing. Diabetic ophthalmoplegia can be bilateral and recurrent and can occur in the absence of other manifestations of diabetic neuropathy.

The bandlike thoracic or abdominal pain of diabetic truncal neuropathy or radiculopathy is often misdiagnosed as an acute intrathoracic or intra-abdominal emergency. Femoral neuropathy in diabetic patients often involves motor and sensory deficits at the sacral plexus and femoral nerve. The relative excess of motor versus sensory involvement differentiates diabetic femoral neuropathy from that seen in other conditions. Other mononeuropathies mimic the compression neuropathies seen in nondiabetic individuals, e.g., carpal tunnel syndrome. All of these focal neuropathic syndromes mimic

Dr. Greene is Professor of Internal Medicine and Director of the Michigan Diabetes Research and Training Center at the University of Michigan, Ann Arbor, MI.

Table 38.1. **CHARACTERISTICS OF NEUROPATHIES**

Neuropathy Type	Nerves Commonly Involved	Treatment
Cranial neuropathy	Oculomotor (III), abducens (VI)	Resolves spontaneously over several months
Mononeuropathy or mononeuropathy multiplex	Median, radial, ulnar, lateral cutaneous, peroneal	Improved glucose control, relief of pressure (surgical, conservative)
Radiculopathy	Intercostal, truncal	Resolves spontaneously over 6–24 mo
Plexopathy	Femoral	Improved glucose control supportive

similar neurological conditions of nondiabetic origin. Thus, diagnosis should be made from recognition of signs and symptoms, and specialized neurological and other diagnostic tests, e.g., electromyography, computerized tomography (CT), and magnetic resonance imaging in consultation with appropriate neurological/neurosurgical experts.

PATHOGENESIS

The typically acute onset and complete or partial recovery suggest a vascular or traumatic basis. Because of their rarity, self-limited course, and inaccessibility to biopsy, focal diabetic neuropathies have rarely been explored histologically. The presumed vascular basis of focal diabetic neuropathy is most convincingly demonstrated for isolated third nerve palsy, which has revealed focal acute demyelinating lesions in the intracavernous watershed area between the intracranial and extracranial vascular beds in association with local thickening of arterioles. Central nerve fibers were most heavily damaged and demyelinated with distal Wallerian degeneration, whereas superficial fibers (thought to innervate the pupil) were relatively spared. Both fusiform lesions were associated with significant disease of the vasa nervorum, although frank vascular occlusion was not documented. Multiple microinfarcts of bridging nerve fascicles of the obturator, femoral, sciatic, and posterior tibial nerves, with vessel-wall thickening and occlusion of the vasa nervora are also possible. These isolated reports have associated the focal neuropathies with acute infarctions within peripheral nerves.

CRANIAL NEUROPATHY

Isolated cranial neuropathies occur frequently in elderly but rarely in young diabetic patients. Signs and symptoms of more generalized diabetic neuropathy may be absent, although the cranial palsies can be recurrent or bilateral. The third cranial nerve is most commonly involved, characteristically with pupillary sparing (in contrast to vascular oculomotor compression palsy, where pupillary dilation is usually an early feature).

Patients present with headache and unilateral ophthalmoplegia sparing lateral eye movement. The accompanying pain is typically intense and referred above or behind the eye but may be mild or absent in 50% of cases. Progressive diminution of pain and return of oculomotor function is the rule, even in elderly patients. The responsible nociceptors may be either perineurial or in the adjacent first and second divisions of the trigeminal nerve, because the third nerve is purely motor.

Differential diagnosis includes lesions of the midbrain and posterior orbit, aneurysm of the internal carotid, cavernous sinus lesions, and tumors at the base of the brain. After consultation with a specialist, appropriate CT scans and arteriography are indicated when the diagnosis is questionable. Other cranial nerves less commonly involved include the sixth, fourth (usually in combination with other cranial nerves), and seventh (presumably on a vascular basis). Other than the third and sixth cranial nerves, there is little evidence to suggest that cranial nerve palsies occur more frequently in diabetic individuals. Once other disease processes (e.g., vascular or space-occupying lesions) are excluded, the treatment of diabetic cranial neuropathy is merely expectant and palliative because these conditions are generally self-limited.

MONONEUROPATHY OR MONONEUROPATHY MULTIPLEX

Isolated peripheral nerve palsies occur more commonly in diabetes; however, causal and coincidental relationships are difficult to differentiate. Forty percent of unselected patients with overt diffuse diabetic neuropathy have either electrophysiological or clinical evidence of superimposed focal nerve damage at common entrapment or compression sites (e.g., median nerve at wrist and palm, radial nerve in upper arm, ulnar nerve at elbow, lateral cutaneous nerve of the thigh, and peroneal nerve at fibular head), suggesting that diffuse diabetic neuropathy predisposes to focal nerve damage. This is further supported by evidence that the risk of developing carpal tunnel syndrome is more than doubled in diabetic subjects. Nerves not commonly exposed to compression or entrapment damage occasionally demonstrate focal impairment in patients with diabetes, but this may reflect coincidental occurrence of diabetes and compression neuropathy. Thus, the diagnosis of mononeuropathy or mononeuropathy multiplex should be confirmed by electrodiagnostic studies.

Nondiabetic causes of mononeuropathy and/or mononeuropathy multiplex should be excluded, e.g., vasculitides, acromegaly, coagulopathies, and hypothyroidism. Compression and entrapment palsies in diabetic patients respond to standard conservative or surgical management, i.e., protection against additional mechanical trauma or surgical release procedures. Treatment of other mononeuropathies is similar for nondiabetic mononeuropathy and is essentially supportive.

RADICULOPATHY

Diabetic radiculopathy (intercostal and truncal neuropathy) presents with dermatomal pain and loss of cutaneous sensation. Although usually singular and unilateral, the syndrome may involve multiple dermatomal levels and may be bilateral in some patients. Hypesthesia or paresthesia may be inapparent initially but usually develop during the course of the disorder. Most frequently, the symptoms are attributed to a compressive lesion, such as a herniated nucleus pulposus, but radiographic studies and myelography are negative. When pain is prominent and hypesthesia subtle, truncal neuropathy is frequently misdiagnosed as an acute intrathoracic or intra-abdominal visceral emergency (e.g., myocardial infarction, cholecystitis, peptic ulcer, or appendicitis).

Electromyographic studies of the paraspinal muscles are usually diagnostic. Signs of diffuse distal symmetrical polyneuropathy are often present. Spontaneous resolution of both symptoms and signs is the rule, usually within 6–24 mo.

PLEXOPATHY

Nondiabetic femoral neuropathy arises from unilateral injury to the femoral nerve or its origins within the lumbar plexus, usually in association with pelvic or abdominal surgery, parturition, or various bleeding disorders. Pain and sensory impairment in the distribution of the femoral nerve (anterior thigh and medial calf) accompany disabling weakness of thigh flexion and knee extension.

In diabetes, the syndrome occurs spontaneously, and sensory loss is usually less marked. Pain, which classically extends from the hip to the anterior and lateral surface of the thigh, may radiate into the foot or originate in the sacroiliac region and extend dorsally down the leg. The pain may develop insidiously or episodically and may be worse at night. Muscle weakness most often involves the iliopsoas, quadriceps, and adductor muscles but usually spares the hip extensors and hamstrings. The anterolateral muscles in the calf may also be involved, mimicking an "anterior compartment syndrome." The plantar response may be extensor and areflexia is present. There may be a slight elevation in the cerebrospinal fluid (CSF) protein content. Distal symmetrical polyneuropathy is almost always present. Nearly complete recovery is the rule, and the syndrome may persist for several years or recur. The syndrome may be distinguished from sciatic neuropathy by a normal straight-leg–raising test. Because of the similarities between the diabetic femoral nerve syndrome and that occurring in association with other conditions, diabetic plexopathy remains a diagnosis of exclusion; space-occupying lesions, trauma, nondiabetic vasculopathies, and skeletal abnormalities must be carefully excluded in consultation with a specialist.

Treatment for the diabetic plexopathy syndrome is supportive pending spontaneous recovery. The beneficial effect of improved diabetes control remains unsupported.

CSF protein is usually elevated, suggesting proximal involvement, i.e., cord or plexus. However, femoral nerve conduction velocity is also prolonged, implying some damage to peripheral nerve motor fibers as well. Unequivocal histopathological evidence of the putative vascular basis of diabetic femoral neuropathy remains elusive, but the disorder is still generally considered to have a vascular basis, probably involving the femoral nerve and/or sacral plexus.

SUGGESTED READING

1. Asbury AK: Focal and multifocal neuropathies of diabetes. In *Diabetic Neuropathy*. Dyck PJ, Thomas PK, Winegrad AI, Porte D, Eds. Philadelphia, PA, Saunders, 1987, p. 45–55
2. Greene DA, Sima AAF, Pfeifer MA: Pathophysiology of diabetic neuropathy. In *Ellenberg and Rifkin's Diabetes Mellitus*. 4th ed. Rifkin H, Porte D, Eds. New York, Elsevier, 1990, p. 710–55
3. Thomas PK, Eliasson S: Diabetic neuropathy. In *Peripheral Neuropathy*. Dyck PJ, Thomas PK, Lambert EM, Eds. Philadelphia, PA, Saunders, 1975, p. 956–81

39. Gastrointestinal Disturbances

JEFFREY L. BARNETT, MD, and AARON I. VINIK, MD, PhD

Gastrointestinal disturbances caused by autonomic neuropathy are a common and often disabling complication of diabetes. Diabetic involvement of the gastrointestinal (GI) tract extends from the esophagus to the anorectum, and clinical presentation ranges from silent to life threatening.

PATHOGENESIS

Gastrointestinal complications of diabetes appear to be more common in patients with long-standing disease and poorly controlled blood glucose levels. The most important GI complications of diabetes mellitus are motility disturbances of the gut, which probably result from widespread autonomic neuropathy. Many patients with enteropathy have long-standing diabetes with somatic and cardiovascular autonomic neuropathy. The clinical features of certain diabetic enteropathies resemble those caused by surgical resection of the nerves supplying that organ. Unfortunately, convincing morphological demonstration of gross nerve pathology in human diabetic enteropathy is lacking, and correlation of GI symptoms with other signs of end-organ neuropathic damage is sometimes poor. Microangiopathic changes, as seen in the retina and kidney, do not seem to cause disease in the GI tract. Disturbed release of gut hormones and metabolic abnormalities, such as hyperglycemia and

Dr. Barnett is Assistant Professor of Internal Medicine at the University of Michigan, Ann Arbor, MI. Dr. Vinik is Director of The Diabetes Research Institute, Norfolk, VA.

electrolyte imbalances, undoubtedly play at least a contributory role in the disruption of GI motility in diabetes. Clinically, this is most apparent when diabetic ketoacidosis occurs and the typical features of anorexia, nausea, vomiting, and abdominal pain develop. As the metabolic derangements are controlled, the GI symptoms resolve. Even acute hyperglycemia alone may inhibit GI motility.

ESOPHAGEAL DISORDERS

Esophageal motor disorders have been described by cineradiography or manometrics in ~75% of people with diabetes. Delayed esophageal transit, demonstrated by nuclear scintigraphy, is also common. In most patients, however, esophageal dysfunction is mild and nonspecific and does not produce symptoms. Therefore, symptoms of dysphagia and chest pain must be as aggressively evaluated in these patients as in nondiabetic patients. Poor peristalsis and diminished lower esophageal sphincter tone predispose to gastroesophageal reflux. These findings, in addition to delayed gastric emptying, may cause a particularly severe ulcerative esophagitis leading to bleeding or stricture formation. People with diabetes are also prone to *Candida* esophagitis, which should be suspected if odynophagia develops or if pyrosis responds poorly to standard antireflux therapy.

GASTRIC DYSFUNCTION

Gastroparesis can be detected in 25% of people with diabetes. Although it is clinically silent in most patients, severe diabetic gastroparesis is the most debilitating of all the GI complications of diabetes. Liquid emptying is controlled by the proximal stomach (fundus) and is dependent on the volume of gastric contents. Solid-phase emptying is determined by powerful circular contractions of the distal stomach (antrum). These contractions grind and mix solid food into particles ≤1 mm in size, so that they may pass through the pylorus into the duodenum. Particles too large to escape through the pylorus during the postprandial period must be emptied during the stomach's interdigestive phase. During periods of fasting, a coordinated wave of activity, known as the migrating motor complex (MMC), sweeps through the stomach and small bowel every 90 min or so to clear the gut of indigestible debris and to prevent bacterial overgrowth.

With diabetic gastroparesis, normal antral contractility is lost; therefore, there are particular problems with solid-food emptying. Loss of gastric MMC activity also occurs, leading to gastric stasis and possible bezoar formation. Recent evidence suggests that patients with this condition may also experience prolonged pylorospasm, which further impairs gastric emptying.

Symptoms

Typical symptoms of gastroparesis (Table 39.1) include

- Nausea
- Vomiting
- Early satiety
- Abdominal bloating
- Epigastric pain
- Anorexia

Classically, patients vomit undigested food consumed many hours or even days previously. Postprandial vomiting is the rule, but morning nausea and "dry heaves" may also occur. Symptoms of gastroparesis are usually not disabling and may consist only of mild early satiety and nausea. Even with mild symptoms, gastroparesis interferes with nutrient delivery to the small bowel and therefore upsets the relationship between glucose absorption and exogenous insulin administration. The result may be wide swings of glucose levels and unexpected episodes of postprandial hypoglycemia. In its most troublesome form, chronic nausea and anorexia are punctuated by bouts of prolonged vomiting requiring hospitalization because of dehydration and uncontrolled hyperglycemia. Inexplicably, symptoms are variable and may fluctuate markedly over a period of weeks to months.

Acute hemorrhagic gastritis is common in patients with repeated vomiting due to gastroparesis or ketoacidosis. Bleeding is usually mild and self-limited. Chronic gastritis with gastric atrophy and hypochlorhydria may also be seen, especially in people with type I (insulin-dependent) diabetes with autoimmune disorders such as pernicious anemia and hypothyroidism. An awareness of the association is important because replacement treatment with vitamin B_{12} and thyroxine may be necessary. Hypochlorhydria predisposes to bacterial overgrowth but is otherwise usually clinically insignificant.

Diagnosis

Upper GI symptoms should not be attributed to gastroparesis until conditions such as gastric ulcer, duodenal ulcer, severe gastritis, and gastric cancer have been excluded. An esophagogastroduodenoscopy or a high-quality upper-GI barium series should be performed. The finding of retained food in the stomach after an 8- to 12-h fast, in the absence of obstruction, is diagnostic of gastroparesis; however, the lack of this finding does not rule out the diagnosis. Often, a nuclear solid-phase gastric-emptying study is useful. This noninvasive simple technique determines the rate of gastric emptying after ingestion of a standard radiolabeled meal. Gastroduodenal manometrics are a helpful complementary study but are more cumbersome and are usually available only in selected research settings.

Table 39.1. GI DISTURBANCES IN DIABETES

Condition	Symptom	Treatment
Esophageal dysfunction	Dysphagia	Metoclopramide
Gastroparesis	Nausea, vomiting, early satiety, anorexia, epigastric pain	Blood glucose control Care with hypoglycemia Bethanecol Metoclopramide Domperidone Cisapride Erythromycin
Hemorrhagic gastritis	Repeated vomiting and hematemesis (ketoacidosis and gastroparesis)	Treat cause
Cholelithiasis	Gallstone biliary colic, cholecystitis	Dissolution therapy, lithotripsy, or surgery
Pancreatic insufficiency	None—steatorrhea	Enzyme replacement
Diabetic diarrhea	Paroxysmal, nocturnal, painless, explosive, diarrhea	Gluten-free diet, pancreatic enzymes, antibiotics, cholestyramine, diphenoxylate, loperamide, Sandostatin (Octreotide, Sandoz)
Fecal incontinence	Soiling without awareness	Treat diarrhea Biofeedback training
Constipation	Infrequent bowel actions, abdominal pain	Improve toilet habits Increase fluid intake Psyllium

Treatment

The initial treatment of diabetic gastroparesis is careful attention to blood glucose control. Hyperglycemia, even acute, may interfere with gastric contractility and the occurrence of MMC. Physiological control of blood glucose levels may improve gastric motor function. Care must be exercised, however, in attempting to attain physiological control when gastric emptying is impaired because of the danger of severe hypoglycemia. Patients who complain of early satiety and bloating may benefit from a low-fat diet and several small meals throughout the day. Fibrous vegetables and poorly digestible solids should be avoided because of their predisposition to bezoar formation.

Pharmacological therapy is usually necessary in patients with clinically significant gastroparesis.

1. Metoclopramide is the drug of choice for gastroparesis. It acts centrally and peripherally and has both cholinergic and anti-dopaminergic properties. Metoclopramide increases the amplitude and frequency of gastric antral contractions in a coordinated manner and stimulates MMC activity. Furthermore, its centrally mediated action on the chemoreceptor trigger zone in the floor of the fourth ventricle give it important antiemetic properties. Controlled trials documenting the efficacy of metoclopramide are not always able to show an improvement in gastric emptying rates, so its efficacy may be partly due to its antiemetic actions. Unfortunately, despite the efficacy of metoclopramide, side effects in nearly 20% of patients limit its utility. Drowsiness, lethargy, and depression are most commonly seen, especially at higher doses. Anxiety, galactorrhea, and extrapyramidal symptoms are also noted, and tardive dyskinesia after long-term use is particularly disturbing. The usual dose is 5–20 mg 0.5 h before meals and at bedtime.

2. Bethanecol is a cholinomimetic agent that increases the amplitude of gastric antral motor activity in a nonspecific manner. Limited efficacy and cholinergic side effects hinder its usefulness.

3. Domperidone, not available in the United States except on a compassionate-use basis (Janssen, Piscataway, NJ), does not readily cross the blood-brain barrier and therefore does not have most of the serious side effects seen with metoclopramide. However, it still has antiemetic actions because of its affect on the chemoreceptor trigger zone. The usual dose is 10–20 mg 0.5 h before meals and at bedtime. Uncommon side effects include headaches and galactorrhea. It appears to be most useful for patients who have had a good response to metoclopramide but are unable to take it because of side effects.

4. Cisapride, also not available in the U.S. except on a compassionate-use basis (Janssen), is the newest and most potent prokinetic agent. It appears to act by releasing acetylcholine

from the myenteric plexus in the gut wall. The usual dose is 10–20 mg 0.5 h before meals. Side effects of headaches, diarrhea, and abdominal cramping are rare. Cisapride may prove to be a very effective drug even in patients who have failed standard agents.

5. Erythromycin (250 mg 0.5 h before meals) and its derivatives that duplicate the action of the motility hormone motilin (the hormone probably responsible for MMC activity) may be useful for patients with gastroparesis.

Severe, disabling symptoms refractory to pharmacological therapy may require placement of a jejunostomy feeding tube. This provides for prolonged stomach rest. A constant-drip delivery may be given overnight, facilitating insulin delivery and freeing the patient for daytime activity. Surgical procedures, such as pyloroplasty and partial gastrectomy, have been disappointing and are rarely recommended.

BILIARY DISEASE

Although the data are controversial, people with diabetes carry a slightly elevated risk for gallstone formation, with a reported incidence 1.5 times that of the general population. The high incidence of type II (non-insulin-dependent) diabetes in populations at high risk for cholelithiasis (women, the obese, and hyperlipoproteinemics) makes it difficult to identify diabetes as an independent risk factor. Theoretically, diabetes predisposes to gallstone formation because of diminished gallbladder contractility, leading to stasis in those with autonomic neuropathy and increased secretion of bile supersaturated with cholesterol. The role of prophylactic cholecystectomy in diabetic patients with asymptomatic gallstones is controversial, but analyses support a hands-off approach. Therefore, routine screening for gallstones is also not necessary. The mortality rate and risk of postoperative complications after emergent cholecystectomy for acute cholecystitis in the diabetic patient exceeds that of the general population. This risk is probably related to diseases associated with diabetes, e.g., renal insufficiency and cardiovascular disease, and not to diabetes itself.

Medical treatments for cholesterol gallstones such as dissolution therapy and lithotripsy (and even laparoscopic cholecystectomy) are attractive alternatives to surgery in the patient with symptomatic gallstones. These treatment alternatives perhaps should be considered for the high-risk diabetic patient with asymptomatic gallstones as well.

PANCREAS

Exocrine pancreatic function is reduced in >50% of people with type I diabetes, and the degree of impairment progresses with increasing duration of the disease. This may be the consequence of chronic insulin deficiency and resultant autonomic neuropathy. However, because 90% of enzyme output must be destroyed before steatorrhea occurs, clinically significant pancreatic insufficiency is rare.

SMALL AND LARGE BOWELS

Diarrhea

The incidence of diarrhea in the general diabetic population is ~5%, but prevalence of >20% has been reported. Diarrhea is typically frequent and watery and may be persistent, intermittent, or alternating with constipation. Mild steatorrhea is common. Patients typically awaken at night to find they have soiled their bedclothes.

The pathogenesis of diabetic diarrhea remains unclear. Small-bowel malabsorption of bile salts producing diarrheagenic effects on the colon is one proposed mechanism. However, therapeutic trials of the bile acid binder cholestyramine are not generally successful. A small subset of patients will have celiac sprue, pancreatic insufficiency, or bacterial overgrowth. These conditions, although uncommon, must be carefully sought if steatorrhea is present. Tests should include

- Specialized breath-hydrogen tests for bacterial overgrowth
- Tests of pancreatic function
- A small-bowel biopsy

Usually, these diseases are not identified, and autonomic neuropathy is presumed to be the etiology. Fecal incontinence seen in these patients is also caused by neuropathic damage, with loss of internal sphincter control and anorectal sensation. Autonomic neuropathy may cause diarrhea by virtue of its effects on gut motility or on enterocyte absorption. Although gut dysmotility makes sense and has been the most widely accepted explanation for diabetic diarrhea, motility testing and small-bowel transit studies have produced variable and inconsistent results. Adrenergic nerve dysfunction interferes with normal electrolyte and fluid absorption by the enterocyte.

Treatment of diabetic diarrhea should address the specific etiology. Celiac sprue and pancreatic insufficiency are treated with a gluten-free diet and pancreatic enzyme supplements, respectively. A trial of antibiotics is appropriate if bacterial overgrowth is found or cannot be ruled out (Table 39.2). A hydrophilic fiber supplement (i.e., psyllium) may be useful especially if diarrhea is mild and alternates with constipation. Chelation of bile salts with cholestyramine may reduce the bile acid component of diarrhea. Standard synthetic opiates such as diphenoxylate and loperamide are potent nonaddicting antidiarrheals that should be tried before agents such as clonidine. Clonidine, an α_2-agonist, may reverse adrenergic nerve dysfunction and improve diarrhea. However, clonidine has potent

Table 39.2. DRUG THERAPY FOR DIABETIC DIARRHEA

Drug	Starting Dose
Psyllium (sugar free)	1 tsp to 1 tbsp 1–3×/day
Kaolin + pectin (mixture)	2 Tbsp 2×/day
Cholestyramine	1 packet (4g) 1–6×/day
Tetracycline	250 mg 4×/day
Ampicillin	250 mg 4×/day
Pancreatic enzymes	2–4 tablets or capsules with meals + snacks
Diphenoxylate	2.5 mg 2×/day
Loperamide	2 mg 2×/day
Clonidine	0.2 mg 2×/day
Sandostatin	50 μg 3×/day

antimotility effects on the gut, which may also explain symptomatic improvement in some patients. Begin treatment with 0.1 mg and increase to 0.4–0.6 mg 2×/day over several days. The long-acting somatostatin analogue Sandostatin (Octreotide, Sandoz) may be effective in patients with severe refractory symptoms.

Fecal Incontinence

Treatment of fecal incontinence should first be directed toward improvement of the diarrhea. Loose stools are always more difficult to retain than solid stools. Sometimes, a combination of a fiber supplement and an antidiarrhea agent such as loperamide (beginning with 2 mg 2×/day) best accomplishes this purpose. Sphincter-strengthening exercises should be encouraged and practiced. Anorectal manometrics with biofeedback is a simple operant conditioning technique that has nearly a 70% success rate in those with intact rectal sensation.

Constipation

Constipation is the most common GI complication, affecting nearly 25% of the diabetic population and >50% of those with neuropathy. Severe problematic constipation is seen in 20% of people with diabetes with neuropathy. Constipation is assumed to be caused by generalized autonomic neuropathy. Myoelectric studies of the colon have demonstrated diminished motility in response to ingestion of a standard meal (gastrocolonic reflex). Cholinergic agents stimulate colonic motility, suggesting a defect in neural control of the smooth muscle. Severe constipation may be complicated by stercoral ulceration, perforation, barium impaction, and fecal impaction. Fecal impaction may cause overflow diarrhea and fecal incontinence and so must be considered in the differential diagnosis of diabetic diarrhea. Long-standing constipation with straining predisposes to stretch injury of the nerves supplying the anal sphincter musculature and may lead to fecal incontinence. A barium enema or colonoscopy should be performed in the patient with recent-onset or problematic constipation to eliminate the possibility of a structural lesion such as a stricture or tumor.

Treatment should begin with an emphasis on good toilet habits, postprandial timing of defecation, regular exercise, and maintenance of adequate hydration. Many constipated patients will respond to a high-insoluble-fiber diet supplemented with a daily hydrophilic colloid (1 tsp to 1 tbsp psyllium $1-3 \times$/day). The intermittent use of saline or osmotic laxatives (e.g., 30–60 mg milk of magnesia may be required for those with more severe symptoms, but stimulant laxatives should be avoided because of their tendency to damage the colonic myenteric plexus after long-term use. Magnesium-containing agents must be used with caution if renal insufficiency exists.

ABDOMINAL PAIN

Autonomic neuropathy may present with abdominal pain, and special consideration should be given to such diagnoses as acute cholecystitis, pancreatitis, gastroparesis, and diabetic ketoacidosis. Occasionally, a patient will present with chronic severe epigastric pain not attributable to any of these conditions. When signs of neuropathy are present, the most likely diagnosis may be diabetic radiculopathy. Symptoms of severe anorexia and weight loss cause this condition to be easily confused with gastroparesis or pancreatic carcinoma. For unclear reasons, symptoms usually resolve after many months.

SUGGESTED READING

1. Achem-Karam SR, Funakoshi A, Vinik AI, Owyang C: Plasma motilin and migrating motor complex in diabetic gastroparesis. *Gastroenterology* 88:492–94, 1985
2. Fedorak RN, Field M, Chang EB: Treatment of diabetic diarrhea with clonidine. *Ann Intern Med* 102:197–99, 1985
3. Jacober SJ, Vinik AI, Narayan A, Strodel WE: Jejunostomy feeding in the management of gastroparesis. *Diabetes Care* 9:217–19, 1985
4. Rothstein RD: Gastrointestinal motility disorders in diabetes mellitus. *Am J Gastroenterol* 85:782–85, 1990
5. Sack TL, Sleisenger NH: Effects of systemic and extraintestinal disease on the gut. In *Gastrointestinal Disease*. 4th ed. Sleisenger NH, Fordtran JS, Eds. Philadelphia, PA, Saunders, 1989, p. 488–528
6. Schiller LR, Santa Ana CA, Schmulen AC, Hendler RS, Harford WV, Fordtran JS: Pathogenesis of fecal incontinence in diabetes mellitus. *N Engl J Med* 307:1666–71, 1982
7. Tsai ST, Vinik AI, Brunner JF: Diabetic diarrhea and somatostatin. *Ann Intern Med* 104:894, 1986
8. Vinik AI, Glowniak JV: Hormonal secretions in diabetic autonomic neuropathy. *NY State J Med* 82:871–78, 1982
9. Yang R, Arem R, Chan L: Gastrointestinal tract complications of diabetes mellitus. *Arch Intern Med* 144:1251–56, 1984

40. Bladder Dysfunction

STEVEN A. KAPLAN, MD

The neuropathy related to diabetes mellitus also affects the genito-urinary system, which is particularly true in the urinary bladder. Diabetic cystopathy refers to the spectrum of voiding dysfunction in patients with diabetes mellitus. The hallmark of diabetic cystopathy is its insidious onset and progression with minimal symptomatology. The incidence of diabetic cystopathy ranges from 27 to 85%. The incidence of cystopathy correlates strongly with both the duration of the disease and the presence of peripheral neuropathy. Severity of disease is a less useful clinical predictor of voiding dysfunction.

It is rare for the clinical symptom complex to manifest in a patient who has had diabetes mellitus for <10 yr. Initial symptoms are usually related to impaired bladder sensation, which may be secondary to injury to visceral afferent fibers within the bladder wall. The impairment of bladder sensation causes a gradual change in the patient's voiding pattern. As the intervoiding interval increases, the patient may void only once or twice daily. With progressive deterioration of bladder sensory function, the patient may experience increasing difficulty in initiating and/or maintaining micturition. Notable is the need to strain abdominally with resulting slow urinary stream and terminal dribbling. This may eventually lead to urinary incontinence. As decreased bladder sensation progresses, resultant impaired bladder contractility ensues. This is usually secondary to a local muscle overstretch injury.

There is no one test that is pathognomonic for the diagnosis of diabetic cystopathy. Quantitative measures of bladder capacity and uroflow are difficult to extrapolate from one series to another. Given

Dr. Kaplan is Director of the Prostate Center at the College of Physicians and Surgeons of Columbia University, New York, NY.

Table 40.1. **MANIFESTATIONS OF DIABETIC CYSTOPATHY**

Clinical
- Poor urinary stream
- Feeling of incomplete bladder emptying
- Straining to void
- Hesitancy
- Infrequent voiding

Urodynamics
- Increased bladder capacity ($>$1000 ml)
- Impaired bladder sensation
- Increased postvoid residual urine ($>$200 ml)
- Decreased bladder contractility (voiding pressure $<$40 cmH$_2$O)
- Acontractile detrusor
- Impaired urinary flow ($<$10 ml/s)

these limitations, the urodynamic abnormalities seen in diabetic cystopathy include

1. Increased bladder capacity ($>$1000 ml)
2. Impaired bladder sensation (first sensation of bladder filling at 500 ml)
3. Increased postresidual urine ($>$200 ml)
4. Decreased bladder contractility, which may progress to detrusor areflexia (voiding pressure $<$15 cmH$_2$O)
5. Impaired urinary flow ($<$10 ml/s)

A patient should not be categorized as having cystopathy based on only one or two of these criteria. The combination of patient history, symptom complex, and basic urodynamic parameters signifies the diagnosis of diabetic voiding dysfunction (Table 40.1).

DIFFERENTIAL DIAGNOSIS

The most important differential diagnosis and one that frequently coexists with diabetic cystopathy is bladder-outlet obstruction, usually caused by benign prostatic hyperplasia (BPH). An important caveat to clinicians caring for this group of patients is that neither diminished uroflow nor increased postvoid residual is useful in distinguishing between bladder-outlet obstruction and diabetic cystopathy. This can be done only by the simultaneous measurement of urinary flow rate and detrusor pressure (P_{det}) ($P_{det} = P_{ves} - P_{abd}$, where P_{ves} is total intravesical or bladder pressure [consisting of inherent bladder pressure and abdominal straining], and P_{abd} is abdominal pressure measured via rectal tube).

TREATMENT

Treatment is predicated on a clear understanding of the underlying pathophysiology that results in diabetic cystopathy (Table 40.2).

Table 40.2. TREATMENT OF BLADDER DYSFUNCTION

Asymptomatic diabetic cystopathy
- Timed voiding
- Double voiding
- Abdominal straining

Symptomatic diabetic cystopathy
- Self–intermittent catheterization
- Bethanechol

Reduction of bladder-outlet obstruction
- Surgical
  - Transurethral resection of the prostate
  - Open prostatectomy
  - Transurethral incision of the prostate
  - Laser transurethral resection
- Nonsurgical
  - Pharmacological
  - Balloon dilation
  - Hyperthermia
  - Prostatic stents
- Reduction cystoplasty

Investigational
- Aldose reductase inhibitors
- *myo*-Inositol

This entails the exclusion of bladder-outlet obstruction as the cause of the voiding dysfunction.

Asymptomatic Patients With Diabetic Cystopathy

There are few short-term complications associated with diabetic cystopathy. Therefore, it is justifiable to treat conservatively with reversible and noninvasive therapy. Scheduled voiding, i.e., having the patient void every 3–4 h, is an easy and effective method for dealing with infrequent bladder emptying caused by impaired bladder sensation. Double or tripple voiding is useful to reduce large postvoid residual volumes. This is done by having the patient void and then repeat in 5–10 min to assist in bladder emptying. Careful consideration should be given when considering the use of abdominal straining or the Crede maneuver to help bladder emptying because it is not physiological. The patient is trying to void against a fixed resistance (the external urinary sphincter), which may prove more deleterious than helpful. Any patient who demonstrates a decrease in uroflow with straining should be specifically cautioned not to strain during micturition.

Symptomatic Patients With Diabetic Cystopathy

The hallmark of therapy in patients with diabetic cystopathy is self–intermittent catheterization. Symptomatic or febrile infections should be treated with culture-specific antibiotics. However, infection should be differentiated from bladder colonization. About 30% of patients on self–intermittent catheterization have positive urine cultures but are asymptomatic, and treatment with antibiotics will result in the proliferation of resistant organisms.

Several treatment regimens have been proposed to treat patients with diabetic cystopathy. However, most have little benefit, and positive results are anecdotal. Bethanechol chloride is a parasympathomimetic, which stimulates bladder contractility in laboratory animals; however, the effect is much less pronounced in humans. The efficacy of bethanechol chloride is predicated on the integrity of the lower motor neuron being intact allowing for reflex bladder function. Therefore, patients with lower motor neuron lesions, such as those with diabetes, are not good candidates for this therapy. Reports demonstrating efficacy are limited to either high oral or subcutaneous dosages.

Nonsurgical management of bladder-outlet obstruction caused by BPH includes

1. Pharmacological: α adrenergic blockers (prazosin, terazosin, doxazosin) and 5α-reductase inhibitors (finasteride)
2. Balloon dilation of the prostate
3. Local hyperthermia
4. Prostatic stents

Table 40.3. **ALTERNATIVE THERAPY FOR BENIGN PROSTATIC HYPERPLASIA**

Modality	Advantage	Disadvantage
Pharmacological		
α-Blockers (1–5 mg/day)	Reversible, prompt response	Postural hypotension effect in some patients
Prazosin		
Terazosin*	Taken once daily	
Doxazosin*	Taken once daily	
5α-Reductase inhibitor (finasteride* [1–5 mg/day])	Few side effects, taken once daily	Takes at least 3 mo to work
Balloon dilation	Minimal anesthesia, short hospital stay, antegrade ejaculation	Unknown durability of response
Hyperthermia*	No anesthesia, outpatient, no side effects	Unclear if effective
Prostatic stents*	Minimal anesthesia, outpatient	Unknown long-term complications

*Under investigation for the treatment of benign prostatic hyperplasia, monitored by the Food and Drug Administration.

When used with cholinergic-type agents, such as bethanecol chloride, these methods may promote bladder emptying. There are few reports to support their use in patients with diabetic cystopathy. However, in patients with concomitant bladder-outlet obstruction, use of these nonsurgical regimens may alleviate some of the patient's voiding symptoms. Recommended dosage regimens, along with advantages and disadvantages of each, are presented in Table 40.3.

Although there have been reports of transurethral prostatic or bladder neck resection to reduce residual urine in diabetic patients, patients with impaired bladder contractility and impaired voiding rarely benefit from a procedure solely designed to reduce bladder-outlet obstruction. Another surgical procedure advocated to reduce the large capacity and low pressure associated with diabetic cystopathy is reduction cystoplasty. However, the major difficulty with this procedure is that the original presurgical bladder recurs within a year.

The value of aldose reductase inhibitors, *myo*-inositol, and γ-linoleic acid remains to be defined.

PATIENT REFERRAL

Patients with large bladder capacities and high postvoid residual urine volumes should undergo a baseline urodynamic evaluation. This is particularly true in patients with concomitant urologic conditions, including bladder-outlet obstruction, neurogenic bladder from other causes such as stroke, poor bladder compliance (high filling pressure), or vesicoureteral reflux. These conditions all predispose the patient to upper-tract deterioration and should be aggressively treated when present.

SUGGESTED READING

1. Blaivas JG: Nontraumatic neurogenic voiding dysfunction in the adult. II. Multiple sclerosis and diabetes. *AUA Update Ser* 12:2–7, 1985
2. Ellenberg M, Weber H: The incipient asymptomatic diabetic bladder. *Diabetes* 16:331–35, 1967
3. Frimodt-Moller C: Diabetic cystopathy. I. A clinical study on the frequency of bladder dysfunction in diabetics. *Dan Med Bull* 23:267–75, 1976
4. Kaplan SA, Blaivas JG: Diabetic cystopathy. *J Diabetic Complications* 1:133–39, 1988
5. Kaplan SA, Blaivas JG: Benign prostatic hypertrophy. *Hosp Pract* May:77–86, 1990

41. Impotence

MICHAEL A. PFEIFER, MD

Impotence is one of the most common complaints among diabetic men. Its prevalence has been reported to be as high as 60%. Attention to this complaint may have a very positive impact on the patient's quality of life.

PATHOPHYSIOLOGY

Impotence can be psychogenic or organic in origin. As a complication of diabetes, it is usually the result of impairment in both the nervous and vascular systems. Unlike many of the complications of diabetes, impotence does not seem to be related to duration, although it is more likely to occur in men with symptoms of peripheral neuropathy.

SYMPTOMS AND DIAGNOSIS

The onset of organic impotence is gradual and progresses in severity. The earliest symptom is generally decreased rigidity and reduced frequency of erection, followed by incomplete tumescence and eventually complete loss of erectile function. Libido generally remains unchanged in diabetic patients.

The neurological component of impotence seems to be due to autonomic nerve-mediated decreased penile smooth muscle relaxation. Microvascular and macrovascular disease has been associated

Dr. Pfeifer is Director of the Diabetes Center for Excellence, Humana Hospital Lexington, and of the Diabetes Research and Analysis Association, Inc., Lexington, KY.

with impotence and may be a combination of arterial stenosis and venous leaks. Internal pudendal artery stenosis seems to be the most common cause of arterial problems. Doppler ultrasound measurements provide a reliable index of blood supply. The penile-brachial pressure index is the most common measure of the degree of vascular disease. An index <0.7 indicates diminished blood supply. Patients may have normal penile blood pressure while at rest but a significant decrease in pressure after exertion, termed *pelvic steal syndrome*. The patient will be unable to maintain an adequate erection. Venous leaks need to be evaluated by penile sonography.

The diagnosis of neurogenic impotence is one of exclusion; therefore, it is important to determine the etiology of impotence to select appropriate treatment. Figure 41.1 is an algorithm to aid in the determination of etiology.

Psychological factors such as stress and emotional disturbances may cause or contribute to impotence and are as common among diabetic men as among the general population. In addition, fear of diabetic impotence may induce impotence. The possibility of psychogenic impotence should be eliminated. The most obvious symptom of psychogenic impotence is sudden onset and/or complaints related to isolated situations or individuals. The Derogatis and Lopez sexual inventory questionnaire may be useful in identifying psychogenic impotence. Monitoring of nocturnal penile tumescence is a useful objective tool in determining whether the patient is physically capable of having an erection. Commercially available devices measure nocturnal erections that require intact neural and vascular mechanisms. If psychogenic impotence is confirmed, the patient should be referred to a therapist with expertise in treating sexual dysfunction.

TREATMENT

Some factors that may contribute to organic impotence must be evaluated and treated (Table 41.1). Impotence is a side effect of many commonly prescribed drugs, e.g., antihypertensives, antidepressants, and tranquilizers. A change in prescription is recommended if current drug therapy is suspected as a potential cause.

In patients with vascular insufficiency, yohimbine (2.5 mg 3×/day; may be increased to 5.0 mg 3×/day) may increase rigidity, but it may also aggravate hypertension. Vasoactive agents can produce erection when injected directly into the corpora cavernosa. Side effects include bruising and priapism. Vascular surgery may correct reduced blood supply or repair venous leaks in some cases. Patients should be referred to a specialist for injection treatment or evaluation for vascular surgery.

Several mechanical devices are commercially available that can produce an erection. These devices create a vacuum to draw blood into the penis and a band to prevent venous return. These devices are particularly useful when venous leaks contribute significantly to

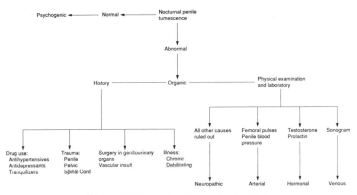

Figure 41.1. Evaluation of impotence.

impotence. The only complication of these devices is that necrosis may develop if the band is left on too long.

Improved glycemic control can improve erectile function in those patients with very poor control. Education and intensive insulin management are recommended.

Pelvic or spinal trauma from surgery or an accident may also cause impotence and may be excluded by a thorough history. Rarely, testosterone deficiency may cause impotence. If serum testosterone is abnormal, prolactin, follicle-stimulating hormone, and luteinizing hormone should be measured.

For patients in whom other treatments are not effective or acceptable, penile prosthesis is an alternative. There are several types available. Prosthesis is complicated by infection, inappropriate placement or size, and pain. Patients should be referred to a urologist for prosthesis.

Table 41.1. TREATMENT METHODS FOR IMPOTENCE

Cause	Treatment
Prescription drugs: antihypertensives, antidepressants, tranquilizers	Change to drug with lower or no incidence of impotence
Poor glycemic control	Education and glucose regulation
Hormonal abnormalities	Correct abnormality
Vascular insufficiency	Yohimbine given orally may be helpful for early loss of penile rigidity or pelvic steal syndrome
	Intracorporal injection of papaverine, phentolamine, or prostaglandins before sexual activity
	Vascular surgery
	Penile prostheses
Venous leaks	Mechanical devices
	Penile prostheses

SUGGESTED READING

1. Buffum J: Pharmacosexology update: prescription drugs and sexual function. *J Psychoact Drugs* 18:97–106, 1986
2. Cyrus J, Broadstone VL, Pfeifer MA, Greene DA: Diabetic peripheral neuropathy. II. Autonomic neuropathy. *Diabetes Educ* 13:111–15, 1987
3. Derogatis LR, Meyer JK, Dupkin CN: Discrimination of organic versus psychogenic impotence with the DSFI. *J Sex Marital Ther* 2:229–40, 1976
4. Kaiser FE, Korenman SG: Impotence in diabetic men. *Am J Med* 85 (Suppl. 5A):147–52, 1988
5. Schiavi R, Hogan B: Sexual problems in diabetes mellitus: psychological aspects. *Diabetes Care* 2:9–17, 1979

42. Female Sexual Disorders

LESLIE R. SCHOVER, PhD

SEXUAL PROBLEMS IN WOMEN WITH DIABETES

Although erectile dysfunction is a common diabetic complication in men, there is not a strong association in women between diabetes and sexual problems. Nevertheless, research suggests that diabetes increases the risk of sexual dysfunction at least in older women.

PATHOPHYSIOLOGY AND RATIONALE FOR TREATMENT

Women's sexual problems can be categorized as affecting desire, arousal, and orgasm or pain with sexual intercourse. In general, premenopausal women with type I (insulin-dependent) diabetes do not have higher rates of sexual problems than healthy women of similar backgrounds. At most, some case series have found that young diabetic women are more likely to complain of inadequate vaginal lubrication. Poor lubrication is the problem that most closely parallels erectile dysfunction in men, in that both aspects of the sexual response depend on genital vasocongestion with sexual arousal. Along with vaginal dryness and lack of expansion, an inadequate genital vasocongestive response could cause irritation or pain with sexual activity. Few differences were found between premenopausal diabetic and control women whose vasocongestion was measured directly by monitoring labial temperature during sexual arousal. Some diabetic women had abnormally high resting labial temperatures, however, obscuring the changes expected with sexual arousal to watching an erotic film. This unusually high baseline may be a sign in itself of subtle autonomic disregulation.

Dr. Schover is Staff Psychologist at The Cleveland Clinic Foundation, Cleveland, OH.

A comparison of older type II (non-insulin-dependent) diabetic women with age-matched healthy control women revealed a greater sexual impact of the disease. Type II diabetic women had more problems with low sexual desire, poor vaginal lubrication, dyspareunia, and difficulty reaching orgasm than did the healthy group. Damage to the vasocongestive component of sexual arousal may be too subtle in young women to be a handicap. As menopause approaches and the vagina loses a degree of elasticity and lubrication, however, the effects of diabetes may become more apparent. The average age of the older groups in the study was 46 yr, and ~50% of the diabetic women were postmenopausal. The greater impact of diabetes on older women's sexual function could result from premature loss of vaginal vascularity, poor vasomotor responsiveness, or even depletion of neurotransmitters in the genital tissue. Pain and difficulty reaching orgasm are perhaps secondary to diminished genital vasocongestion.

ASSESSMENT OF SEXUAL DYSFUNCTION

In a busy clinic, assessment of sexual problems is easily overlooked. Female patients, especially older ones, are often reluctant to ask about their sexual concerns. Male physicians may also feel embarrassed about raising this topic with a female patient, perhaps even fearing that a question will be misinterpreted as an improper advance.

A dignified way to ask about sexuality is to make a practice of including the following question in the section of an interview that assesses signs of diabetic complications: "Diabetes also may interfere with a woman's sexual response. Have you noticed any changes in your sex life that could be related to your diabetes?"

If the woman responds affirmatively, further questions can be asked:

- Some women notice a decrease in their sexual desire or interest. Has that been a problem for you? Do you feel pleasure and excitement once sexual activity begins?
- A common problem for diabetic women is vaginal dryness or tightness with intercourse. Have you experienced this?
- Have you had pain or discomfort with intercourse? Does this include pain at penetration, with deep thrusting, or soreness and irritation after sexual activity?
- Is it more difficult for you to reach an orgasm than in the past?
- Have you had recent problems with repeated infections in your vagina or urinary tract?
- Do you have concerns or questions about contraception and diabetes?

With most women, a brief sexual assessment will only add a minute or two to the interview. The questions should be put into the context that sexual health is a legitimate part of general health. It helps to preface these questions with a normalizing statement, i.e., "It is not unusual for diabetes to cause some mild problems in a woman's sexual function." The physician can even introduce the topic by saying, "As part of the history (or follow-up), I always ask about your sexual health, because that is one important part of your quality of life."

The woman's spouse or sexual partner can also play an important role in sexual assessment or counseling. If the partner is present, the interviewer should ask for his/her viewpoint on any sexual problems discussed. In older couples, a woman may be more concerned about her husband's waning erectile capacity than about any dysfunction of her own.

THERAPY AND EXPECTED RESULTS

If a woman's sexual problem is mild, began recently, or appears to have a strong diabetes-related cause, some practical and brief interventions by the health-care team may be effective. Loss of desire for sex is often related to depression. If a woman also has disturbed sleep, a change in her appetite for food, depressed mood, chronic fatigue, somatic symptoms without clear organic cause, and trouble with concentration or memory, she probably could benefit from treatment for depression. Antidepressant drugs and brief symptom-focused psychotherapy are both effective. A young woman who has lost her ovarian function because of bilateral oophorectomy or pelvic radiotherapy for cancer may experience less desire for sex because of a hormonal deficiency. Estrogen replacement can improve vaginal elasticity and lubrication, but additional supplementation with androgens is more likely to directly increase sexual desire. Although androgen therapy has been helpful to women who undergo surgical menopause, it has no documented benefit for premenopausal women with low sexual desire or for women who are menopausal but still have their ovaries. Diabetic women with end-stage renal disease may be hyperprolactinemic. The resulting loss of sexual desire sometimes improves with a dopamine agonist, erythropoietin therapy, or a kidney transplant.

The arousal-phase problem of poor vaginal lubrication with its attendant side effects of vaginal irritation and pain with sexual activity is often easy to treat. A woman who has low estrogen levels can use replacement estrogen as a pill, patch, or vaginal cream. The estrogen can actually reverse vaginal atrophy within a few months. The pH of the vagina normalizes. For premenopausal diabetic women, or for those postmenopausal patients who have risk factors preventing estrogen replacement, vaginal lubricants are quite helpful. One new product, Replens (Columbia Laboratories, nonprescription), contains polymers that bind to vaginal mucin, hydrating the mucosa and helping to maintain a favorable vaginal pH. Because many diabetic women have recurrent monilial infections, Replens used three times weekly may prevent chronic irritation. Replens has not yet been tested in the diabetic population, however, and is a fairly expensive product. For sexual activity, the physician can recommend a water-based gel lubricant, e.g., Today Personal Lubricant. For women with very severe dryness, a vaginal suppository (Condom Mate or Lubrin, Upsher Smith) can also be inserted before foreplay.

To minimize coital pain, a woman should learn to relax the pubococcygeal muscles. She can identify the muscles by contracting them during urination and noticing that the flow stops. Women who feel comfortable putting a finger inside of their vaginas can also squeeze the muscles and feel the slight vaginal contraction. Once the woman has found the muscles, she can practice squeezing them for a count of 3 and then releasing them, 10 times in a row. If vaginal penetration for intercourse feels tight and painful, a woman can tense and relax the muscles before and during the process. In general, patients who have pain on penetration or with deep thrusting should use coital positions that give the woman more control. These include the woman sitting or kneeling over her partner or both partners lying on their sides facing each other.

Some diabetic women have lost a leg or have limited mobility. For them, a physical therapist may have suggestions on positioning for intercourse, perhaps with pillows as an aid to comfort or stability. Women with neurogenic bladder should try to empty their bladders before sexual activity, with self-catheterization if needed. This can help prevent stress incontinence during intercourse or orgasm and help avoid urinary tract infections.

A decrease in orgasmic capacity is not common as an isolated problem in diabetic women. Rather, it is often a product of lessened desire and excitement or physical discomfort during sex. Before assuming that trouble with coital orgasm is related to diabetic neuropathy, ask if the woman is still orgasmic with clitoral stimulation (i.e., by her hand, vibrator, or from a partner). Many healthy women have a difficult time reaching orgasm from penile-vaginal thrusting alone.

It is also important to know whether concerns about pregnancy are affecting a couple's sex life. Infertility treatment often temporarily disrupts sexual pleasure. On the other hand, fear of pregnancy can interfere with sexual desire and activity.

REFERRAL TO SPECIALIST

A referral to a specialist in sexual problems is indicated under the following conditions:

- The sexual problem is severe or has been present for several years.
- The problem does not respond to primary-care team intervention.

- In addition to having a sexual problem, the patient is poorly adjusted psychologically or has a highly conflicted close relationship.

For most women's sexual problems, the referral of choice is to a mental-health professional who has special training in treating sexual dysfunctions. Probably the most common causes of sexual problems in diabetic women are psychological, e.g., anxiety about attractiveness, poor sexual communication, relationship conflict, or a history of a traumatic sexual experience. The best way to find a competent specialist is to refer only to a fully qualified social worker, psychiatrist, or psychologist who has specialty training at the postgraduate level. These professionals can often be located on the faculty of a local psychology department or medical school. County or state mental-health organizations can also provide referrals.

A gynecologist with special expertise in treating sexual problems is especially helpful with dysfunctions related to menopause or to genital pain.

The gynecological examination should include assessment of tenderness around the vaginal vestibule, the condition of Bartholin's glands and the vaginal mucosa, and the presence of pain deep in the vagina or pelvis with pressure or movement of the cervix and uterus. Women who have vulvar tenderness, burning, and pain at the introitus with sexual stimulation sometimes have a syndrome known as vulvar vestibulitis. Inflammation of numerous glands around the vestibule can be diagnosed with colposcopy. Common causes of coital pain only on deep thrusting include endometriosis, pelvic adhesions, abnormalities of the uterine ligaments, or ovarian cysts. However, none of these gynecological problems has been associated with diabetes.

SUGGESTED READING

1. Jensen SB: Sexual dysfunction in insulin-treated diabetics: a six-year follow-up study of 101 patients. *Arch Sex Behav* 15:271–83, 1986
2. Schover LR, Jensen SB: *Sexuality and Chronic Illness: A Comprehensive Approach*. New York, Guilford, 1988
3. Schreiner-Engel P, Schiavi RC, Vietorisz D, Smith H: The differential impact of diabetes type on female sexuality. *J Psychosom Res* 31:23–33, 1987
4. Slob AK, Koster J, Radder JK, van der Werff ten Bosch JJ: Sexuality and psychophysiological functioning in women with diabetes mellitus. *Sex Marital Ther* 16:59–69, 1990
5. Tyrer G, Steel JM, Ewing DJ, Bancroft J, Warner P, Clarke BF: Sexual responsiveness in diabetic women. *Diabetologia* 24:166–71, 1983

43. Postural Hypotension

ITALO BIAGGIONI, MD

Maintenance of upright posture is made possible by instantaneous cardiovascular adaptation that depends primarily on an intact autonomic nervous system. When this system fails, as may occur in long-standing diabetes mellitus, orthostatic hypotension ensues. The importance of these cardiovascular adaptation processes are not apparent until the incapacitating symptoms of patients with autonomic failure are observed. The cardiovascular autonomic neuropathy seen in patients with diabetes mellitus shares common features with primary autonomic failure. Features pertinent to diabetic autonomic neuropathy are emphasized herein.

PATHOPHYSIOLOGY

When a normal individual stands, up to 700 ml of blood pools in the legs and lower abdominal veins. Venous return decreases, resulting in a transient decline in cardiac output. The reduction in central blood volume and arterial pressure is sensed by cardiopulmonary volume receptors and arterial baroreceptors. Afferent signals from these receptors reach vasomotor centers in the brain stem. Efferent fibers from these centers reduce parasympathetic output and increase sympathetic outflow. Norepinephrine is released from postganglionic sympathetic nerve terminals at target organs, resulting in an increase in heart rate and cardiac contractility, partial restoration of venous return and diastolic ventricular filling by venoconstriction, and an increase in peripheral resistance by arteriolar

---

Dr. Biaggioni is Assistant Professor of Medicine and Pharmacology at Vanderbilt University, Nashville, TN.

vasoconstriction. As a net effect of these adaptive mechanisms, cardiac output remains reduced by 10–20%, systolic blood pressure is reduced by 5–10 mmHg, diastolic blood pressure increases by 2–5 mmHg, mean blood pressure remains almost unchanged, and heart rate increases by 5–20 beats/min.

DEFINITION

Orthostatic hypotension is arbitrarily defined as a decrease in systolic blood pressure >30 mmHg or any fall in diastolic blood pressure on standing. It is best characterized clinically as any decrease in arterial blood pressure that produces symptoms such as lightheadedness, blurry vision, and pain in the back of the neck, finally leading to transient loss of consciousness. Symptoms never occur while supine but usually occur shortly after standing and are always relieved immediately on sitting or lying down. Failure to meet these criteria should make the physician rule out other causes of syncope that may occur in diabetic patients (e.g., hypoglycemia, arrhythmias, or transient ischemic attacks).

DIAGNOSIS

Subclinical cardiovascular autonomic neuropathy is relatively common, but overt orthostatic hypotension usually appears as a late complication. The diagnosis of cardiovascular autonomic neuropathy can be easily done with simple measurements of heart rate and blood pressure (Table 43.1).

Autonomic failure is not always the cause of orthostatic hypotension in diabetic patients. Patients with severe autonomic neuropathy lack the compensatory increase in heart rate and plasma norepinephrine that should accompany orthostatic hypotension. In patients with significant orthostatic tachycardia, factors should be ruled out that may precipitate orthostatic hypotension in patients with borderline autonomic function, e.g., hypovolemia or pharmacological agents (Table 43.2).

Two additional factors may precipitate hypotension in patients with autonomic failure. Meals lower blood pressure dramatically in patients with primary autonomic failure. Likewise, insulin lowers blood pressure in diabetic patients with autonomic neuropathy and has no effect in those without autonomic neuropathy. This effect may be more pronounced if hypoglycemia is present. The incidence and magnitude of these problems is small in most patients, but the possibility exists.

TREATMENT

In general, a stepwise approach to treatment is preferable according to the severity of the symptoms (Table 43.3). These should be

Table 43.1. ASSESSMENT OF AUTONOMIC FUNCTION: BEDSIDE PHYSIOLOGICAL TESTS

Posture
- Measure blood pressure (BP) and heart rate (HR) after patient has been supine 15 min and standing 5 min.
- Express as supine − standing values.
- Normal response: systolic BP = 0 to −15 mmHg, diastolic BP = −5 to 5 mmHg, HR = 0−15 beats/min.

Sinus arrhythmia (SA) ratio
- Have patient breathe deeply 6×/min while monitoring HR in continuous strip.
- Measure longest R-R interval during expiration and shortest R-R interval during inspiration. Take average of 6 breaths.
- SA ratio = $R\text{-}R_{exp}/R\text{-}R_{insp}$.
- Normal response: ≥1.2.

Valsalva ratio
- Use 6- to 12-ml syringe barrel as mouthpiece connected to sphygmomanometer.
- Ask patient to blow mercury column to 40 mmHg for 15 s while monitoring HR in continuous strip. Repeat 4×. Make sure effort is barred by thorax and not mouth.
- Measure shortest R-R during strain and longest R-R after release.
- Valsalva ratio = $R\text{-}R_{release}/R\text{-}R_{strain}$.
- Normal response: ≥1.4.

Cold pressor test
- Measure baseline BP and HR. Have patient place hand in ice water for 1 min. Measure BP and HR at end of minute.
- Normal response: rise in systolic BP >15 mmHg.

considered general guidelines, and treatment should be individualized. Some recommendations may actually be contraindicated in a given patient.

Nonpharmacological Therapy

In patients with persistent symptoms, conservative nonpharmacological therapy is indicated. Medical therapy includes the following (Table 43.3):

Table 43.2. DRUGS THAT MAY PRECIPITATE OR WORSEN ORTHOSTATIC HYPOTENSION IN PATIENTS WITH AUTONOMIC FAILURE

- Diuretics
- Tricyclic antidepressants
- Phenothiazides
- Venodilators (nitrates)
- Antihypertensives (α-blockers, guanethidine)
- Insulin

Table 43.3. STEPWISE APPROACH TO MANAGEMENT OF ORTHOSTATIC HYPOTENSION

1. Remove aggravating factors
   - Volume depletion
   - Anemia
   - Drugs*
   - Prolonged bed rest/deconditioning
   - Alcohol
2. Medical treatment
   - Liberalize salt intake, salt supplements
   - Head-up tilt during the night
   - Waist-high support stockings
   - Exercise as tolerated
3. Pharmacological treatment†
   - Fludrocortisone
   - Short-acting pressor agents

* See Table 43.2.
† See Table 43.4.

- Increase salt intake: Patients with autonomic failure may be unable to conserve sodium, and liberalization of sodium intake is generally recommended.
- Avoid supine diuresis: These patients have exaggerated nocturnal diuresis with relative hypovolemia and worsening of orthostatic hypotension early in the morning. To minimize exaggerated nocturnal diuresis, patients should elevate the head of the bed with 6- to 9-inch blocks.
- Decrease venous pooling: During the day, wear waist-high custom-fitted elastic support stockings that will exert pressure on the legs and reduce venous pooling (some patients find them cumbersome to wear, and sensory neuropathy or vasculopathy may limit their use).
- Avoid wearing support stockings while supine because they may contribute to diuresis and supine hypertension.

Pharmacological Therapy

Some patients may require pharmacological therapy in addition to nonpharmacological therapy. At this stage, the goal of treatment is to minimize symptoms rather than to normalize an upright blood pressure:

- Fludrocortisone: Therapy is usually initiated with fludrocortisone acetate at a low dose (0.1 mg/day) and increased slowly to 0.4 mg/day if needed. A weight gain of 1–2 kg and mild ankle edema may be desirable in these patients. However, hypokalemia, supine hypertension, and pulmonary edema may occur, and patients must be monitored carefully.

- Pressor agents: It may not be possible to keep severely afflicted patients symptom free throughout the day. A more realistic goal may be to provide them with some periods when they can remain upright. This is probably best achieved by adding short-acting pressor agents.

Most of the agents listed in Table 43.4, if effective in a given patient, will increase blood pressure for 2–3 h. In general, these agents are preferably given before exertion, and their continued use is discouraged to avoid side effects and the potential development of tolerance. Patients should also avoid lying down for 4–5 h after taking these drugs to prevent supine hypertension; these drugs have negligible effects in normal subjects. The increase in blood pressure seen in patients with autonomic failure is a reflection of their extreme hypersensitivity to most pressor and depressor agents. For this reason, treatment should be started at very small doses and should be individualized. This is best done by measuring blood pressure at 15- to 30-min intervals for 2–3 h after administration of the first dose of each drug tried. Note that some of these agents may be contraindicated in patients with other diabetic complications. Some patients may benefit from short periods of hospitalization to regulate treatment with these agents.

Treatment of Related Conditions

Many patients may also have supine hypertension resulting from preexisting essential hypertension and/or the lack of autonomic buffering mechanisms that maintain normal blood pressure. In occasional patients, significant hypertension may be present even in the seated position. During the day, supine hypertension is best managed by simply avoiding the supine position. At night, it is often necessary to give vasodilators at bedtime, after which the patient should be advised against getting up during the night without assistance. The following agents have been used with some success:

- Hydralazine hydrochloride (25–100 mg)
- Minoxidil (1.25–5 mg)
- Very low doses of nitrates as transdermal preparations (e.g., ¼ of a Nitropatch applied at bedtime and removed on arising)

Patients with angina may also be difficult to manage. Nitrates and other venodilators may produce dramatic hypotension in patients with autonomic failure. Conversely, angina may be precipitated by postural hypotension and relieved by resuming the supine position. β-Blockers may be an alternative treatment in these patients if no contraindication to their use exists. Propranolol (20–60 mg/day) and pindolol (15 mg/day) will probably not worsen orthostatic hypotension and may actually improve it in some patients.

Table 43.4. PHARMACOLOGICAL AGENTS IN TREATMENT OF ORTHOSTATIC HYPOTENSION

Drug	Initial Dose	Side Effects	Contraindications
NaCl (enteric coated)	2 g/day	Nausea, diarrhea	
Fludrocortisone (Florinef)	0.1 mg/day	Hypokalemia	Congestive heart failure
		Supine hypertension	
Phenylpropanolamine (Propagest, Propradine)	12.5 mg*	Anorexia	
		Nervousness	
Yohimbine (Yocon)	2.5 mg*	Nervousness, tremor	
Ergotamine (Medihaler)	1 puff (0.36 mg)*	Gastrointestinal discomfort	Coronary artery disease
			Peripheral vascular disease
Indomethacin (Indocin)	25 mg*	Gastrointestinal discomfort	Peptic ulcer

Please refer to more detailed sources for complete list of side effects and contraindications.

*A dose of these short-acting pressor agents, given before exertion, will improve orthostatic symptoms for 2–3 h. In general, administration of >3 doses/day is discouraged to avoid side effects and development of tolerance.

SUGGESTED READING

1. Bannister R (Ed.): *Autonomic Failure: A Textbook of Clinical Disorders of the Autonomic Nervous System*. 2nd ed. Oxford, UK, Oxford Univ. Press, 1988
2. Christensen NJ: Acute effects of insulin on cardiovascular function and noradrenergic uptake and release. *Diabetologia* 25:377-81, 1983
3. Cryer PE: Disorders of sympathetic neural function in human diabetes mellitus: hypoadrenergic and hyperadrenergic postural hypotension. *Metabolism* 29:1186-89, 1980
4. Paul S, Zygmunt D, Haile V, Robertson D, Biaggioni I: Chronic orthostatic hypotension. *Compr Ther* 14:58-65, 1988

44. Sudomotor Dysfunction and Dark Vision

MICHAEL A. PFEIFER, MD

The pupils and sweat glands are both innervated by autonomic nerves, and their functions may be compromised by diabetic neuropathy. Although these may seem minor complications of diabetes, impairment of both can greatly impede the activities of daily living, and sudomotor dysfunction may even result in life-threatening situations.

SUDOMOTOR DYSFUNCTION

As many as 60% of diabetic patients may eventually experience sudomotor dysfunction. As in other forms of diabetic neuropathy, the longer nerves tend to be impaired before shorter nerves, resulting in anhidrosis in the lower extremities. There is a compensatory hyperhidrosis in the upper body.

Sudomotor function is regulated by a complex pathway that includes the sympathetic nervous system. Functionally, the ability to regulate core temperature at an appropriate level is compromised. Loss of the ability to regulate core temperature can result in heat exhaustion and heat stroke. Symptoms of sudomotor dysfunction include excessive perspiration on the trunk and face. Sudomotor impairment may occur before any other signs or symptoms of sensory or motor impairment.

Dr. Pfeifer is Director of the Diabetes Center of Excellence, Humana Hospital Lexington, and of the Diabetes Research and Analysis Association, Inc., Lexington, KY.

Treatment

Parasympathetic stimulants will often result in increased sudomotor function in the lower extremities; however, the side effects from these agents (increased salivation and sweating on the trunk and face) are often intolerable. Therefore, the most beneficial therapy may be education about the causes of the increased upper-body sweating and awareness of the risk of heat exhaustion and heat stroke. Anhidrosis in the lower extremities may contribute to development of foot and leg ulcers (see chapt. 47).

DARK VISION

Parasympathetic and sympathetic nerves work antagonistically to adapt pupil size to the level of illumination. Sympathetic nerves dilate the pupil, and parasympathetic nerves constrict the pupil. Autonomic neuropathy of the nerves to the pupil causes reduced pupil size probably from sympathetic impairment, resulting in an inability to adapt pupil size to changes in illumination, and reduces the ability to maintain contraction in continuous bright light. These patients may fail to dilate adequately with atropine. Decreased pupil diameter has been associated with reduced anterior chamber depth, which is thought to predispose to the development of glaucoma. Symptoms include night blindness and poor dark adaptation.

Treatment

Therapy consists primarily of education about the problems associated with night blindness and poor dark adaptation. Patients should be closely monitored for glaucoma.

SUGGESTED READING

1. Hreidarsson AB, Gundersen HJG: Reduced pupillary unrest: autonomic nervous system abnormality in diabetes mellitus. *Diabetes* 37:446–51, 1988
2. Kennedy WR, Navarro X: Sympathetic sudomotor function in diabetic neuropathy. *Arch Neurol* 46:1182–86, 1989
3. Moore MV, Jeffcoate WJ, Haworth S: Autonomic neuropathy and the pathogenesis of glaucoma in diabetes mellitus. *Diabetic Med* 6:717–19, 1989
4. Pfeifer MA, Cook D, Brodsky J, Tice D, Parrish D, Reenan A, Halter JB, Porte D Jr: Quantitative evaluation of sympathetic and parasympathetic control of iris function. 5:518–28, 1982
5. Pfeifer MA, Greene DA: Diabetic neuropathy. *Curr Concepts* Nov.:36–37, 1985

45. Cardiac Denervation Syndrome

MICHAEL A. PFEIFER, MD

Cardiac denervation syndrome is a severe expression of cardiovascular autonomic neuropathy (CAN). The natural history and prevalence of diabetic cardiac denervation are not well defined. Table 45.1 lists some known consequences of cardiac denervation syndrome.

Figure 45.1 illustrates the effect of autonomic neuropathy on heart rate. Loss of autonomic nerve function is progressive and selective. A decrease in parasympathetic function has been documented within 12 mo of the diagnosis of diabetes and is lost long before sympathetic function is completely lost. Cardiac denervation syndrome is manifested by a fixed heart rate of 80–90 beats/min that does not respond to stress, mild exercise, sleep, or postural changes.

THERAPY

There is no treatment for diabetic autonomic neuropathy. However, it is important to identify patients with CAN because there are interventions that can reduce the associated morbidity and mortality. CAN has been associated with a higher incidence of painless ischemia that precedes more severe cardiac events, i.e., myocardial infarction and sudden death. It is also associated with a decreased survival rate after myocardial infarction and increased mortality over 5 yr.

Dr. Pfeifer is Director of the Diabetes Center of Excellence, Humana Hospital Lexington, and of the Diabetes Research and Analysis Association, Inc., Lexington, KY.

Table 45.1. CONSEQUENCES OF CARDIAC DENERVATION SYNDROME

- Increased incidence of sudden death
- Increased silent myocardial ischemia and infarction
- Increased incidence of cardiac arrhythmias
- Poor exercise tolerance
- Cardiovascular lability during anesthesiology
- Denervation hypersensitivity to autonomic drugs or medicines that contain autonomic drugs (e.g., Novocaine with epinephrine)
- Poor survival after myocardial infarction
- Increased morbidity during pregnancy
- Poor prognosis for 5-yr survival

DIAGNOSIS

An algorithm, with measures of CAN, has been proposed as a method of identifying patients at risk for painless myocardial ischemia (Fig. 45.2). Measurements of R-R variation and evaluation of heart-rate responses to the Valsalva maneuver are simple, reliable, and noninvasive tests with which to screen patients for CAN.

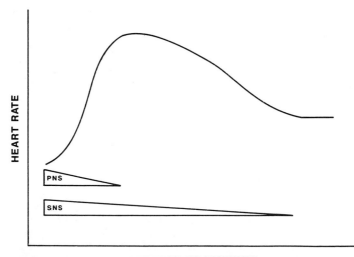

Figure 45.1. Effects of autonomic neuropathy on heart rate in diabetic patients. As duration of diabetes lengthens, heart rate increases (due to decrease in parasympathetic nervous system [PNS] tone) and then decreases (due to continued loss of PNS/sympathetic nervous system [SNS]). Finally, when heart is denervated, fixed heart rate is present (1). From Genovely and Pfeifer (3). © 1988. Reprinted by permission of John Wiley & Sons Ltd.

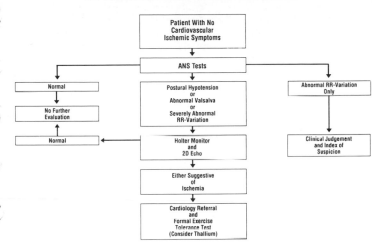

Figure 45.2. Clinical algorithm for screening diabetic patients for painless myocardial ischemia. From Pfeifer (5). © 1990 by the American Diabetes Association. Reprinted with permission.

R-R Variation

R-R variation refers to the difference in time between *R* waves of the QRS complex due to sinus arrhythmia. Chemical blockade has shown that this difference is primarily a result of parasympathetic regulation. This test requires the patient to breathe at a fixed rate (5–6 breaths/min) for a specified period (4–6 min). Commercially available devices are used to perform and analyze the results of this test. Figure 45.3 shows the results of this test in normal and

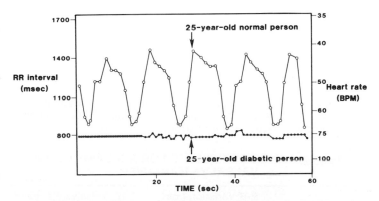

Figure 45.3. R-R variation and effect of cardiac autonomic neuropathy. Changes in heart rate during deep breathing in normal and diabetic subjects. Variation in heart rate (sinus arrhythmia) during breathing is termed *R-R variation*. Both patients were breathing at fixed rate of 5 breaths/min. From Pfeifer and Peterson (6).

diabetic patients. A quantitative value, $\overline{R}$, is calculated by a vector analysis technique and is based on the magnitude of the heart-rate swings during exhalation and inhalation (sinus arrhythmia). Table 45.2 lists the range of values.

Valsalva Maneuver

The Valsalva maneuver quantitates the change in heart rate during and after the patient blows against a standardized pressure. A complex reflex arc regulates the heart-rate changes produced by a Valsalva maneuver and thus is a more general measure of autonomic function. Figure 45.4 illustrates the effect of a Valsalva maneuver on heart rate in a nondiabetic and a diabetic patient. A Valsalva ratio (slowest heart rate after Valsalva maneuver/fastest heart rate during Valsalva maneuver) quantitates the change (Table 45.2).

Holter Monitoring

Patients with abnormal R-R variation and Valsalva maneuver, an R-R variation <10, or postural hypotension may lack the ability to feel pain and should be evaluated further for heart disease. Holter monitoring of the S-T segment for 48 h is one mechanism of evaluation.

ADDITIONAL COMPLICATIONS

Diabetic patients with autonomic neuropathy experience a higher incidence of cardiovascular lability during anesthesia. Before any surgical procedure, diabetic patients should be evaluated for CAN, and the anesthesiologist should be informed. Atropine treatment may be necessary before anesthetic induction to avoid severe bradycardia. Propranolol administration postoperatively will help prevent catecholamine-induced tachycardia in the recovery room. Diabetic patients also respond to atropine and epinephrine in an unpredictable manner. Adrenergic agonists should be avoided when autonomic neuropathy is suspected.

An exercise stress test should be performed before patients with autonomic neuropathy begin an exercise program. Patients may fatigue easily and/or experience painless ischemia. Painless ischemia would preclude participation in strenuous exercise.

Table 45.2. **RANGE OF RESULTS FOR R-R VARIATION AND VALSALVA MANEUVER**

	R-R Variation (ms)	Valsalva Maneuver
Abnormal	<20	<1.50
Borderline	20–30	
Normal	>30	>1.50

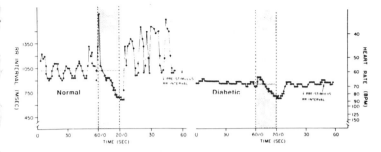

Figure 45.4. Heart-rate responses to Valsalva maneuver. *Shaded areas* represent Valsalva maneuver of 40 mmHg for 20 s. In nondiabetic subject, during Valsalva period, heart rate gradually increases (shorter R-R intervals). After Valsalva period, baroreflex-mediated bradycardia is observed. Diabetic subject with clinical evidence of autonomic neuropathy has no evidence of R-R variation or reflex bradycardia. From Pfeifer and Peterson (6).

SUGGESTED READING

1. Burgos LG, Ebert TJ, Asiddao C, Turner LA, Pattison CZ, Wang Cheng R, Kampine JP: Increased intraoperative cardiovascular morbidity in diabetes with autonomic neuropathy. *Anesthesiology* 70:591–97, 1989

2. Ewing DJ, Campbell IW, Clarke BF: Assessment of cardiovascular effects in diabetic autonomic neuropathy and prognostic implications. *Ann Intern Med* 92:308–13, 1980

3. Genovely H, Pfeifer MA: RR-variation: the autonomic test of choice in diabetes. *Diabetes Metab Rev* 4:255–71, 1988

4. Hilsted J, Richter E, Madsbad S, Tronier B, Christensen NJ, Hilderbrandt P, Damkjer M, Galbo H: Metabolic and cardiovascular responses to epinephrine in diabetic autonomic neuropathy. *N Engl J Med* 317:421–26, 1987

5. Pfeifer MA: Cardiovascular autonomic neuropathy. *Diabetes Spectrum* 3:45–48, 1989

6. Pfeifer MA, Peterson H. Cardiovascular autonomic neuropathy. In *Diabetic Neuropathy*. Dyck PJ, Thomas PK, Asbury AK, Winegrad AI, Porte D Jr, Eds. Philadelphia, PA, Saunders, 1987, p. 122–33

7. *Physician's Guide to Non-Insulin-Dependent (Type II) Diabetes: Diagnosis and Treatment*. 2nd ed. Lebovitz H, Ed. Alexandria, VA, Am. Diabetes Assoc., 1988

46. Angina and Congestive Heart Failure

ALAN J. GARBER, MD, PhD

Ischemic symptomatology as the result of coronary artery insufficiency produces characteristic symptoms of substernal tightness or heaviness, which are generally precipitated by exercise and relieved promptly by rest. This substernal precordial pain may radiate to the left arm or shoulder and the elbow and wrist. Alternatively, there may be exertional pain in the jaw, back, or abdomen. Whereas >95% of nondiabetic patients have characteristic exertional symptomatology, only ~70% of diabetic patients experience such characteristic anginal symptomatology. In diabetic patients, atypical locations may include epigastric, neck, or jaw discomfort with or without precordial prominence. When present, fatigue is an ominous prognostic symptom because it indicates a marked fall in cardiac output as the result of global rather than localized myocardial ischemia. Stable angina is the form precipitated by exercise and is generally the result of a fixed atherosclerotic lesion in one or more coronary arteries. Unstable angina can occur with exercise or at rest. This form of angina is also probably the result of a fixed atherosclerotic lesion, but the presence of rest pain suggests a considerable spastic component to the pathogenesis of the ischemia. Variant angina is precipitated at rest and generally reflects a primary pathophysiological role for coronary arterial spasm. This differentiation of rest- versus exercise-associated angina pertains equally to diabetic and nondiabetic patients. Again, however, the atypical nature of symptomatology in patients with diabetes makes this differentiation clinically more difficult.

Dr. Garber is Professor of Medicine, Biochemistry, and Cell Biology at the Baylor College of Medicine and Chief of the Diabetes Metabolism Unit at The Methodist Hospital, Houston, TX.

DIAGNOSTIC TESTING FOR CORONARY ARTERY INSUFFICIENCY

In patients with diabetes, the suspicion of coronary artery insufficiency in the presence of atypical symptoms or even in the absence of symptoms should be pursued vigorously, particularly in patients with diabetes of >20 yr duration, >40 yr of age, or with multiple risk factors for coronary atherosclerosis including

- Concurrent hypertension
- Smoking
- Obesity
- Hyperlipidemia
- Dyslipidemia
- Type A personality

Exercise testing with a standardized Bruce protocol suffers from some interpretive difficulties in female patients, in patients with rather profound hypertension, and in patients with concurrent digitalis administration. On the other hand, thallium perfusion with exercise has a much lower false-negative or false-positive rate than routine exercise stress testing. However, in patients with diffuse triple-vessel disease, which is likely to be more frequent in diabetes, a uniformly depressed thallium uptake may produce interpretive difficulties because no localized lesion will be evident.

Coronary arteriography should be performed in all patients with diabetes and one or more additional risk factors for coronary atherosclerosis. In addition, all patients failing a trial of medical management or having unstable angina or variant angina at the time of presentation also require a precise definition of coronary anatomy. In view of the asymptomatic or atypical symptom pattern of patients with diabetes mellitus, a reliance on symptomatology as a justification for visualization of the anatomy is impractical and potentially unwise. Therefore, patients with diabetes who are already at high risk should have a precise definition of coronary anatomy at the outset of therapy. Patients generally present with triple-vessel disease at the time of initial diagnosis. Double- or single-vessel disease is encountered less often. Left-main disease is significantly more common in the diabetic than the nondiabetic population. There may also be a slightly greater frequency of concomitant distal disease in patients with diabetes mellitus. Such distal disease can strongly influence the outcomes of invasive surgical and nonsurgical treatments. Careful attention must be paid to the complication of radiocontrast-induced nonoliguric renal failure in patients with diabetes.

NONPHARMACOLOGICAL THERAPY

Because angina results from an acute imbalance between myocardial oxygen consumption and the ability of the coronary arteries to supply the amounts of oxygen required, therapies that tend to reduce myocardial oxygen consumption are of primary importance for the medical management of angina pectoris. These include such obvious maneuvers as the normalization of systolic and diastolic blood pressures, cessation of cigarette smoking, and weight reduction for obesity. Prevention of significant hyperglycemia and hypoglycemia is essential to avoid the adverse hyperadrenergic consequences of poor glucose regulation and its attendant burden on myocardial function. An exercise program designed and supervised by an approved cardiac rehabilitation program is also useful in assisting weight loss and glucose control and improving cardiovascular function.

PHARMACOLOGICAL THERAPY

Nitrates

Nitroglycerin works acutely by decreasing myocardial oxygen consumption, in terms of both preload and afterload reduction. Nitrates also improve myocardial oxygen availability by dilating epicardial coronary vessels, decreasing coronary arterial resistance, and improving collateral blood flow (Table 46.1). Nitrates are a specific therapy for coronary vasospasm and are essential to the management of any form of angina that is the result, at least in part of

Table 46.1. PHARMACOLOGICAL THERAPY FOR ANGINA PECTORIS

Agents	Dosage	Advantages/Disadvantages
Nitrates (nitroglycerin)		
Sublingual	0.15−0.6 mg as needed	Short acting, 30-min duration, headache
Ointment	0.5−2 inches every 4−6 h	Long acting, orthostasis
Transdermal patch	2.5−15 mg every 2−4 h	Long acting, orthostasis
β-Adrenergic antagonists Nonselective		
Propranolol	40−120 mg 4×/day	Antiarrhythmic hyperlipidemia, erratic kinetics
Cardioselective		
Atenolol	50−100 mg 2×/day	Less metabolic disturbance, low antiarrhythmic potential
Metoprolol	50−200 mg 4×/day	Less metabolic disturbance, low antiarrhythmic potential
Ca^{2+} slow channel entry antagonists		
Nifedipine	20−30 mg 4×/day	Marked vasodilation, flushing, hypotension
Diltiazem	60−90 mg 4×/day	Moderate vasodilation, decreased arteriovenous conduction, bradycardia
Verapamil	80−120 mg 4×/day	Moderate vasodilation, decreased arteriovenous conduction, bradycardia

spasm, of an element of its pathogenesis. Nitrates have several adverse effects that may limit their usefulness. The most prominent of these is hypotension. Nitrates will reduce blood pressure in patients who are both normotensive and hypertensive. However, in patients with autonomic neuropathy, small doses of nitrates may produce disabling orthostatic hypotension that precludes their use. In addition, rapid-acting nitrates, e.g., sublingual nitroglycerin, tend to produce headaches and palpitations. Although nitroglycerin is itself the most rapid acting, it also has the shortest duration of action. Pharmacological modifications of this agent, e.g., isosorbide, have a greater duration of action but tend to produce a similar pattern of side effects, particularly prominent headache. Longer-acting forms of nitroglycerin via transdermal routes of administration by ointment, paste, or patches produce better results. Dosage is determined by the amount of skin exposed to the agent. There appears to be little or no consequence of nitrate therapy, acutely or chronically, on diabetes control, lipid metabolism, or insulin sensitivity. Nitrates are not contraindicated in patients with congestive heart failure, a unique characteristic not shared by β-blockers or Ca^{2+} slow channel entry antagonists.

β-Adrenergic Blockers

β-Adrenergic antagonists are effective therapy for chronic coronary insufficiency because they decrease myocardial oxygen consumption as the result of a diminution of heart rate, cardiac contractility, and systolic blood pressure (the latter particularly on exercise). β-Adrenergic antagonists available for clinical therapeutic use include nonselective β-antagonists, selective β_1-antagonists, and adrenergic antagonists with intrinsic sympathomimetic activity (Table 46.1). In addition to the beneficial effects on myocardial metabolism by systemic β_1-blockade, benefits such as renin suppression and reduced free–fatty acid levels also result. However, blockade of the β_2-receptor produces deleterious systemic consequences such as bronchospasm, vasoconstriction, and an increased frequency and severity of insulin-induced hypoglycemia. Because the perception of oncoming hypoglycemia is adrenergically mediated, these counterregulatory mechanisms may be blunted or even eliminated by large doses of nonselective β_2-adrenergic antagonists. In contrast, selective β_1-adrenergic antagonists such as atenolol and metoprolol at high doses have much greater nonselectivity than is generally appreciated. Thus, only the lowest dose of cardioselective β_1-antagonists should be chosen for insulin-requiring diabetic patients with coronary artery insufficiency. Atenolol and metoprolol differ from one another with regard to intrinsic membrane stabilizing activity and hence their antiarrhythmogenic potential. In this category, metoprolol has much greater activity than atenolol, albeit at sufficiently high doses as to override its cardioselectivity. A similar loss of cardioselectivity at these high doses is observed with atenolol, although membrane-stabilizing activity is not observed.

β-Blockers are contraindicated in patients with overt heart failure, cardiogenic shock, disturbances in cardiac rhythm such as significant sinus bradycardia, sick sinus syndrome, and second- or third-degree heart block. Patients who are heavy cigarette smokers or have a history of bronchospasm should not be given β-adrenergic antagonists.

Ca²⁺-Channel Blockers

Ca^{2+} slow channel entry antagonists are effective therapy for coronary ischemia because they decrease myocardial oxygen consumption by a diminution of cardiac afterload and, to a lesser extent, cardiac preload and cardiac contractility. These antagonists also increase myocardial oxygen delivery by decreasing coronary vascular resistance and preventing coronary arterial spasm. Therefore, Ca^{2+}-channel blockers are useful in all forms of coronary ischemia complicated by coronary arterial spasm, particularly if the spasm is inadequately or incompletely treated by nitrates. Ca^{2+}-entry antagonists are also indicated for therapy of angina when β-adrenergic antagonists are contraindicated or if they produce debilitating adverse reactions. Nifedipine, diltiazem, and verapamil are the most widely available Ca^{2+}-channel blockers for the therapy of coronary ischemia (Table 46.1).

Ca^{2+}-channel blockers have several undesirable side effects, e.g., hypotension at doses necessary for adequate relief of coronary ischemic symptoms. All three agents may exacerbate congestive heart failure and result in edema, and constipation. The tendency toward edema and worsening of congestive heart failure may require concurrent diuretic therapy, usually with a loop diuretic such as furosemide. Therefore, Ca^{2+}-channel blockers should not be used in patients with acute congestive heart failure, serious disease of the conduction system, or hypotension, especially in diabetic patients with previously determined autonomic neuropathy in whom orthostasis would be worsened considerably in the presence of these drugs.

SURGICAL THERAPY FOR CORONARY ISCHEMIA

Surgery or invasive nonsurgical management by techniques such as percutaneous transluminal coronary angioplasty should be considered in all patients failing an adequate trial of pharmacological management. The risks of coronary artery surgery are not adequately balanced by the gains obtained in patients with single-vessel disease, unless it is a left-main lesion. However, in patients with significant proximal lesions in two or three vessels, coronary artery bypass graft placement, internal mammary artery insertion for myocardial revascularization, or a combination of both processes produces a significant improvement in long-term survival. Because of the frequency of atypical angina in diabetic patients, coronary artery bypass surgery should be considered in patients with left-main disease or severe triple- or double-vessel disease with large areas of the myocardium at clear-cut risk. Successful surgery depends on the presence of bypassable proximal lesions with adequate distal runoff. The quality of the distal runoff must be ascertained before surgery by adequate arteriography.

Percutaneous transluminal coronary angioplasty should always be considered in single-vessel disease or proximal multiple-vessel disease, which might otherwise be treated with coronary artery bypass procedures. The morbidity and mortality rates from angioplasty are significantly less than that of surgery, and it should therefore be considered as the initial form of therapy, particularly in patients for whom surgery might have a somewhat higher risk.

Regardless of the form of therapy used, coronary ischemia as manifested by angina pectoris must be adequately diagnosed and satisfactorily tested to prevent myocardial infarction or particularly the multiple small infarctions characteristic of so-called diabetic cardiomyopathy. Either or both of these outcomes produce loss of myocardial muscle and ultimately become the antimortum event responsible for the death of at least 60% of all patients with diabetes mellitus. A comprehensive therapeutic program should aggressively address concurrent atherosclerotic risk factors in addition to hyperglycemia in each patient.

TREATMENT OF CONGESTIVE HEART FAILURE

In patients surviving one or more myocardial infarctions, congestive heart failure is a likely event as the result of inadequate myocardial function. It is a lethal disease with a 2-yr mortality approaching 30%. In these patients, symptoms of heart failure at rest and persistent hyponatremia are ominous prognostic signs. The pathogenesis of congestive heart failure involves an inadequacy of peripheral circulation, oxygenation, and metabolite delivery so that irreversible circulatory compensations arise that further complicate the congestive state, ultimately resulting in increased morbidity and mortality. The primary compensation is the development of hyperreninemic hyperaldosteronism.

Although digitalis and diuretic administration have been the cornerstone of therapy for congestive heart failure, neither deals satisfactorily with the underlying pathogenesis of the disease or the important element of hyperreninemia, which considerably complicates the course of congestive failure. Although digitalis or diuretics are themselves not contraindicated in patients with diabetes, these agents may not be suitable first-choice therapy for congestive heart failure. Instead, angiotensin-converting enzyme (ACE) inhibitors reduce the mortality from congestive heart failure by at least 50% and dramatically improve both symptoms and functional capacity of patients with this debilitating disease (Table 46.2). In general,

Table 46.2. ANGIOTENSIN-CONVERTING ENZYME INHIBITORS: THERAPY FOR CONGESTIVE HEART FAILURE

Agent	Dosage (mg)	Advantages/Disadvantages
Captopril	12.5–50 2×/day	Short half-life, preferred in azotemic subjects
Enalapril	5–20 1 or 2×/day	Longer half-life, may require only once-daily administration, potential hypotension, potential hyperkalemia

patients do better with shorter-acting ACE inhibitors, e.g., captopril, particularly if the serum creatinine level is elevated as the result of intrinsic renal disease or chronically poor renal perfusion. Captopril, in doses of 12.5–50 mg twice daily, should be adequate in most patients. Reversal of hyponatremia is an excellent prognostic sign regarding the efficacy of ACE-inhibitor therapy for congestive failure. Congestive heart failure may also be an important concurrent symptomatology for coronary ischemia in patients with diabetes. Therapy for this ischemia or angina in its most atypical form may therefore focus on the treatment of exercise-induced congestive failure and should also rely on ACE inhibitors whenever possible.

SUGGESTED READING

1. CONSENSUS Trial Study Group: Effects of enalapril on mortality in severe congestive heart failure: results of the Cooperative North Scandinavian Enalapril Survival Study (CONSENSUS). *N Engl J Med* 316:1429–35, 1987
2. Shub C: Stable angina pectoris. 3. Medical treatment. *Mayo Clin Proc* 65:256–73, 1990

47. Myocardial Infarction

ALAN J. GARBER, MD, PhD

Atherosclerosis is the most important of all chronic diabetic complications because it accounts for ~80% of total diabetic mortality. Seventy-five percent of that mortality occurs as the result of markedly accelerated coronary artery disease. As a consequence, 77% of all hospitalizations for diabetic complications are accounted for by the general category of coronary atherosclerosis. Although diabetes itself accelerates atherosclerosis 200–400%, diabetic patients are often afflicted with multiple risk factors for atherosclerosis, including such important concomitant or related disorders as hypertension, hyperlipidemia or dyslipidemia, and obesity. At least 75% of all patients survive their first myocardial infarction. Their long-term survival, however, depends primarily on the prevention of recurrent infarction, with sudden death or the resulting loss of muscle mass sufficient to produce chronic congestive heart failure.

DIAGNOSIS

Painless myocardial infarction is more common in patients with diabetes than in the nondiabetic population. Often, the so-called painless infarction is actually symptomatic, with various but markedly atypical nonclassic presentations. Diabetic patients with acute infarction present with characteristic substernal and left arm pain in ~66–80% of cases reviewed. On the other hand, atypical locations for pain, particularly of a lesser intensity, range from the angle

---

Dr. Garber is Professor of Medicine, Biochemistry, and Cell Biology at the Baylor College of Medicine and Chief of the Diabetes Metabolism Unit at The Methodist Hospital, Houston, TX.

of the jaw or the neck to epigastric pain associated with vomiting. Few patients have painless presentations, although even these may be suspected by florid symptoms of congestive dysfunction with shortness of breath, cough, and other pulmonary complaints. In general, the counterregulatory anti-insulin hormonal response with the resulting loss of diabetes control is out of proportion to the severity of the presenting symptomatology. Thus, diabetic patients can present in severe diabetic ketoacidosis with minimal or no symptomatology pointing to the underlying acute myocardial infarction as the precipitating cause of illness. Diabetic patients are also more likely to have silent ischemia during electrocardiographic (ECG) monitoring.

Diagnostic Testing

ECG diagnosis of acute myocardial infarction is complicated considerably in patients with diabetes mellitus. Approximately 25–35% of diabetic patients have a tendency toward multiple, small, nontransmural infarctions that are non–Q wave in character. Nonetheless, most diabetic patients present with characteristic ECG findings of Q waves and S-T elevation with T-wave inversion. In patients with small non–Q-wave infarctions, more subtle changes may require comparison with prior ECGs or may even yield indeterminate results based on ECG evaluation. In no instance should an absence of characteristic ECG findings be allowed to otherwise exclude a diagnosis of myocardial infarction in patients with long-standing diabetes mellitus, particularly if the patients have additional concurrent risk factors for coronary artery disease.

Confirmation of the clinical diagnosis of infarction is best obtained by sequential analysis of creatine kinase levels with particular attention paid to isoenzyme MB subfractions. Other enzyme studies, e.g., lactase dehydrogenase, may be useful adjuncts but are not sufficient for diagnosis. Sequential evaluations of subtle changes in ECGs may also reinforce the diagnostic impression provided by creatine kinase analysis.

TREATMENT OF MYOCARDIAL INFARCTION AND RELATED DISORDERS

Glucose and Ketone Control

Because of the metabolic response to stress and the increased counterregulatory hormone output that characterize the internal milieu of diabetic patients immediately postinfarction, a loss of diabetes control with hyperglycemia and even ketosis is common. Patients with previous ketosis-resistant type II (non-insulin-dependent) diabetes mellitus may present in overt ketoacidosis as the result of myocardial infarction. Under most circumstances, blood glucose levels should be maintained at 100–150 mg/dl (5.5–8.3 mM), although the risks of hypoglycemia in the immediate postinfarction period are considerable. Bursts of catecholamine release provoked by insulin hypoglycemia have an arrhythmogenic potential that may be lethal during the period of myocardial irritability immediately after acute infarction. Intermittent subcutaneous insulin administration by sliding scale may not be wise in this population of patients. Instead, continuous intravenous insulin infusion at rates of 1–4 U/h for treatment of hyperglycemia and rates of 4–8 U/h for ketosis or ketoacidosis may be necessary initially. In such patients, particularly if they are taking nothing by mouth, the use of a concurrent infusion of glucose (5–7.5 g/h) is extremely useful in avoiding hypoglycemia and minimizing the development of ketosis in type II previously non-insulin-dependent or insulin-requiring patients. In these patients, return to diet or oral-agent control should not be attempted before the 5th day after the myocardial infarction or any other complicating intercurrent complications attendant to the infarction.

Thrombolytic Therapy

In any myocardial infarction, a central zone of necrotic tissue is surrounded by one or more zones of ischemic myocardium that may retain functional characteristics and viability. A critical period of 2–6 h appears to exist in which some, if not all, of the ischemic myocardium may be restored to viability by reperfusion of the coronary channel occluded during the period of acute infarction. Data from various trials clearly indicate that thrombolytic therapy with tissue plasminogen activator, streptokinase, or a combination of both agents is associated with ~50% reduction in peri-infarction mortality rates in patients with acute myocardial infarction. To maximize the benefits of such therapy, an interval of optimally not more than 2 h and preferably not more than 6 h should have transpired from the time of presumed onset of the myocardial infarction as judged by symptomatology.

The coronary anatomy should be visualized as soon as possible during the acute infarction period. In reasonably stable patients with acute infarction, percutaneous transluminal coronary angioplasty may be combined with thrombolytic therapy to reduce or eliminate the ulcerated complicated plaque and the superimposed thrombosis. This recommendation pertains to patients with one- or two-vessel disease. In patients with high-grade stenosis in three or more vessels, coronary artery bypass graft placement should be considered and performed as soon as possible to prevent further muscle loss and the resulting chronic congestive failure (see chapt. 46).

Medical Management During Peri-Infarction Period

Routine antiarrhythmic and antihypertensive therapy in diabetic patients may be used as in nondiabetic patients. There are, however, two general precautions that apply to patients with diabetes. First, the use of β-adrenergic antagonists, particularly nonselective antagonists, increases the risks of insulin-induced hypoglycemia in patients administered high-dose nonselective or selective β-blockage. As an alternative, calcium slow channel entry antagonists may produce antiarrhythmogenic effects similar to β-blockers without the potential for worsening of hypoglycemia. Second, there is a potential for adrenergic antagonists to redirect splanchnic blood flow in an adverse fashion. As the result of antiarrhythmic or antihypertensive therapy, patients may have variable insulin response and sensitivity and variable rates of glucose production depending on delivery of peripheral substrates to the liver for gluconeogenesis. This variable response to exogenous insulin when using intensified therapy can cause considerable instability in their blood glucose, particularly when cardiac output is rather unstable in the peri-infarction period.

PREVENTION OF RECURRENT INFARCTION

Atherosclerosis, tends to progress relentlessly in the coronary and peripheral circulation and almost always involves pathology in multiple vessels. Definitive therapy to arrest or reverse coronary atherosclerosis and to prevent recurrence of infarction has not been identified, although the outlines of such a program have begun to emerge from the Cholesterol-Lowering Atherosclerosis Study regarding reversal of atherosclerotic regions in nondiabetic patients. In nondiabetic patients, low-density lipoprotein cholesterol levels of <80–100 mg/dl (<2.08–2.6 mM) seem important for atherosclerotic reversal in nondiabetic patients. A similar requirement is likely in diabetic patients. Combinations of HMG-CoA reductase inhibitors and a bile salt sequestrant are required for such profound therapeutic reductions. Pravastatin (20 mg) or Lovastatin (40 mg/10 g) plus colestipol (2×/day) are generally recommended. Efforts should also be made to raise the otherwise relatively low high-density lipoprotein concentrations seen in patients with diabetes. Although success in raising these high-density lipoprotein levels to normal levels may be difficult if not impossible to obtain, hypolipidemic agents and ancillary therapies such as diet and exercise may be useful.

The question of glycemic control in the progression of atherosclerosis remains unresolved, although the threshold for the acceleration of atherosclerosis seems to occur with minimal postprandial hyperglycemia, even before fasting hyperglycemia is observed. This suggests that aggressive glycemic control may be a rational form of therapy in the outpatient setting after myocardial stability is obtained in the postinfarction period. Regardless, attention to obvious risk factors and the mild dyslipidemia associated even with well-controlled diabetic patients is essential to prevent recurrent infarction and particularly to reverse diffuse disease in clinically inoperative situations.

SUGGESTED READING

1. Stone PH, Muller JE, Hartwell T, York BJ, Rutherford JD, Parker CB, Turi ZG, Strauss HW, Willerson JT, Robertson T, Braunwald E, Jaffe AS, MILIS Study Group: The effect of diabetes mellitus on prognosis and serial left ventricular function after acute myocardial infarction: contribution of both coronary disease and diastolic left ventricular dysfunction to the adverse prognosis. *J Am Coll Cardiol* 14:49–57, 1989

2. The TIMI Study Group: Comparison of invasive and conservative strategies after treatment with intravenous tissue plasminogen activator in acute myocardial infarction: results of the Thrombolysis in Myocardial Infarction (TIMI) Phase II Trial. *N Engl J Med* 320:618–27, 1989

48. Peripheral Arterial Disease and Intermittent Claudication

MARVIN E. LEVIN, MD

Peripheral vascular disease is common in diabetic patients, particularly those with type II (non-insulin-dependent) diabetes. At diagnosis, 8% of type II patients have clinical evidence of peripheral arterial disease (PAD).

PAD contributes significantly to amputation. Half of all nontraumatic amputations in the United States occur in diabetic patients. At early stages, peripheral neuropathy causes an insensate foot, allowing painless trauma, ulceration, and infection. Poor circulation then compromises the delivery of oxygen, nutrients, and antibiotics, which ultimately leads to amputation. The outlook for the diabetic patient with an infected foot ulcer and significant PAD is poor.

RISK FACTORS

Risk factors for PAD are listed in Table 48.1. They vary in importance from patient to patient.

Cigarette Smoking

Of the treatable risk factors, smoking is the most important. Smokers have a much lower mean age at amputation. A single cigarette can cause spasm of the arteries and a reduction of blood flow lasting

Dr. Levin is Professor of Clinical Medicine at the Washington University School of Medicine, St. Louis, MO.

Table 48.1. RISK FACTORS FOR DIABETIC MACROVASCULAR DISEASE

Not treatable
- Genetic
- Age
- Duration of diabetes

Treatable
- Smoking
- Hypertension
- Hypercholesterolemia
- Hypertriglyceridemia
- Hyperglycemia
- Hyperinsulinemia
- Obesity
- Miscellaneous
  - Inotropic drugs
  - β-Blockers

≥1 h. Cigarettes reduce high-density lipoprotein cholesterol, increase platelet aggregation and fibrinogen levels, and decrease erythrocyte flexibility.

Hypertension

Hypertension is a significant risk factor for PAD. More than 50% of type II diabetic patients have hypertension, compared to 20% of nondiabetic individuals. In addition to hypertension, drug therapy can worsen peripheral circulation. For example, β-blockers cause unopposed α-vasoconstriction and therefore should be avoided in patients with PAD.

Hyperlipidemia

Hyperlipidemia occurs in 44% of type II diabetic patients compared with 23% of nondiabetic individuals. Obesity, often associated with type II diabetes, is an independent risk factor, because it is associated with insulin resistance and hyperinsulinemia.

Hyperglycemia

Hyperglycemia per se is probably not a major risk factor for PAD, although patients who have impaired glucose tolerance but normal fasting blood glucose and glycosylated hemoglobin may have evidence of macrovascular disease.

DIABETIC VS. NONDIABETIC PAD

There are several differences between diabetic and nondiabetic PAD. The content of the atherosclerotic plaque is not qualitatively different in terms of the content of calcium, cholesterol, lipids, platelets, and smooth muscle cells. Important differences are noted in Table 48.2.

SIGNS AND SYMPTOMS OF PAD

Intermittent Claudication (IC)

Signs and symptoms of PAD are listed in Table 48.3. One of the most common is IC, which affects 2% of the population and may be present in up to 10% of those over age 65 yr. Although the degree of ischemia may be severe enough to cause claudication, many of these patients may not have symptoms because of peripheral neuropathy and the inability to detect pain.

The pain or discomfort associated with IC is characterized by a cramping or aching sensation, most often in the calf. It occurs with walking and is relieved when the individual stops to rest, without the need to sit down. Higher vascular obstruction, e.g., in the aorta, will cause claudicatory pain in the buttocks and upper thighs and is frequently accompanied by impotence. Obstruction of the iliac arteries will cause pain in the lower thigh.

This pain should be differentiated from similar but nonischemic pain, which may also be induced by walking. Nonischemic leg pain, or pseudoclaudication, can be caused by arthritis, muscular or radicular disorders, spinal cord compression, anemia, phlebitis, or even myxedema. The patient experiencing pseudoclaudication will usually have to sit, and the pain may last 15–20 min before disappearing. Patients with arthritically induced symptoms will frequently bend over or stretch their backs to obtain relief.

The distance a person can walk before experiencing claudication will vary. Pain occurs after a shorter distance if a person is walking fast, uphill, or on a hard surface. Over time, discomfort develops

Table 48.2. DIFFERENCES IN DIABETIC AND NONDIABETIC PERIPHERAL ARTERIAL DISEASE

	Diabetic	Nondiabetic
Clinical	More common, younger patient, more rapid	Less common, older patient, less rapid
Male:female	2:1	30:1
Occlusion	Multisegmental	Single segment
Vessels adjacent to occlusion	Involved	Not involved
Collaterals	Involved	Usually normal
Lower extremities	Both	Unilateral
Vessels involved	Tibials, peroneals, smaller vessel	Aortic, iliac, femoral
In-hospital mortality with amputation	1.5–3.0%	Significantly less

Table 48.3. **SIGNS AND SYMPTOMS OF PERIPHERAL ARTERIAL DISEASE**

- Intermittent claudication
- Cold feet
- Nocturnal pain
- Rest pain
- Nocturnal and rest pain relieved with dependency
- Absent pulses
- Blanching on elevation
- Delayed venous filling after elevation
- Dependent rubor
- Atrophy of subcutaneous fatty tissues
- Shiny appearance of skin
- Loss of hair on foot and toes
- Thickened nails, often with fungus infection
- Gangrene
- Miscellaneous: blue toe syndrome, acute vascular occlusion

after walking a shorter distance. However, use of walking distance to determine the degree of occlusion is not always reliable, because it is dependent on these other variables. When evaluating deterioration or improvement in an exercise program, all of these conditions must remain constant.

Examination of the patient with IC involving the calf muscle may reveal both femoral and pedal pulses but no popliteal pulse. Pedal pulses are present due to collateral arteries around the knee. However, after a brisk walk, the foot will become pale and pulseless, because blood bypasses the skin of the foot and flows instead to the skeletal muscles of the calf. IC usually results from a single arterial block. However, with multiple areas of vessel involvement in the diabetic patient, tandem occlusions may be present.

Some patients with symptoms of IC have normal pulses at rest; therefore, it is of value to subject these patients to standardized treadmill testing. Exercise will lead to decreased pulse pressure and significant diminution or disappearance of the pulses. The drop in ankle pressure may require several minutes to return to normal. Patients with normal circulation have no drop in their ankle pulse pressures with exercise. Note that many of these patients have coronary artery disease, and electrocardiographic monitoring may be indicated.

Other Signs and Symptoms

The sensation of cold feet may also be due to peripheral neuropathy. Nocturnal and rest pain are ominous signs and are an indication for vascular surgery. Nocturnal pain may also occur secondary to peripheral neuropathy. Patients with nocturnal or rest pain with ischemia can obtain relief by keeping the legs in a dependent position and frequently sleeping sitting up in a chair. Delayed venous filling is a simple bedside test. The patient's legs are raised 45° until they blanch. The patient is then asked to sit upright with the legs dependent. Venous filling should occur within 15 s. Delayed filling of 15–25 s indicates moderate ischemia; >25 s indicates severe ischemia.

Dependent rubor may also occur in patients with varicose veins. Shiny appearance of the skin and loss of the hair on the dorsum of the foot are classic signs of severe PAD. Atrophy of the subcutaneous tissues makes it appear that the skin is pulled tight around the foot. Thickened nails can be indicative of PAD. The blue or purple toe syndrome is important to recognize because it is a surgically treatable condition. It results from cholesterol emboli from an ulcerated more proximal plaque. There is frequently a livido reticularis pattern of the foot and petechiae. Patients often complain of myalgias because of the emboli to the muscular arteries. Removal of the ulcerated plaque will prevent further embolization and may save the foot.

A sudden onset of leg pain with accompanying paleness, paresthesias, paralysis, pulselessness, and a cold leg indicates acute thrombosis or embolus to a peripheral artery. This is a surgical emergency. The clot must be removed within 4–6 h, or peripheral nerves and muscles may be lost.

TREATMENT OF PAD AND IC

The mainstay of treatment for diabetic PAD is cessation of smoking, exercise, pharmacological therapy, and when indicated, vascular surgery.

Exercise

The improvement in walking seen with exercise training is not related specifically to increased blood flow or to the development of collateral vessels but rather to the clearance of metabolic end products from ischemic muscles. If IC improves with exercise, continue treatment. If not, the use of a hemorrheologic agent, pentoxifylline, is indicated. IC rarely requires vascular surgery. The long-term outlook for patients with IC is relatively good with conservative management. Most patients who have been followed for a long time remain stable or improve if they stop smoking and participate in a supervised exercise program. Vascular surgery is indicated in the presence of severe ischemia.

Vasodilators

In obstructive arterial disease, vasodilators are of no value and may be contraindicated. Raising systemic blood pressure is one of the most effective means of increasing collateral blood flow. However, most vasodilators tend to lower systemic pressure. They are not effective in the treatment of either IC or the ischemic symptoms of rest pain, and they fail to increase blood flow in most patients with ischemic limbs. Remember that the arteries in the diabetic patient are sclerosed and have little vasospastic disease. In fact, vasodilators can worsen an ischemic area by causing the "steal effect," in which dilation of the healthy vessels steals blood away from the sclerosed vessels and the tissues they supply.

Sympathectomy

Sympathectomy is rarely of any benefit in diabetic PAD. These vessels are sclerosed with very little capability of dilation. Because of involvement of the autonomic nervous system, many of the patients also have preexisting autosymphathectomy.

Antiplatelet Drugs

Because diabetic patients have increased platelet adherence and aggregation that contribute to atherosclerosis, some physicians have considered the use of antiplatelet drugs (dipyridamole and aspirin) to reduce the incidence of gangrene and amputation. The efficacy of this has not been confirmed in clinical trials.

Hemorrheologic Agents

Factors influencing blood flow through blood vessels include hematocrit values, plasma viscosity, platelet activity, and erythrocyte and probably leukocyte deformability. Diabetes is a hypercoagulable state with increased blood viscosity, which is caused by increased fibrinogen, von Willebrand factor, platelet adhesion and aggregation, and decreased flexibility of erythrocytes. The only hemorrheologic agent approved for use in the U.S. for the treatment of IC is pentoxifylline. However, its true efficacy in this setting is unclear.

Pentoxifylline has also been approved for the treatment of chronic occlusive PAD of the extremities by the Canadian Health Protective Branch. In the U.S., several anecdotal reports have found it beneficial in the treatment of ischemic ulcers of the toes in patients who are not candidates for vascular surgery.

Peripheral Vascular Surgery

Indications for peripheral vascular surgery include

- Nocturnal pain
- Rest pain
- Foot ulcers unresponsive to treatment
- Infection unresponsive to treatment
- Incipient gangrene
- Severe disabling IC

Surgery is rarely indicated for IC and then only if the patient is severely disabled or his/her livelihood depends on walking or vigorous use of the legs, e.g., a mail carrier or drivers of clutch vehicles. Other indications include patients with cardiac disease or post–cardiac bypass who require an exercise program.

Transcutaneous angioplasty can be beneficial. However, this procedure is less effective in diabetic patients because its greatest applicability is in the larger vessels, and PAD in diabetes occurs most often, although not exclusively, in the smaller vessels below the knee.

Laser therapy is still experimental. Injury to the endothelium by percutaneous angioplasty or laser therapy may stimulate atherosclerotic changes in the long term.

Because classic peripheral vascular findings involve the vessels below the trifurcation, artificial grafts are not used. The most successful surgery consists of in situ surgery, where the vascular surgeon uses the patient's own saphenous vein. The only postsurgical medication is 1 aspirin/day.

Not all patients with significantly impaired peripheral blood flow are candidates for vascular surgery. This can occur either because the preoperative angiograph indicates that the vascular obstruction cannot be bypassed or the patient's general condition prohibits surgery.

In the inoperable patient with ischemic foot changes, pentoxifylline may be beneficial. Many nursing home patients with these conditions who are deemed inoperable by a vascular surgeon might qualify for this treatment. If improvement or stabilization is achieved, the drug should be continued indefinitely. Pentoxifylline should be given 400 mg 3 ×/day with meals, and physicians should encourage patients not to skip doses.

WHEN TO REFER

Definite and urgent indications for referral of patients with PAD are rest pain or night pain due to PAD, evidence of cholesterol emboli or acute vascular occlusion. Patients with ulcers that will not heal, incipient gangrene, and infection resistant to treatment should have vascular surgical consultation.

Patients with mild PAD should be carefully followed with a peripheral vascular examination every 3–4 mo. Patients with moderate PAD should have vascular laboratory evaluation as a baseline. Patients should be referred to the vascular surgeon for further evaluation if they begin to exhibit signs of

- Decreased circulation
- Increased IC
- Decreased pulses
- Loss of hair on the dorsum of the feet
- Delayed venous filling time on dependency
- Dependent rubor

SUGGESTED READING

1. Bild D, Selby J, Sinnock P, Browner W, Braveman P, Showstack J: Lower-extremity amputation in people with diabetes: epidemiology and prevention. *Diabetes Care* 12:24–31, 1989
2. Brand, FN Abbott RD, Kannel WB: Diabetes, intermittent claudication, and risk of cardiovascular events: the Framingham study. *Diabetes* 38:504–509, 1989
3. Hiatt WR, Regensteiner JG, Hargarten ME, Wolfel EE, Brass ER: Benefit of exercise conditioning for patients with peripheral arterial disease. *Circulation* 81:602–609, 1990
4. Levin ME, Sicard GA: Peripheral vascular disease in the person with diabetes. In *Diabetes Mellitus: Theory and Practice*. 4th ed. Rifkin H, Porte D Jr, Eds. New York, Elsevier, 1990, p. 768–91
5. Schwartz RN, Logan NM, Johnson PJ, Strodel WE, Fine JG, Kazmers A, Hyde GL: Pentoxifylline increases extremity blood flow in diabetic atherosclerotic patients. *Arch Surg* 124:434–37, 1989

49. Foot Ulcers and Infections

GARY W. GIBBONS, MD, and FRANK W. LOGERFO, MD

For most people with diabetes, amputation is a significant concern; most major amputations in this country are performed on diabetic patients. Many of these could be avoided with appropriate treatment.

PATHOPHYSIOLOGY

Minor trauma leading to cutaneous ulceration is the precipitating event for diabetic foot problems. The presence of neuropathy, vascular insufficiency, and an altered response to infection makes the diabetic patient uniquely susceptible to foot problems.

Neuropathy includes sensory loss and loss of position sense of the foot. Motor neuropathy affects all of the muscles of the foot and leads to the characteristic deformities. Autonomic neuropathy results in a falsely warm foot secondary to altered blood flow. Reduction in sweating causes abnormally dry skin that fissures and cracks easily.

Peripheral vascular occlusive disease has important distinctions in diabetic patients. The intima and media of diabetic arteries frequently contain extensive calcium (Monckeberg's sclerosis), making them rigid and noncompressible. Results of noninvasive vascular laboratory tests are thus often incorrect or misleading. Surgical manipulation of these calcified vessels is delicate, and laser therapy of distal calcified vessels is contraindicated. Development of collateral circulation around occlusions and stenoses is poor, especially

---

Drs. Gibbons and Logerfo are Associate Professors of Surgery at the Harvard Medical School, Boston, MA.

in diabetic patients who smoke, with resulting limb-threatening consequences (rest pain or tissue loss). Diabetic macrovascular disease frequently involves the tibial/peroneal vessels between the knee and the foot. However, the foot vessels are usually spared; thus, modern treatment approaches to ischemic diabetic foot ulcers should no longer be based on the concept of small-vessel disease.

Infections are often undetected until limb and sometimes life are threatened. Diabetic patients do not feel the progression of ulceration, and the signs and symptoms of infection (i.e., temperature, tachycardia, elevation of leukocyte count) are not manifest until late. The first sign of serious infection may be loss of blood glucose control or a flulike syndrome. Any patient reporting this must be carefully evaluated for infection.

PREVENTION

Patient education is essential. The following instructions may help patients avoid foot ulcers and infections.

Shoes

* Wear well-fitting shoes even if they are not stylish.
* Change shoes during the day to relieve pressure areas.
* Try running or walking shoes for everyday wear.
* Select dress shoes of soft leather and have them fitted carefully.
* Use orthotics to solve fitting problems.
* Break in new shoes slowly.
* Shake shoes out and inspect them before wear for areas that might cause blisters or rubbing.

Foot Hygiene

* Wash feet daily with mild soap. Rinse and dry thoroughly, especially between the toes.
* Apply moisture-restoring creams once or twice daily except between the toes.
* Wear clean intact socks appropriate for the shoes being worn.
* Avoid astringents and all over-the-counter preparations for calluses, corns, nails, etc.
* Trim nails with a slightly rounded edge.
* Avoid "self-bathroom surgery." Seek a qualified professional for treatment of all foot problems.
* Do not use foot soaks.
* Do not use heating pads or sleep next to space heaters or stoves; hot or cold sensations in the feet result from neuropathy not poor circulation.
* Wear socks if feet feel cold.
* Never go barefoot.

Problems to Report to Doctor

- Cuts or breaks in the skin.
- Ingrown nails.
- Changes in color or discoloration of the foot.
- Change in sensation or pain.
- Change in architecture of the foot.

Clinical Management

It is important for patients to control weight and blood pressure, eliminate smoking, and exercise daily. Careful evaluation for infection is mandatory in diabetic patients who suddenly lose control of their blood glucose.

The patient's legs and feet, including the heels and the areas between the toes, should be examined at regular intervals, and neurological and vascular examinations should be conducted. Table 49.1 lists the clinical signs of vascular insufficiency, and their presence indicates the need for noninvasive testing and a consultation with a vascular specialist.

Skin changes, callus formation, or foot deformities should be evaluated and shoes inspected for appropriateness, excessive wear, and foreign bodies. Patients at high risk for developing foot ulcers may need to be seen more frequently or referred to a specialist for particular problems (Table 49.2).

MANAGEMENT

The severity of the infected foot ulcer will determine the proper course of treatment. A major decision is whether the patient can be initially treated as an outpatient or needs to be admitted to the hospital. Early superficial ulcers with minimal cellulitis (<2 cm) may be treated at home if there is no evidence of systemic toxicity and the patient is compliant, reliable, and has a vigilant support system. Hospitalization is indicated if there is no significant improvement within 24–48 h.

Inspection of the wound to determine the extent of tissue destruction and sepsis is the first step: Carefully cleanse the area with

Table 49.1. CLINICAL EVIDENCE OF ARTERIAL INSUFFICIENCY

- Diminished or absent pulses
- Absent hair from forefoot or toes
- Cornification of nails
- Atrophic skin and subcutaneous tissue
- Decreased skin temperature
- Pallor on elevation
- Dependent rubor
- Venous filling time >25 s

Table 49.2. **PATIENTS AT HIGH RISK FOR ULCERATION**

- History of previous ulcer
- Neuropathy: sensory, motor, autonomic
- Peripheral vascular disease
- Structural changes:
  - Hammertoes
  - Bunions
  - Charcot's foot
  - Pes cavus or planus
  - Other pathological changes in shape
- Callus formation
- Bleeding into callus or under a nail
- Skin changes
  - Dyshidrosis
  - Ingrown nails
  - Mycotic toenails
  - Evidence of poor hygiene
  - Fissuring
  - Chronic tinea pedis
  - Chronic skin infections
- Abnormal gait
- Abnormal patterns of wear on shoes

an antiseptic solution, and, with a sterile probe, forceps, and scissors, unroof all encrusted areas. Inspect the wound to determine the extent of tissue destruction and possible bone and joint involvement. Little or no anesthesia is required because most of these patients have neuropathy. Figures 49.1 and 49.2 are algorithms for treating superficial uncomplicated ulcers and deep ulcers with limb-threatening potential.

Treatment of Superficial Uncomplicated Ulcers and Infections

In addition to the guidelines in Fig. 49.1:

- Apply plain gauze sponges wetted with diluted isotonic antiseptic solutions (wet to dry dressings) to open ulcer once or twice a day.
- Treat fissures or cracks in the skin with an antibiotic ointment and a plain gauze outer dressing.
- Treat athlete's foot (with superficial bacterial superinfection) with local antifungal cream or solution on plain gauze and an oral antibiotic.
- Weight bearing is avoided until healing is assured and then resumed gradually. If weight bearing progresses too rapidly, acute Charcot's foot (neuropathic joint disease) may result.
- Footwear should be modified to protect sensitive high-risk areas.

Once healed, these patients are regarded as high risk, and careful follow-up, including modification of footwear and orthotics, is recommended.

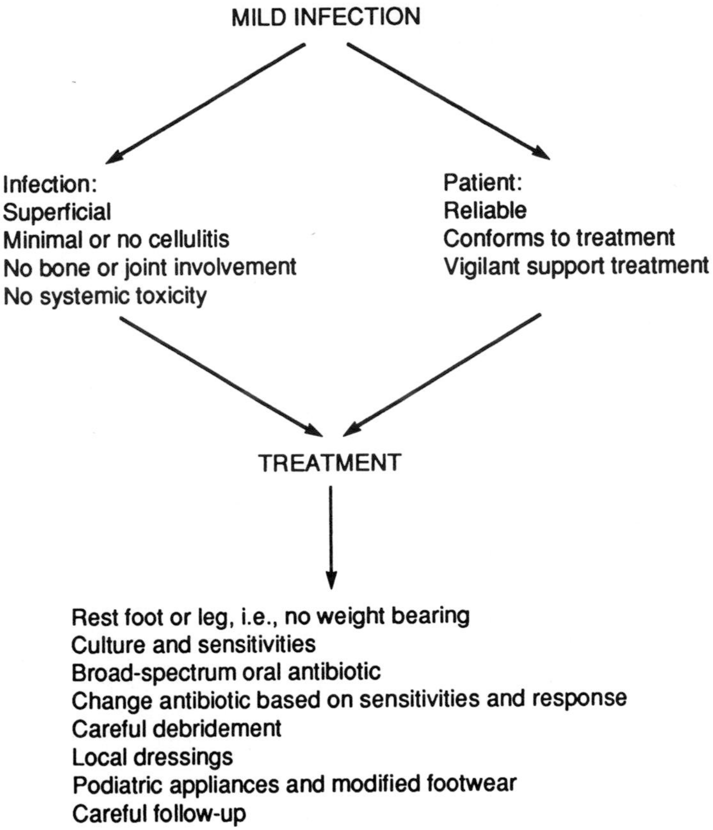

MILD INFECTION

Infection:
Superficial
Minimal or no cellulitis
No bone or joint involvement
No systemic toxicity

Patient:
Reliable
Conforms to treatment
Vigilant support treatment

TREATMENT

Rest foot or leg, i.e., no weight bearing
Culture and sensitivities
Broad-spectrum oral antibiotic
Change antibiotic based on sensitivities and response
Careful debridement
Local dressings
Podiatric appliances and modified footwear
Careful follow-up

Figure 49.1. Management of mild-infection foot ulcer.

Treatment of Limb-Threatening Infections

The treatment of limb-threatening infections is outlined in Fig. 49.2. Surgical intervention, especially in a patient with systemic toxicity, should not be delayed even if the patient has not yet been stabilized medically and blood glucose is not controlled. Blood glucose control often requires the use of insulin.

Proper antibiotic therapy and wound care are essential to limb salvage. Whenever possible, deeply infected tissue or bone should be cultured. Initial use of intravenous broad-spectrum antibiotics is justified by the polymicrobial nature of these infections. Absorption of oral antibiotics may be inhibited by associated gastroenteropathy, especially in hyperglycemic seriously ill patients.

Choice of an initial antibiotic or combination depends on

- Local bacterial resistance patterns
- Prior antibiotic history

- Gram stain of deep exudate
- Appearance of wound and pus
- Allergies
- Associated renal, hepatic, and cardiac impairment

Changing antibiotics and the duration of therapy depends on bacterial sensitivities and the response of the wound to surgical management.

To determine the extent of tissue destruction or bone or joint involvement, plain X rays (plus/minus magnification views) are helpful initially but are not definitive. Scans and magnetic resonance may be useful in the differential diagnosis of osteomyelitis versus acute Charcot's disease. In difficult cases, consult with an experienced radiologist.

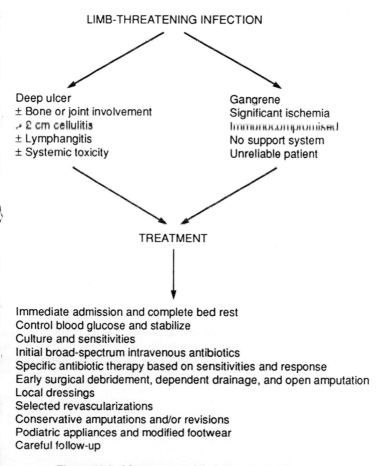

LIMB-THREATENING INFECTION

Deep ulcer
± Bone or joint involvement
↗ 2 cm cellulitis
± Lymphangitis
± Systemic toxicity

Gangrene
Significant ischemia
Immunocompromised
No support system
Unreliable patient

TREATMENT

Immediate admission and complete bed rest
Control blood glucose and stabilize
Culture and sensitivities
Initial broad-spectrum intravenous antibiotics
Specific antibiotic therapy based on sensitivities and response
Early surgical debridement, dependent drainage, and open amputation
Local dressings
Selected revascularizations
Conservative amputations and/or revisions
Podiatric appliances and modified footwear
Careful follow-up

Figure 49.2. Management of limb-threatening foot ulcer.

Surgical management of potentially serious foot ulcers in diabetic patients requires debridement that is extensive enough to ensure there is no undrained pus or necrotic tissue left. It is a misconception that treatment of infections in diabetic patients should be limited to antibiotics and small incisions for drainage. Diabetic patients do not tolerate undrained infection, but they heal well if the infection is completely resolved and circulation is adequate.

Dressings are begun with the initial surgical management and should consist of diluted isotonic antiseptic solutions or saline applied to plain gauze and packed into the wound 1–3×/day. Soaks, heat, whirlpools, astringents, full-strength solutions, or harsh medicines should be avoided. Standard wet-to-dry dressings are the most effective means for mechanically debriding the wound and permitting continual wound observation.

Assessment of the vascular status of the involved extremity is needed once sepsis is controlled. Because of the peculiarities of diabetic peripheral vascular disease, noninvasive laboratory testing plays only a complementary role to clinical evaluation and judgment. No one should accept the notion of small-vessel disease in the diabetic foot, and complete up-to-date arteriography should be done. This procedure should include visualization of the foot vessels in patients who are definitely ischemic or in cases where there is question. Vascular reconstruction, especially pedal artery bypass grafting, is successful in almost 90% of extremities with limb-threatening ischemia. After revascularization, revisions or more distal forefoot-saving amputations can be carried out with the ultimate achievement of limb salvage.

SUGGESTED READING

1. Gibbons GW: The diabetic foot: amputation and drainage of infection. *J Vasc Surg* 5:791–93, 1987
2. Gibbons GW, Eliopoulos G: Infections of the diabetic foot. In *Management of Diabetic Foot Problems*. Kozak GP, Hoar CS Jr, Rowbotham JL, Wheelock FC Jr, Gibbons GW, Campbell DR, Eds. Philadelphia, PA, Saunders, 1984, p. 191
3. Logerfo FW, Coffman JD: Vascular and microvascular disease of the foot in diabetics: implications for foot care. *N Engl J Med* 311:1615–19, 1984
4. Logerfo FW, Gibbons GW: Ischemia in the diabetic foot: modern concepts and management. *Clin Diabetes* 7:72–74, 1989
5. Pomposelli FB, Jepson SJ, Gibbons GW, Campbell DR, Freeman DV, Logerfo FW: Efficacy of the dorsalis pedis bypass for limb salvage in diabetic patients. *J Vasc Surg* 6:745–52, 1990

Index

About the American Diabetes Association

The American Diabetes Association (ADA) is the nation's leading voluntary health organization dedicated to improving the well-being of all people affected by diabetes. Equally important is its unceasing support for research to prevent and cure this chronic disease that affects some 14 million Americans. ADA carries out this important mission through the efforts of thousands of volunteers working at state affiliates and local chapters in more than 800 communities throughout the United States.

Membership in ADA puts you in contact with a network of more than 270,000 caring people throughout the country. Affiliates and chapters offer support groups, educational programs, counseling, and other special services. Membership also brings 12 issues of the lively patient education magazine *Diabetes Forecast*.

In addition, ADA publishes an array of materials for every age-group on topics important not just to the individual with diabetes but to the entire family. Considerable effort is also devoted to educating health-care professionals and building public awareness about diabetes.

ADA also distributes a free quarterly newsletter with practical advice and helpful hints on living with diabetes. To receive a copy, call the toll-free number listed below.

Information on ADA membership and programs is available through the state affiliates (listed in the white pages of the telephone book) or through the American Diabetes Association, Diabetes Information Service Center, 1660 Duke Street, Alexandria, VA 22314; 1-800-ADA-DISC.

Essential Information for Health-Care Professionals

Physician's Guide to Insulin-Dependent (Type I) Diabetes: Diagnosis and Treatment

This authoritative *Guide*, written by a diverse committee of experts, covers treatment advice about all areas of type I diabetes. A "highlights" section precedes each chapter to help you preview key concepts and understand important points.   1988.   152 pages.   Spiral bound.   #PTIPG
Nonmember: $19.95   Member: $17.95

Physician's Guide to Non-Insulin-Dependent (Type II) Diabetes: Diagnosis and Treatment. 2nd Ed.

Essential for professionals who treat patients with type II diabetes, the *Guide*'s easy-to-use format provides you with the latest knowledge in the areas of classification and pathogenesis, treatment, and complications. Like the *Type I Guide*, a "highlights" section precedes each chapter.   1988.   112 pages.   Spiral bound.   #PTIIPG
Nonmember: $19.95   Member: $17.95

Goals for Diabetes Education

Presented in a convenient checklist format, this 48-page book provides you with a logical, thorough approach to both the initial and in-depth phases of patient education. A *must* for all professionals involved in education!   1986.   48 pages.   Softcover.   #PEGDE
Nonmember: $5.00   Member: $4.50

Nutrition Guide for Professionals: Diabetes Education and Meal Planning

This publication helps you use the *Exchange Lists for Meal Planning* effectively. An excellent reference for professionals who teach dietetics or need a comprehensive understanding of nutrition principles. Chapters cover everything from creating meal plans for varied needs and life-styles to the complete data bases of nutrients that form the basis for the *Exchange Lists*.   1988.   92 pages.
Softcover.   #PNNG
Nonmember: $12.95   Member: $11.00

Exchange Lists for Meal Planning

Here's the preferred system for diabetes meal planning. Colorful charts, helpful tips on good nutrition, and the six easy-to-use food *Exchange Lists* show your patients how to balance their diet and gain control over diabetes.   1989.   32 pages.   Softcover.
#CELMP
Nonmember: $1.30   Member: $1.10

ADA PROFESSIONAL JOURNALS

Diabetes

Original research about the pathophysiology and treatment of diabetes.   12 issues per year plus supplements.
#SUBSCRIPTION1
1 year: $90

Diabetes Care

Clinical research journal for professionals who diagnose and treat patients with diabetes and its complications.   12 issues per year including 4 topical review issues plus supplements.
#SUBSCRIPTION2
1 year: $65

Diabetes Spectrum: From Research to Practice

Each issue provides a practical interpretation of a current topic in diabetes research by experts in that field.   6 issues per year.
#SUBSCRIPTION3
1 year: $30

Clinical Diabetes

This easy-to-read bimonthly publication provides the most current medical information about diabetes and its treatment for the pri-

mary-care physician.   6 issues per year.   #SUBSCRIPTION4
1 year: $15

IDF Bulletin ⌐

The official publication of the International Diabetes Federation, this journal reviews diabetes research worldwide and provides insights into treatment in different socioeconomic environments and cultures.   Published for the IDF by ADA.   3 issues per year. #SUBSCRIPTION5
1 year: $15

Join the leading professional network for diabetes information.

From research to practice—the American Diabetes Association *Professional Section* offers health-care professionals and researchers the information and interdisciplinary contacts they need to stay on the cutting edge of advances in the diabetes field.

We invite you to become a *Professional Section* member—it's an investment in your career and in your community.   For more information, call toll-free 1-800-ADA-DISC.

How to Order Any or All of These Publications

On a piece of paper

1. Write your name and address.
2. Write the "ship to" name and address (if it is different from your own).
3. Write the item name, item number, quantity, appropriate unit price, and total for each item.
4. Add on 4.5% state sales tax if you are a Virginia resident (subscriptions are not taxable).
5. Add on shipping and handling charges using the publication total and the chart below:

Shipping and Handling

up to $5.00...........$1.75	$25.01–$50.00 ....$5.50
$5.01–$10.00........$3.00	over $50.00 .....10% of order
$10.01–$25.00 ......$4.50	

All orders are shipped either 1st Class Mail (if total weight is under 1 lb) or UPS (regular, ground service).
6. Add $3.00 to shipping and handling for each additional shipping address.
7. If the "ship to" address is outside the United States, please add $15 per "ship to" address for airmail shipments. Overseas express air service is not available. Payment for foreign orders must be made in U.S. funds, drawn on a U.S. bank.

8. Send your check or money order (official purchase orders are accepted for orders greater than $25.00) to the following address:

American Diabetes Association
1970 Chain Bridge Road
McLean, VA 22109-0592

Prices are subject to change without notice. Please allow 6–8 weeks for normal domestic delivery.

If you have any questions about how to order, please call 1-800-ADA-DISC, ext. 363, and we will be glad to help you.